D0793859

stutter

stutter

Marc Shell

HARVARD UNIVERSITY PRESS
CAMBRIDGE, MASSACHUSETTS
LONDON, ENGLAND
2005

Printed in the United States of America

Library of Congress Cataloging-in-Publication Data

Shell, Marc.
Stutter / Marc Shell.
p. cm.
Includes index.
ISBN 0-674-01937-7 (alk. paper)
1. Stuttering. I. Title.
RC424.S564 2005
616.85′54—dc22 2005051264

Acknowledgments

My speech therapist at Montréal's Royal Victoria Hospital in the 1950s was the kindly Marie Cardoza; I thank her for allowing me into the medical library at the Speech Clinic when I was only ten years old. My high school chums Steven Springer, Rhona Prupas, and Elyse Vaintrub taught me about friendship and conversation. I owe special thanks to my high school buddies Michael Krashinsky and David Caplan, who risked losing debating tournaments when they chose me as their partner. Although my psychology professor at Stanford was a positivist, he allowed me to write my term paper on theories of stuttering—"much against my better judgment," said he. René Wellek and Geoffrey Hartman, my teachers at Yale, allowed me to get by the Ph.D. oral examination without my speaking fluently. Neil Schmitz, my colleague at SUNY/Buffalo, was especially heartening to me by virtue of his courage in writing about stuttering. My sometime collaborator and department associate Peter Fenves, now at Northwestern, has offered brilliant advice. Many of my colleagues at Harvard have been profoundly helpful in aiding me to think through problems in articulation: Dan Albright, Maria Ascher, David Elmer, Jorie Graham, John Hamilton, Carmen Gloria Iguina, Barbara Johnson, Elaine Scarry, Werner Sollors, Doris Sommer, Evangeline Stefanakis, and Lindsay Waters. Dr. David B. Rosenfield of the Speech and Language Center at the Baylor College of Medicine has made a generous contribution. Students in three Harvard seminars have been extraordinarily giving and forgiving. Mihaela Pacurar and Casiana Ionita have assisted with myriad research issues.

During our thirty-five-year friendship, Stanley Cavell has pressed me often, by speech and action. I am not the first to block on his question: Must we mean what we say?

Stuttering is a family affair. My wife, the philosopher Susan Meld Shell, has put up with my talk for decades. Our daughter, the historian of science Hanna Rose Shell, claims not to hear me stutter. Our son, the urban historian Jacob Adam Shell, is the only person I know who counts himself free to tease me about my speech.

All have a bona fide say in *Stutter.*

Contents

Illustrations

stutter

Prologue

> Friedrich [Nietzsche] was singing—enunciating clearly, though when he talked he used to stutter—he was singing a poem, which was unknown to us, and it was his latest poem, "Venice." I do not like Friedrich's compositions. They are mediocre. Nevertheless, this song . . . well, by God, it was sublime.
>
> —André Malraux, *The Walnut Trees of Altenburg,* trans. A. W. Fielding[1]

Clinicians and therapists know how intractable a practical problem stuttering is for the fifty million stutterers worldwide.[2] Neurologists, physiologists, and evolutionary biologists know likewise how fascinating stuttering is for understanding what a human being is. Students in the humanities, though, often seem to know more about metaphors and themes of stuttering in the arts than about stuttering itself and its actual bearing on aesthetics. A few cultural histories of stuttering include lists of artists and celebrities who have stuttered, but few literary critics and humanists deal directly with its relevance—with the way it involves elementary and motivating matters essential to literary language, human psychology, and the general representations that inform artful production.

The pan-global and pan-cultural phenomenon of stuttering "literalizes" in the human body and spirit many of the key notions that humanists deal with—imitation, representation, doubling, synonymy, punning, inexpressibility, and metrics. Yet stuttering is not much looked into. Why not? One answer is that literary criticism and book lovers prefer literature featuring characters that the reader can pity. Even the most "politically correct" person, however, would have to admit that at times he has laughed at the stutterer. Stuttering thus gives us "sensitive souls" a problem—as in the case of Porky Pig. It gives us "ugly feelings" about ourselves that we do not want to face. Many of the central legends of our religious, literary, and popular culture are stutterers—including Moses, Hamlet, and Marilyn Monroe, all of whom, and others, we shall consider in chapters that follow. Yet, in almost all such cases, our celebration of these persons is inseparable from how and why we ignore, or remain ignorant of, the stuttering that is generally integral to what they accomplished.

Laughter is no small matter here. When a stutterer speaks, he often feels *gagged* (in the sense of "stoppered"). Throat-constriction and breathing difficulty suffocate or choke him.[3] Child stutterers thus often depict themselves as strangulated and out of breath.[4] By the time they are adults, however, stutterers know that gags (in the sense of "mouth-stoppers") are also technical instruments. Their elocution teachers use gags to help improve speaking and singing[5] even as surgeons and torturers use gags to correct offensive physical and political behavior.[6] One of those instruments, branks, have a sharp metal gag, or bit, that enters the mouth and painfully restrains the tongue.[7] The rest is silence. The stutterer in this tongue-stocks is, of course, already the quintessential, laughing-stock for gags (in the sense of "humorous remarks or situations"). After all, the same word, *gag,* means both "stopper" *and* "joke." What has gagging (meaning "shutting up") to do with gagging (meaning "joking around")? In *Stutter,* we shall consider how gags gag; likewise we shall demonstrate how verbal wit arises from the same involuntary blockages of meanings and shifting of terms that inform stuttering.[8] The *gaga* is no simple madman, and in the 1950s, the most celebrated television star was Milton Berle, known as "The Thief of Bad Gags."[9] Berle's routines featured punning malapropisms (*bad gag* for *Baghdad*) and stumbling stutters *(da da da da)*. Berle made people laugh, often against their will, as on a fast laugh track with "NO EXIT" signs. I thought the laughers in his television studio suffered from the same symptoms as stutterers: spasmodic utterances, inarticulate sounds, facial distortions, shaking of the sides, and loud, distressful whoops at inhalation. Their maniacal movements and sounds reminded me of Bumpo in *The Voyages of Dr. Doolittle* (1922).[10] Bumpo overdoses on "laughter-beans" and then, stutterer-like, he almost dies of laughter.

Do people laugh at the stutterer in an involuntary way that uncannily duplicates the involuntariness of the stuttering itself? Or is the laughter somehow also voluntary? Stuttering opens up for reflection this gap between the involuntary and the voluntary so fundamental to twentieth century aesthetics. Likewise, as we shall see, it provides access to the neurological and evolutionary roots of human language, the history and purpose of song, and the roots of legislation. By looking at stuttering in this way, we examine issues ranging from the political uses of language to the individual's inability to speak, from bodily movement to verbal fluidity, and from animal physiology to the intellectual achievements of speaking animals.

Stuttering involves spiritually and physiologically inescapable ways of human articulation. At the same time, it pertains to the problem of the unspeakable or what remains unspoken. One of the pressing problematic undertakings of literature and literary studies in the wake of Walter Benjamin's study of Goethe's *Elective Affinities* (1924–1925)[11] is how to think the inexpressible—or speak the unspeakable. The problem is also an American conundrum. Ralph Waldo Emerson writes in his essay "Goethe; Or, the Writer" (1850), "Whatever can be thought can be spoken, and still rises for utterance, though to rude and stammering organs. If they can not compass it, it waits and works, until at last it moulds them to its perfect will and is articulated."[12] It would be an optimistic opinion: that whatever can be spoken waits until a person's stammering organs are molded so as to become adequate to speak it.

The plenitude of my *Stutter*'s paratactic em-dashes (—) are the symptoms merely of an already anticipated failure.[13] On the other hand, *Stutter*'s elisions (. . .) usually indicate "a passing over in silence," as when one might omit pronouncing a vowel in spoken discourse.[14] My words fly up, my thoughts remain below. "What signifies," asks Emerson, "that he trips and stammers; that his voice is harsh or hissing; that his method or his tropes are inadequate? That message will find method and imagery, articulation and melody. Though he were dumb, the message would speak. If not,—if there be no such God's word in the man,—what care we how adroit, how fluent, how brilliant he is?" Nietzsche, whose ghost plays the singing stutterer in André Malraux's novel *The Walnut Trees of Altenburg* (1948), wrote in *Thus Spake Zarathustra* (1884): "Let your virtue be too exalted for the familiarity of names, and if you must speak of it, be not ashamed to stammer about it."[15]

I have taken thirty-five years to publish a book on *speaking* block. But the wait is the result neither of writing block[16] nor of publishing block. Writer's block may involve a "heightened sense of perfection" or terror of "having nothing to say," but it is better understood as a sign of trying to articulate what one cannot express. Often, like stuttering, writer's block is best treated, in the short run, by switching languages. Publication block, or fear of publishing,[17] kicks in when, or if, a manuscript is "complete." Some persons associate publication block with fear of criticism or of mockery, but they miss the right diagnosis by an ell. The optimistic, blue-eyed son in Bob Dylan's anthem "It's a Hard [—It's a Hard—It's a Hard—It's a Hard] Rain's a-Gonna Fall" (1963) sees "ten thousand talkers whose tongues were all broken." That son finally manages to croak out, barely well enough, the last words of the ballad: "I'll know my song well before I start singing."

One might also include here such diagnostic terms with neurological implications as *agraphia* (an "Inability to write [as a manifestation of brain-disease] that may be appropriately enough allowed to include *incoordinate* as well as *paralytic* defects in the power of mental expression by Writing," as Bastian puts it in *The Brain as an Organ of Mind* [1888])[18] and *dysgraphia* (an "Inability to write coherently [as a manifestation of brain damage]") because both of these writing-diseases are often linked with stuttering.[19]

One name for the condition where a speaker repeats his own words, phrases, or sentences is *palilalia*. This term inhabits textbooks in both rhetoric and neurology. So, properly fascinating to literary theorist as well as medical doctor are the Mosaic God, who calls himself "*I am—I am,*" and Marilyn Monroe, who reiterates "*da—da—da,*" and Shakespeare's Hamlet, who verbigerates "*Well—well—well.*" Ongoing puzzles in neurology concomitantly lend themselves to rhetorical analysis: Why does palilalia disappear when stutterers chant? How does singing put to rest the verbal tics of Tourette's Syndrome?[20] Enduring mysteries in poetics accordingly involve neurological investigation: Why does the zebra finch stammer? How do poets sing like birds? Thus, the enigma of stuttering moves beyond the province of speech therapy and engages the peculiar knots of mind and body that help define humankind.

1 Preambulations

> The radical cause of the complaint is often attributed to that which . . . merely exacerbates the pain.
>
> —*Art of Preserving the Feet . . . By an Experienced Chiropodist* (London, 1818)

The speech-fluency disorder or disability that I will focus on in this book is stuttering—a communications disorder whose description in most cultures generally involves stumbling in speech.[1] In this disorder, which is (at least initially) involuntary, the flow of speech is broken (or one breaks that flow) in the form of repetition, prolongation, or cessation of sound. The speaker knows what he wants to say but cannot say it. Exemplary for our purposes here would be repetition of the *schwa* vowel with consonants ("d-d-daddy"), reiteration of syllables ("da-da-dada"), prolongations of vowels ("daaaaaad"), and nonstandard stoppages (no sound), as well as an accompanying struggle to speak differently. We say that the break in the flow of speech results from excitement, indecision, or sudden emotion (such as fear, anger, delight, or grief), as well as from constitutional conditions of the organs of speech or of the nervous system. Yet such definition and etiology raise epistemological questions about the distinction between voluntary and involuntary action, as well as between the psychological and biological realms and between a would-be speaker's knowing and not knowing what he intends to say (if anything). They also beg questions about the difference between such polar opposites as flow and stoppage, repetition and prolongation, and sound and silence. Moreover, they adopt the viewpoint of a detective who cannot reliably tell whether a silence he detects in someone else goes along with that person's struggle or refusal to speak or merely attends a normal period of quiet.[2] Refusal to speak is certainly often a sign of stuttering—for example, in James Earl Jones's childhood as reported in his autobiography, *Voices and Silences* (1993), or in Annie Glenn's refusal to do an interview as shown in the movie *The Right Stuff* (1983). "Refusal to speak," however, is not always easy to distinguish from simply "not speaking." A case in point would be the stutterer in the TV program *Tongues of Angels* (an episode of *Studio One* which I watched on March 17, 1958): the stutterer here is so ashamed of his stuttering that he carries a card saying he is mute.[3] In fact, many a stutterer's parent fears that his child will actually *become* mute. Somerset Maugham would sometimes speak whole sentences fluently and then stop midsentence, showing no externally detectible signs of inner conflict.

> Maugham had learned his speech by heart, and everything went well until he came to a passage in which he said: "I have reached the stage where I have absorbed all the philosophy I am capable of absorbing and told all the stories I am able to tell. And I know that anything I may yet have to learn about life will be learned, not from the dusty highways and byways which I frequented in my youth, but a comparatively secure and certainly more comfortable refuge . . . the v—— He stalled at the *v*, and the distinguished assembly sat in silence, staring hypnotized at his lower lip, which desperately sought to make the link with his upper teeth. Instead of

> giving up in confusion, Maugham stood perfectly still, though his fingers were trembling. After a few moments he said, "I'm just thinking of what I shall say next." Then he lapsed into silence again as ashes dropped from poised cigars and smoke drifted around the ancient pictures. "I'm sorry to keep you waiting," Maugham said, and became silent once more. Then suddenly lip and teeth connected and he came out with: "the verandah of a luxury hotel." He finished the speech in style, remaining imperturbable throughout the ordeal, and presenting the dinner guests with a remarkable display of moral courage and self-control.[4]

I myself was a silent stutterer for some years. During that period, I came to know something of stuttering both as a "disability" and as an important factor in "cultural history."[5] Both are concerns of mine in this book—which, like works about stuttering published in the past few decades, is to some small extent a sort of memoir.

Among such memoirs that I do not cite in the main body of *Stutter* are a few which, written during the century before I was born, suggest the sweep of the genre: James Malcolm Rymer's *The Unspeakable; or, The Life and Adventures of a Stammerer* (1855); Benjamin Beasley's *Stammering, Its Treatment; and, Reminiscences of a Stammerer* (1897); Wendell Johnson's *Because I Stutter* (1930); James Sonnett Greene's anthology *I Was a Stutterer: Stories from Life* (1947), with a preface by the literary critic and editor Albert Bigelow Paine; and Charles Pellman's *Overcoming Stammering* (1947), which includes Aaron Pellman's autobiographical sketch "A Glimpse into a Childhood of Stammering."[6] There have been many dozens of autobiographical accounts of stuttering published since the 1950s, many privately printed and most available in major libraries. One good example is Ida E. Witten's book *The Face of All the World Is Changed* (1990).[7] I will cite many others in the following chapters.

In the 1950s, the most widely accepted theory of stuttering in North America had it that stuttering was diagnosis-induced, or identification-induced. Stuttering, said the theorists, was a disease that usually began because young people were made to become too aware of the way they were speaking. This "iatrogenic" theory of stuttering meant that you became a stutterer as a result of being told by your doctor—or teacher or parent—that you stuttered. "Poor mothering" was often blamed—as in Clarice Pont's book *The Immediate Gift* (1961).[8] Presumably this explanation helped also to explain stuttering as the symptom of a "social phobia."[9]

Do you become a stutterer in some sort of hysterical, hypochondriacal, or hypnotic sense? For example, when a hypnotist tells a two-eared person that he has only one ear, the two-eared person begins to act as though he had only one ear, even though he *actually* continues to have two ears. (Many novels and films deal with attempts to cure stuttering through hypnosis; Andrei Tarkovsky's 1974 movie *Zerkalo* is a fine example.)[10] Or, to pursue the analogy with stuttering, does iatrogenic hypnosis mean that you would *actually* lose one of your ears—and thus become the one-eared person that your doctor or teacher or parent said you were? There is a midpoint between these two positions: "Bless thee, Bottom, bless thee! Thou art translated," says Quince when Bottom, in Act 3 of Shakespeare's *A Midsummer Night's Dream,* appears with his head transformed into that of an ass—a blend of two creatures.

I do not want to debate whether the iatrogenic theory is

correct within its own peculiar cultural parameters. (There would be important parallels here to considering stuttering in terms of other psychogenic and sociogenic factors.) Nor do I wish to consider *why* most speech therapists today argue against the iatrogenic view. (They favor the view that very early "intervention" is important—a view which, for them, at least has the advantage of pecuniary self-interest. The proper course of treatment is still much debated among physicians. That 3–4 percent of children but only 1 percent of adults stutter, regardless of intervention in childhood, suggests that there are many other factors besides the various therapies.)[11] Similarly, I will not consider the self-contradicting burdens that the iatrogenic theory puts on parents when it advises them to make a deliberate effort to stop worrying about their child's stuttering. Parents are told to *act as if* they're free from care, while at the same time they're told they should *really* care. This is like telling someone who cannot fall asleep that he should try harder. Finally, I want to set aside the fact that the practical or therapeutic results of the iatrogenic theory for the child were often much kinder than those of most previous theories. Many earlier theories had entailed grueling physical exercises, brutal surgeries, and psychologically intolerable assignments of willfulness to the child and consequent punishments. Many of the surgical treatments, some verging on torture, are detailed in the standard histories of stuttering.[12] By the same token, one might consult the works of the early surgeons themselves—Alfred Post in the United States (1841), for example, and Johann Dieffenbach in Germany (1841).[13] Dieffenbach resected the posterior portion of the tongues of hundreds of stutterers, with the result that "many of his patients died from pharyngeal swelling and suffocation."[14] Did believers in the diagnosis-induced theory of stuttering believe in it mainly because, at least, it did not further torment the stutterer?

There was another reason the first professional proponents of the iatrogenic theory came to believe it was true. They had private knowledge of the results of a disturbing experiment carried out in the 1930s and kept largely secret until the 1980s. The experiment, directed by Wendell Johnson and focusing on twenty-two children aged five to fifteen, took place at the Soldiers' and Sailors' Orphanage in Davenport, Iowa, and was written up in 1939 as a master's thesis by Mary Tudor at the University of Iowa.[15] The experiment showed that "normal" children—children labeled and treated as "nonstutterers"—actually become stutterers by virtue of a process called "evaluative labeling." The experiment showed likewise that "deprogramming" those same children, so that they might resume normal speech, was much more difficult and sometimes impossible. In fact, many of the children showed "stuttering behaviors" several years after the study, despite the original therapists' efforts to "cure" them; and some of the orphans *never* recovered, but became permanent stutterers.[16] (Shakespeare's Bottom in *A Midsummer Night's Dream* was, at least, eventually transformed back to his human form.) The researchers learned "how to make stutterers out of nonstutterers," but they never figured out how to "unmake" them. The psychologists did not discover a cure for stuttering, but they now believed they knew how it started. Its critics hypothesize nowadays that the Iowa experiment was kept secret for decades—until the 1990s—because it showed psychologists in such a negative light: professionals who were causing the very impediment that they sought to study and cure.[17] (What sort of doctors will generate the impediment whose existence guarantees their livelihoods? Doesn't the Hippocratic rule state that a physician should, at a minimum, do no harm? "As to diseases, make a habit of two things—to help, or at least to do no harm [*adikih eirxein*].")[18]

The iatrogenic stuttering experiment is the historical basis for the novel *Abandoned: Now Stutter My Orphan* (1999), by Jerry Halvorson.[19] The plot involves two orphans: a stutterer and a polio survivor. The stutterer is ten-year-old Frank. (He's modeled on Franklin Silverman—who claims, in real life, to be the first to have "unearthed" the experiment.)[20] The polio survivor is nine-year-old Carl. One day stuttering Frank and stumbling Carl are taken to a revival meeting. They come forward to be healed by the minister. Both receive temporary relief from their maladies. But when they return to the orphanage, Frank begins to stutter again and Carl has to put his leg brace back on.

I guess that my own stuttering was only *partly* the result of diagnoso-genesis. On the one hand, I was probably genetically predisposed to stutter. Several family members of mine stutter in some way.[21] And researchers have demonstrated a familial—if not also genetic—predisposition to stutter, as evidenced in an article in the tellingly named Russian journal *Defektologiya* (Defectology).[22] (When discussing genetics in this context, medical scholars sometimes point to similarities between stuttering and Tourette's Syndrome.)[23] In the popular realm—which will be a focus of my meditations here on the sociopathology of stuttering—Porky Pig cartoons make the same point. In the animated features *Porky the Rainmaker* (1936), *Porky's Poppa* (1938), and *Porky and Teabiscuit* (1939), Porky's father, Phineas Pig, stutters badly (worse than Porky does). And in the Dell comic books that I read during the 1950s, Petunia

Pig, Porky's girlfriend, also stutters. (There doesn't seem to be any mention of Porky's mother in the original Porky Pig series.)[24] According to Shell Family myth, my epileptic paternal Uncle Label stuttered for merely neurogenic reasons[25] and genetically based stuttering came down to us children only from the mother's side!

An ancient notion about stuttering holds that it is infectious,[26] so the fact that Petunia Pig stutters, or that Roger Rabbit's brother stutters on the letter *d* in much the way Roger himself stutters on *p*,[27] may not mean that their stutters are genetically based. Petunia, for example, may have contracted her "disease" from friend Porky. The idea goes far back in the medical annals. "If you have one child who stutters, then keep the other children away from him, unless you want them to stutter also": this old rule of thumb, from a nineteenth-century medical text, still has adherents.[28] One relevant story concerns Erasmus Darwin's attitude toward his eldest son, Charles (who, had he lived longer, would have been the uncle of the famous naturalist Charles Robert Darwin, who wrote *On the Origin of Species*). Erasmus, a physician, poet, and botanist, "stammered extremely," to the point where "a high degree of stammering retarded and embarrassed his utterance." His son "had contracted the propensity" to stutter, so Erasmus sent him abroad, "to break the force of habit, formed on the contagion of daily example." It is worth remarking that Erasmus Darwin had "an incurable weakness" in his right leg, much like Carl in Halvorson's novel *Abandoned*. His leg weakness, the result of a "fractured part" of the knee, caused "a lameness" and hence stumbling.[29]

Another example is the seventeenth-century scientist Robert Boyle, alias Philaretus, who wrote of himself: "The second Misfortune that befell Philaretus was his Acquaintance with some Children of his owne Age, whose stuttering Habitude he so long Counterfeited that he at last contracted it."[30] Similarly, the novelist and teacher Edward Hoagland wrote: "Once I imitated a child's stutter at a summer camp, thereby . . . picking up the malady at the age of six."[31] The *Westminster Gazette* of October 6, 1893, likewise mentions "a professor of elocution who has caught a trick of stammering from those whom he has cured of traulism."

I myself felt some of my parents' fear that my traulism (stutter) was "infectious." Was I perhaps to blame for the stuttering of my younger sister Lieba? Had she "learned" it from me? (That Lieba was left-handed—which, according to the literature of the period, apparently predisposed children to stutter—seemed almost to get me off the hook.)[32] Was my brother Brian kept away from me because, though I did not stumble much (compared with other polio survivors), I did stammer a lot (compared with other stutterers)?

Not all people with "predispositions" to stutter end up as stutterers. Likewise, not all people who live around stutterers become stutterers. There are usually "exacerbating factors," both physical and psychological. This was certainly true in my case.

For example, my bout with polio at age six affected me physically and psychologically. First, in the year or two following the illness, paralysis probably affected my physical ability to speak fluently. Emma Luethy Hayhurst, in her memoirs, describes how her crippling polio precipitated a severe stutter: "A side effect of the polio in my case was stammering."[33] The nineteenth-century physician Samuel Potter, himself a stutterer, wrote that *dyslalia* (stuttering) is associable not only with *paralalia* (articulation disorder) but also with *alalia* (language and motor speech disorders arising from motor paralysis).[34] Yet paralytic disease sometimes actually cures stuttering, as in some cases of Landry's Ascending Paralysis, or Guillain-Barré Syndrome, though no one knows why this happens. There is still no reliable research about the relationship between stuttering and such diseases.[35]

Second, the psychosocial and psychological stress of having had polio included, in my case, a fear that often accompanies a paralysis that lingers on. This is the fear of losing whatever ability to move, to be flexible or fluid, that an afflicted person might still have left. Dread of paralysis of both body and speech meant anxiety about both stumbling and stuttering. In his novel *La Parole prisonnière* (Speech Imprisoned), Jean Métellus—who holds degrees in neurology and linguistics—presents stuttering as a "metaphor" for bodily paralysis.[36]

A third exacerbating factor involves the way that poliomyelitic paralysis affects the spirit even as it violently disrupts the link between mind and matter. That stuttering can be brought about by such a spiritual crisis is clear enough from the historical record: the glossoplegia, or tongue paralysis, of the eleventh-century Sufi philosopher Al-Ghazzali was induced by what we now call a *crise de foi* (crisis of faith).[37]

For me, a fourth factor was a rarely articulated fear of being "abandoned." For a polio survivor in the 1950s, to fear that one would be abandoned was common. Such fear was not unjustified for disabled children: first-person narratives like *Abandoned Child* (1995), by the polio survivor Marie Morgart, historical novels like Halvorson's book *Abandoned,* and a rich statistical literature all tell sad stories of parents' abandonment of polio cripples. In any case, such fear makes it even easier to induce stuttering by medical or parental disapproval of physical or linguistic hesitancy.

In fact, the treatment I received was nearly the opposite of the one that Wendell Johnson and his colleagues proposed for young stutterers. Johnson said that parents who feared that their children would stutter should ignore or disregard any speech hesitancy, unless they wanted actually to trigger it. Yet my father's uncontrollable fear that his son was a stutterer (like his brother Label) probably helped to make that son a stutterer. When I was eight years old and recently paralyzed from polio, he would sometimes yell at me because I was not speaking fluidly enough. In later years, I associated my father's anger with the scene in the movie *The Cowboys* where John Wayne turns on a boy who stutters and starts screaming at him. (In those days I myself had a Gene Autry cowboy suit.) Wayne says that the boy could easily stop stuttering, if only he *really* wanted to; and he then goes on to say that the boy should either stop stuttering or leave the group.[38] He might have heeded the advice of the nineteenth-century theologian Frederic Myers: "The father who should impose the obligations of manhood upon a yet lisping son . . . would be as unjust as he would be unwise."[39]

My father's behavior toward me was not unusual in the context of the culture surrounding the polio epidemics. As early as 1949, Elizabeth Rice had written: "Parents seemed to need to discover some obvious deformity" after a child had had poliomyelitis. "If there was no physical deformity and no residual paralysis on which they could concentrate their attention," she wrote, "they recognized personality [and other] changes. . . . Some parents imagined problems that did not exist or exaggerated those that did because of their own state of emotional turmoil or their need for re-

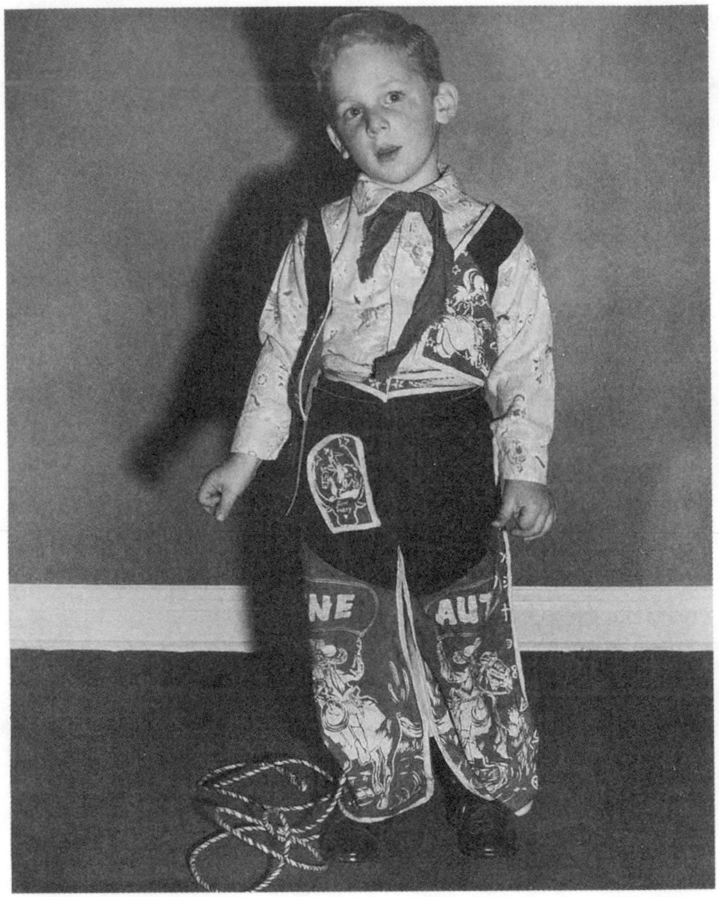

1. The author in Gene Autry costume, 1953. Photo by Bennie Cytrynbaum.

lease when the child was out of danger."[40] So my father, who had been a medical student, uncovered the stuttering in me. From the sequelae of physical paralysis of the legs, he helped to establish—inadvertently and without bad intention—an intermittent paralysis of the vocal chords.

By the time I was nine and in fourth grade, I was failing two subjects in school: Gym (due to my intermittently weak leg) and Reading Out Loud (due to my intermittently blocked speech).[41] One fourth-grade text that I had special difficulty reading aloud was *The Girl Next Door* (1946), an official school-reader about a girl polio survivor who had just moved into a new neighborhood.

I was lucky, perhaps, that I was not asked to leave the public school system, because children who were not "mainstreamed" had a far worse time than I.[42] But I was hurt hard, emotionally, by the mainstream. Being teased in the schoolyard was not the only problem. One day, the school principal, Mr. Webster, asked me into his office. He explained to me that stuttering was a "sure sign" of being mentally deficient, or "retarded." My failure to read aloud properly, said the principal, was not *my* "fault." I wondered, "Who *else*'s failing (but mine) was it?"—without daring even to try to speak the words. "Who *else* (but me) would have to live with this *faillite* [bankruptcy]?" That is how the French Canadian kids named my problem in the playground. I had no words, in those days, to ask anything of Principal Webster.

Principal Webster's notion that stuttering is a sure sign of mental slowness is still a means to tease stutterers[43] in the playground and helps in bullying them.[44] Popular songs employ the same mechanism, as in Bachman-Turner Overdrive's best-selling song "You Ain't Seen Nothing Yet" (1974), which Randy Bachman, a Canadian, wrote in order to mock the stuttering speech-patterns of his brother Gary. (His siblings were actually encouraged to mock the young George VI's stammer.)[45] Even today, children's books and cartoons take up the myth of the unintelligent stutterer.[46] Similarly, many school psychologists and administrators still see stuttering as a symptom of "mental retardation"[47] or as a disabling "nervous condition."[48]

Anyhow, I failed fourth grade because of my stuttering—or, rather, because of the Protestant School Board's official policy toward stuttering.

It is only fair to add that I had a second strike against me, besides stuttering. Some people in the 1950s, including a few family doctors in my hometown of Montréal, believed that the disease polio not only lowered the polio survivor's ability to keep himself from stumbling but also lowered his IQ, or "intelligence quotient."[49] One corollary of Juvenal's adage "Mens sana in corpore sano"[50] ("A sound mind in a sound body")—the only writing engraved in my high school auditorium—was "An unsound body indicates an unsound mind."

The Comparatist's Disease

These days I am a more or less inaudible stutterer, or stammerer. I now tend toward the extreme of regular speaking fluency—and away from that of tongue paralysis, say, or that of the facial paralysis known as Moebius' Syndrome.[51] You might not always know, listening to me, that I am "slow of tongue." But I *do* talk the talk (inwardly). "Am I a stutterer or a person who stutters?"[52]

I am a professor of comparative literature with a concomitant intellectual interest in at least three types of verbal substitution typical among stutterers.

First, there is *translational* or *interlinguistic synonymy,* whereby a word in one language passes for a word in *another language.* When growing up in bilingual Montréal, I used bilingual synonymy as a means to avoid stuttering. Some scholars discuss this strategy in terms of "word switching" and others in terms of "sound-based avoidance."[53] Such avoidance techniques are part of being a "covert" or "closet" stutterer; I like to think of them also in terms of what some researchers call "self-correction."[54] As an example of translational or interlinguistic synonymy, consider how the French word *argent* (literally, "silver") often means pretty much the same as the English word *money.* In officially bilingual Canada, when I lecture at a predominantly anglophone university and feel the approach of a linguistic spasm for the English word *money,* I may switch *legally* to the French *argent.* You might think of this stutter-avoidance technique as a sort of internalized "simultaneous translation." The American novelist Henry James, by the way, stuttered in English but rarely in French; I know many people like that.

Second, there is *intralinguistic synonymy,* whereby a word in one language passes for another word in that *same language.* When lecturing at officially anglophone Harvard or at the officially francophone Sorbonne, I sometimes draw upon a certain facility in intralinguistic synonymy. For example, in a lecture at the Sorbonne on the subject "Comment Penser l'Argent" (How to Think Money), I might take advantage of the fact that the French word *monnaie* ("money") means pretty much the same as the French word *argent.*[55] If, while lecturing in France, I feel a stutter coming on for *argent,* I can switch—unnoticed—to *monnaie.* (Stuttering for money is, of course, another matter. A certain Balbus Blaesius stuttered so severely that the Romans exhibited him in a locked cage, and people would pass coins to him in return for his stuttering. [The name Blaesius still informs Romance-language words for "stuttering" and "lisping."] The very word *begging* is associated with stuttering: the mendicant "lay sisterhood" of the Be-

speak, to stammer."[64] Relatively recent rap music is often associated with stuttering, as in the 1988 song "Stutter Rap": "But I'm under the *hammer* / 'cause all I seem to do is s-s-s-st- . . . / [Chorus:] Come on man! / . . . s-s-s-st-stammer!"[65] Compare the second verse of "Stop Stutterin', Sam," from 1924: "Ev'ry morning early, / He would phone his girlie; / Then he'd *stammer* / And he'd *hammer* / On the telephone / Until poor Ka-Katie / Would lose her head and moan.")[66] Finally, Porky hits his thumb and, in pain, cries out, "O son of a bi-bi-bi, son of a bi-bi-bi, son of a bi-bi- gun!" Then he hams things up. He turns directly to the "camera" and taunts us: "You thought I was going to say 'son of a bitch,' didn't you?" But we still don't know for sure what Porky, the *ham,* originally *meant* to say. We know only what he *actually* said: first *gun* and then *bitch.*

Purposeful stutterers sometimes have much the same effect in public discourse. For example, the classicist Seth Benardete (according to Ronna Burger) reports a gag in the philosopher Leo Strauss's hemming and stuttering introduction of the Jewish scholar Martin Buber. Here's how Benardete says that Strauss used aural anticipation and verbal expectation to put Buber down:

> *Seth [Benardete]:* One spring, Martin Buber came to Chicago. He was to speak at Hillel House, and [Leo Strauss] was asked to introduce him. I was sitting on a couch with Mrs. Strauss. Buber came in, looking very dignified.
>
> *Ronna [Burger]:* Venerable?
>
> *Seth:* Very venerable. He was right next to Strauss, next to the podium. And Strauss began this way: "I have the great pleasure to introduce Martin Buber, who is probably the greatest Jewish thinker since Mmm . . ." And after a long

time, it finally came out "Moses." Then he went on, "since Moses Mmm." Everybody thought—

Ronna: Maimonides, at least.

Seth: Right, But Strauss continued, "Mmm . . ." and at last, "Mendelssohn." I flipped over the back of the chair. I thought it was the funniest thing I had ever heard. What happened was—you could see from Buber's face—when Strauss said "Moses," he blew up like a frog, and then he was slightly deflated when Strauss said "Moses Mmm . . ." and completely so by the end.

Ronna: What happened to Mrs. Strauss when you flipped over?

Seth: She held my hand, I think.[67]

There are often material consequences to a stutterer's choosing to say one word instead of another. For example, the stutterer sometimes gets one thing instead of another. In their didactic novel —*And the Stutterer Talked* (1938), Abraham Kanter and Abe Kohn describe the sort of give-and-take event that most adult stutterers recall from childhood:

> One morning [the mother of the novel's hero, Billy] sent him for lemons, and he returned with a purchase of oranges. Why, she wanted to know, did he bring oranges instead of lemons? "Because the man didn't have any lemons," said Billy. Whereupon she determined to return the oranges herself and give the grocer a piece of her mind. She went and Billy started after her with fear-stricken eyes. Then he hid himself in the bedroom.
>
> "Billy," she said, quite beside herself with anger, when she returned, "why did you lie to me?"

> A flood of pent up tears rushed down Billy's cheeks. The mother gathered him in her arms. "Come, son, she consoled, "tell your mother what is the matter. She knows her little man wouldn't deliberately story to her." And Billy, amid violent sobs, said, "I couldn't say the word."[68]

For the speaker Porky Pig—as well as for his interlocutors—verbal substitution is similarly no small joke when circumlocution is motivated without much regard to originally intended "meaning" but mainly with regard to what is actually "unspeakable."[69] For one thing, a sequence of substitutions such as Porky often creates is usually a tremendous intellectual challenge for the speaker. After all, one originally unintended lexical change leads willy-nilly to others. So, too, do concomitant changes of syntactic construction. What finally comes out can resemble the final utterance in a game of Telephone—the result of what is called, in the title of one cartoon, *Porky's Phoney Express.* (The titles of two other cartoons, *Porky's Bear Facts* [1941] and *Porky Pig's Feat* [1943], indicate the same problem of lost original meanings.) Consequential and unpredictable changes of meanings in my own speaking—and, I daresay, also in my style of writing—often end with "muddled syntax" and neverending, uncontrolled meaning.[70] Oftentimes, by the time *I* am done speaking, the *speaking* has done me in.

Likewise, I wonder: Who, really, is speaking? Is it me—a sort of professional ventriloquist like Edgar Bergen? Or is it me—a carved, wooden persona like Bergen's dummy, Charlie McCarthy? In the end, intralinguistic substitution makes for personal substitution, and vice versa. This, finally, is the real meaning of *Porky's Double Trouble* (1937): the dubbing in doubling, the pun in the stutter.

Some techniques that the stutterer picks up in the process of learning "to *stutter* voluntarily" (versus "to speak without stuttering")[71]—and hence learning "to *speak* relatively fluently"—often amount to "a process akin to learning a second language."[72] "I have learned three foreign languages in my life: English, French, and 'Fluency.'"[73] These techniques include rhetorical stratagems such as "pull-outs," "cancellations," "bounces," and "link[ing] syllables [in a phrase] together as if they formed one long word"—as one student of the Danish-Canadian theorist Einer Boberg summarizes it.[74] In his book *Tongue Wars: Recovery from Stuttering,* William Perkins argues provocatively that "voluntarily controlled fluency is the wrong scientific objective, to say nothing of the wrong treatment objective"; and indeed, "voluntarily controlled fluency"[75] is more a symptom of stuttering—like James Earl Jones's self-imposed silence—than it is a cure for stuttering. Yet mastering these stratagems for attaining pseudo-fluency is as good as learning a second language, both alongside a first language and within that first language.

A doubly forked tongue.

Whatever benefit to his fluency a bilingual stutterer may derive from switching between languages is easily more than offset in the cases of those Montréalers who, like my young self, are anxious not only about how well they do (or don't) *know* a less familiar language but also about how fluently (or haltingly) they speak *any* language.[76] Among the usual factors to consider here would be the diglossic stutterer's age (as argued in such essays as "Stuttering out of Bilingualism")[77] and the particular sociological role of "foreign dialect"[78] in any given geographic locale.[79] In Québec, members of the generally francophone Association des Jeunes Bègues du Québec (Association of Young Stutterers of Québec) switch from French to English; contrariwise, members of the generally anglophone Canadian Association for People Who Stutter switch from English to French. (Below, we will compare stutterers who do not stutter when they sing or speak onstage.)[80]

Oftentimes when growing up in Québec I would "switch" between French and English. As it seemed to me then, my individual pathology of bilingualism reflected the war "between two nations [even races] at war in the bosom of a single state" that Lord Durham had noticed as Canada's main problem.[81] What is more, I thought that bilingual Canada's pathology had a sociolinguistic counterpart in the English language itself. Even today I am not sure whether this was an idle wish on my part or a sort of incipient and perhaps unprovable hypothesis.

I refer here to what was then called "the dualism of [the] elder [French] phraseology" in the English language.[82] I was told by my anglophone teachers that during the bilingual—or Anglo-Norman—period in England, speakers began to provide "practically synonymous word-pairs,"[83] sometimes called "doublets," where one word was originally "Anglo-Saxon" (Germanic) and the other was essentially "French" (Latin), as in the phrases *hue and cry* or *goods and chattel*. We were taught that the existence of these two traditions alongside each other explained why it was "not an infrequent thing in Chaucer for a line to contain a single fact bilingually repeated."[84] This is why English sometimes seems to be a "walking phrase book or dictionary," useful in studying other languages, especially French.[85] My favorite such doublet was the obviously English-French name of the forever linguistically doubling Porky Pig (the word *pork* is of Latin derivation; *pig* is Germanic).[86]

In *Philology of the English Tongue* (1871), which was assigned to our class in the curiously colonial and Victorian high school that I attended, John Earle argued that "this equivalent coupling of words, one English and one French, is no mere accidental or rhetorical exuberance. It sprang first out of the mutual necessity felt by two races of people and two classes of society to make themselves intelligible to one another."[87] I wanted the explanation for this coupling to go beyond historical exigency. So I was happy when I went to college. I learned (at the then similarly Victorian McGill University) that intralingual doubling had been widespread in English even before the Norman invasion in 1066. All this suggested to me that the English, including the anglophone population of Québec ("brittanique de souche"—"British by race"), may always have suffered from a sort of redundancy, or internalized stutter. At the time, I thought that this internalized stutter, a sort of linguistic pathology, helped to explain the brilliance of Humphrey Chimpden Earwicker's remarkable stutter—at least as the anglophone Irishman James Joyce presents him in his forcedly monumental and multilingually crabbed *Finnegans Wake*. (My forthcoming essay "Doublets, Duplicates, and Reiteratives: An Initial Shilly-Shally in the Linguistics and Poetics of Ablaut Epanalepsis in Everyday Language" explores the similar hypothesis that anglophone reduplicative terms like *shilly-shally* and *dilly-dally* play a unique lexical and syntactic role in spoken English.)

Earlier I wondered: Who, really, was speaking? Was that me? Was it some (other) dummy? Not only does the question assume that there is such a thing as a *single* "self"—a not unproblematic hypothesis—but it seems almost to suggest that it might be better for *me,* whoever I am, if I am a stutterer, to talk not at all, or to stay "mum." (That is how the actor James Earl Jones dealt with his stutter during three years of his childhood.)[88] Silence as such should be considered as the sure cure for stuttering. "The only sure *cure* for stuttering is silence."[89] Yet silence is also the stutterer's extreme avoidance technique. Like the substitution of one word for another, and like the evasion strategy that consists of playing hooky from a class where oral performance is required, silence is as much a *symptom* of stuttering as its cure. "But break my heart / For I must hold my tongue," says Hamlet.[90] Muteness is often a clearer symptom of stuttering than audible stammering.[91]

Most stutterers do not triumph in this way, nor can they remain silent for long. If a stutterer must talk, he or she might fluently sing the words as song—or smoothly recite them as poetry. Careful students of elocution, as well as of music- and language-metrics, have remarked rightly that most stutterers cease to stutter when they singsong. In this way stutterers overcome muteness or effective language-removal. At one time, the cat had the stutterer's tongue,[92] but not when the stutterer sings. When singsonging, the stutterer becomes . . . a nightingale! Says T. S. Eliot in *The Waste Land:* "Twit twit twit / Jug jug jug jug jug jug / So rudely forc'd. / Tereu."

In Book 6 of Ovid's *Metamorphoses,* Philomel's enemies amputate her tongue (the same thing happens to Lavinia in Shakespeare's *Titus Andronicus*). Philomel's able art is her compensation for tonguelessness; likewise, her compensation for bodily disability is her artfulness. In the same manner, one may even say that what *sometimes* develops from the mental effort needed to deal with stuttering by way of both intra- and interlinguistic synonymy and personal substitution has certain rewards. After all, "compensating" for the difficulties of dis-ease, if not of dis-ability, is often a precondition for, if not a trigger of, genius.[93] Victor Shklovsky, the Russian Formalist literary critic, claimed that intellectual hurdles can be as good for the mind as physical ones are for the body.[94] Was it Shakespeare's near-inability to *stop* punning that helped make him the writer he was?[95] William Butler Yeats used to say that it was his dyslexia that made *him* the singsong poet he became.[96]

Demosthenes, who is among the most famous of stuttering orators and verbal compensators, used to fill his mouth with pebbles and declaim at the sea's edge.[97] (The young man in Bob Dylan's song "It's a Hard [—It's a Hard—It's a Hard—It's a Hard] Rain's a-Gonna Fall" likewise prepares his song *on* the shore: "And I'll stand on the ocean before I start *sinking* / And I'll know my song well before I start *singing*.") Demosthenes had *rhotacism*—"[a stuttering] difficulty with [the] *r* sound," as Samuel Potter puts it in *Speech and Its Defects* (1882).[98] At the sea's edge, this rhetorician's rhetorician was supposed to have practiced on a well-known tongue-twister: "Rerétoreuka to rerétoreumeno ró." I would translate Demosthenes' words: "I have pronounced as a rhetor [that is, performed the function of a rhetor, or *rhêtoreuô*] the rhetorical *rho*."

The phrase plays on how the perfect tense in the Greek language is formed by the reduplication, or stutter, of the first syllable in *reré-toreu-meno.* It also plays on how pronouncing the phrase "correctly"—which is to say, both palilogically and stutteringly—allows one to render the statement "true" according to the traditional Greek concept of public speaking. That concept sees speaking as actually doing, a theory which is almost a byword these days for what good literature and good literary criticism ought to do.[99] (He might have been surprised, though, by Renaissance theories that associate speech impedance with proximity to flowing water.)[100] No wonder, therefore, that

Demosthenes became the greatest Greek orator. He became the voice of the erstwhile Greek Empire in the fourth century B.C.E., calling the Macedonians "barbarians," just as James Earl Jones—a stuttering actor—is now the voice of America's AT&T.[101] (Concerning rhotacism, Anna Comnena in the twelfth century reported the following incident involving her father, Alexius Comnenus, emperor of Constantinople: "Basilacius [the enemy] came down suddenly upon the army. . . . But as the man he expected to find [Alexius] was nowhere to be seen, . . . [Basilacius] shouted still more loudly, and cried out, 'Where in the world is the Stammerer?' thus in his words too jeering at [Alexius]. For except in one respect, this Alexius, my father, had a very clear utterance, and no one was a better natural orator than he in his arguments and demonstrations, . . . but only over the letter *r* his tongue lisped slightly, and stammered a little, although his enunciation of all the other letters was quite unimpeded.")[102]

The stutterer's sometime muteness, discussed in the previous section, is a particularly poignant situation. The stutterer Edward Hoagland writes that because his father did not want his son to cease speaking, his father "turned over to me at the last [only on his deathbed] an old family history which he'd been hiding, partly because it mentioned a lot of muteness among my ancestors."[103] For me, at least, a situation in which a silent person successfully pretends to be mute instead of "coming out" as a stutterer is like that of a stumbling polio survivor in a plaster leg-cast pretending to be an athlete with a broken leg instead of "coming out" as a polio survivor. In the movie *Lucky Break* (1994), for example, a woman polio survivor actually breaks her leg and is thus enabled to pursue a love affair. Likewise, in the movie *Just the Way You Are* (1984), a paralyzed person has an unneeded leg-cast put on in order to pursue a love affair. I am myself a stuttering stumbler whose limbs were twisted by polio.

Talking the Walk and Walking the Talk

> My strength has gone from my body
> and my heart runs out like water;
> my flesh is dissolved like wax
> and the strength of my loins is turned to fear.
> My arm is torn from its socket
> and I can lift my hand no more;
> My foot is held by fetters
> and my knees slide like water;
> I can no longer walk.
> I cannot step forward lightly,
> For my legs and arms are bound by shackles
> which cause me to stumble.
> The tongue is gone back which Thou didst make
> marvelously mighty within my mouth;
> it can no longer give voice.
> I have no word for my disciples
> to revive the spirit of those who stumble
> and to speak words of support to the weary.
> My circumcised lips are dumb.
>
> —Thanksgiving Hymns, no. 18, *The Dead Sea Scrolls,*
> trans. Géza Vermès

That stumbling and stuttering are somehow the same is, of course, already suggested by most Indo-European languages. For example, the English term *stutter* is cognate with *stumble;* and oral *stammering* often goes together with pedal *stumbling.* Older glossaries discuss both "stammering in speech" and "stammering in going."[104] Other words suggest the same conjunction of stumbling and stammering: *falter, shamble, shrench, stacker, titubate,* and *totter.* So Thomas Elyot reminds us in his *Dictionary* of 1538: "*Titubo:* To stacker in speaking or going, as a man being drunk or sick." And in *Promptorium parvulorum* (1440) we read: "Stakerynge, in mevynge, *vacillacio,*" and "Stackering, in speech (or stammering), *titubacio.*"[105]

Not surprisingly, many writers in English point to the linkage between *stumbling* and *stuttering.* Richard Harvey writes in *Plaine Percevall* (1589): "And so foorth following the Traulila-lilismus, as far as Will Solnes stuttring pronunciation may stumble ouer at a breath. The same illness, we say, leads to both of these afflictions together."[106]

Some writers point to the similar linkage between *stumble* and *stammer.* "Give him a good shock in the mouth, that you may make him stammer and shuffle his legs confusedly together," says Gervase Markham in *Cavelarice* (1607).[107] In his translation of Quevedo's writings (1707), John Stevens says: "My Legs naturally stammer."[108] And the American writer Sylvester Judd says in *Margaret* (1845): "I stuttered up to No. 4 yesterday after the funeral."[109]

Staggering and *stammering* likewise mean both "pedal stumbling" and "verbal stuttering." Thus, Richard Bernard's translation of Terence's play *The Eunuch* reads: "He comes running to me . . . very crooked, staggering and stammering for age."[110]

All these semantic associations of pedal with verbal disability have extensive expressions in the more general cultural and medical realms. In "The Ugliest Girl in the World," Bob Dylan refers to stumbling as stuttering: "Well, the woman that I love / She speaks with a stutter and she walks with a hop / Don't know why I love her, but I just can't stop."[111] Lisping is sometimes grouped together with stuttering and is, like stuttering, often compared with pedal lameness. John Struthers thus writes about "a lisping lamiter of feeble frame" in his poem "The Poor Man's Sabbath" (1850).[112] Many stutterers refer to their speech as lame or paralytic; thus the poet Bianca Plouffe writes, "Un tourbillon de peur, / Me paralyse" ("a whirlwind of fear paralyzes me").[113] Walking badly and talking badly often go together in Shakespeare's works—as in *Henry IV*.[114]

Moreover, some writers make the parallel between stumbling and stuttering the conceptual center of both autobiographical and fictional writing. Thus, Somerset Maugham endows Philip, the main character in his quasi-autobiographical novel *Of Human Bondage* (1915), with a polio-like clubfoot instead of Maugham's own stutter—a pedal defect instead of a speech impediment.[115] About his verbal stumbling, Maugham often used to say: "The first thing you should know is that my life and my production have been greatly influenced by my stammer."[116]

Stuttering polio survivors such as myself are much aware of the association of stumbling with stuttering. In the 1950s, while I was supposed to be recovering from polio, my mother used to call me her "walkie-talkie." (A walkie-talkie is a doll that one can make walk and talk.)[117] But I never learned to walk or talk the way my mother wanted: I was a totterer who stuttered or a stutterer who tottered. Many children's books of the period, such as Alberta Armer's *Screwball* (1963), included characters who were polio stutterers.[118] In Jan Mark's novel *The Ennead* (1976),[119] one of the characters, Isaac, both limps and stutters. I had company.

I recall from Bob Dylan's visit to Montréal in 1962 that he sings about Emmet Till,[120] a celebrated victim during the American civil rights movement. Till was a stutterer who had had polio. Jean Nordhaus, who is a polio survivor, writes in her poem "The Stammer:" "I grapple / With my tongue as Jacob / Wrestled with the angel / For a word." John Tierney, senator for New South Wales in Australia, is a polio survivor who stutters;[121] so too is Luis Fermin, once touted (mistakenly) as "the last polio victim in the Western hemisphere."[122]

Many a paralytic polio survivor refers to his own speech or writing as a form of stuttering. The polio survivor Walter Scott, for example, referred to his "paralytic custom of stuttering with my pen."[123]

The anonymous essay "Psellism" (the word comes from the Greek *psellízein,* meaning "to stammer"), published in Charles Dickens' weekly *Household Words* in 1856, argues that "apoplexy" (paralysis) is often associated with stuttering.[124] We might well ask: Why? Why *do* so many paralyzed polio survivors stutter? The author of "Psellism" suggests that "stammering . . . arises as a barrier by which the sufferer feels that the world without is separated from the world within him."[125] What else might speech "impediment" and "pedal" crippling have in common? Let us set aside—at least for now—the unlikely hypothesis that there is a single "gene" that makes the same person likely both to stutter and to contract paralytic polio. Let us hypothesize instead that stuttering is triggered or exacerbated—whether in those few people who have some genetic predisposition to stutter or in all people—by some sort of psychological trauma in childhood.[126] Polio provides this trauma in the form of the dissociation—or diremption—of body from mind. This amounts to a separation of will from action following suppression of the memory of the extraordinarily painful onslaught of the initial experience. Other physical disabilities, especially those that involve the tongue, would tend to trigger stuttering in much the same way.[127] The analogy with Post-Traumatic Stress Disorder and shell shock is useful here. Vietnam war veterans suffered an extraordinarily high incidence of delayed reactions—including nightmares, flashbacks, survivor guilt, sleeplessness, depression, nervousness, loss of energy, and diminished sexual desire—even years after the horrors they experienced in Vietnam. Among these reactions was stuttering.[128] Paul Hardcastle catches this aspect of the Vietnam War experience in his song "19," with its chorus of singing girls: "All those who remember the war / They won't forget what they've seen / Destruction of men in their prime / whose average was nineteen / Dedededededede-Destruction / Dedededededede-Destruction / War, War / Dededede-Destruction, wa-wa-War, wa-War, War / Dedededededede-Destruction / War, War."[129]

Moreover, physiological changes that occur in the area of the mouth, tongue, and throat during a poliovirus attack sometimes render the polio survivor mute. Muscles and nerves in the lung and throat regions can become useless. Polio thus "causes" speech problems when it affects the mouth or tongue. William Russell MacAusland, in his magisterial medical textbook *Poliomyelitis* (1927), observes that polio survivors manifest "speech disturbances" especially when they try to pronounce labials (sounds that require closure of the lips) and linguals (the vowels and all consonants except the labials and gutturals).[130] Many of the first-person polio narratives that I have read refer to such periods of intermittent bulbar paralysis. For example, Arthur C. Clarke, who went on to write *2001,* reported of his bout with polio: "I think I must have missed an iron lung by the thickness of a nerve fiber. Although I could breathe without much trouble when perfectly relaxed, the slightest exertion left me gasping. I could not speak more than two or three words without panting for breath."[131] Often polio patients are afraid that they will become unable to talk—that they will be left mute. Enid Foster, a writer in Bulawayo, South Rhodesia (now Zimbabwe), reported that her daughter joked with her, "It's a good thing your mouth was never paralyzed, Mummy!"[132]

Dr. MacAusland also discusses the effect of polio on speech after the poliomyelitis attack has subsided. In cases of "cerebral polio," he says, the sequelae often include speech problems.[133] Such effects, if short lived, would make child polio survivors relatively "conscious" of their speech defects. And according to some theoreticians, this consciousness, whether apart from or together with any lingering physical weakness from neuronal damage, would make such children more susceptible than others to becoming stutterers. As mentioned earlier, some researchers believe that "undue" attentiveness to intermittent speech paralysis can trigger the very stuttering it is meant to avoid or repress.

Stutter Writing

> Who cannot stumble in a stuttering stile?
> And shallow heads with seeming shades beguile?
>
> —John Marston, *The Metamorphosis of Pygmalion's Image* (London, 1598)

> I don't think anyone has ever done a study of speech difficulties specific to writers. . . . Did any of these take to text

> because of their difficulties with *parole?* Was their literary style affected by the nature of their impediment?
>
> —MARGARET DRABBLE, "Public Speech and Public Silence," address to the British Stammering Association, 2001

Speakers and writers often use the term *stuttering* metaphorically to refer to something other than the actual "speech impediment." (Likewise they often use the dozens of synonyms for *stuttering* that I employ in this book.) Even theorists who claim vociferously that they would never use neurophysiological and medical conditions "metaphorically" nevertheless use stuttering as such. One example would be Susan Sontag. On the one hand, Sontag claims—in *Styles of Radical Will*—that Samuel Beckett has an "ontological stammer." On the other hand, she harshly criticizes—in *Illness as Metaphor* and *AIDS and Its Metaphors*—just such metaphorical or rhetorical "misappropriations."[134] Elsewhere I have written about this sort of unwitting contradiction between stated purpose and actual practice, and about its consequence for the theory of metaphor and for the cultural history of medicine.[135] In the present instance, we need merely to underscore that such contradiction is especially common when it comes to quasi-philosophical expressions of stuttering. Gilles Deleuze is a case in point when he uses the terminology of *speech* impediment to characterize *writing* excellence. He praises Ghérasim Luca and Charles Péguy because "they stutter when they write."[136] Deleuze follows the lead of Marcel Proust, Walter Benjamin, and Paul de Man in arguing that every great writer creates a foreign language inside his or her own language.[137] In *What Is Philosophy?* Deleuze explains philosophy as "that which stutters" and hence saves words by creating a "perpetual disequilibrium in language"; it is a system that "overstrains itself [and so] begins to stutter, to murmur, or to mumble."[138] For Deleuze, parataxis is thus the finest trope, since it produces apparent fissures in language.[139] Whether philosophy is more or less successful a fissuring agent than, say, poetry or music is a driving question for Friedrich Nietzsche's various investigations.[140] Whether such representations of stuttering in *writing* are adequate to the thinking about stuttering as a *speech* impediment is a question perhaps best left to thinkers who, like Johann Georg Hamann, have the purported advantage of actually stuttering when they speak.

On the more "literal" level, then, we ask with Margaret Drabble: Why are there so many professional writers who *really* stutter when they speak?

One answer to this question, Hoagland surmises, is that writing is the best way for the stutterer to escape his prisonhouse of silence: "Being in these vocal handcuffs made me a desperate, devoted writer."[141] (Some stutterers write in order to be silent: "Ecrire, c'est se taire"—to write is to keep silent.)[142] This is an attractive explanation. After all, Charlotte the spider in E. B. White's *Charlotte's Web* takes to spinning out her words as text precisely because, although she can spin silk as well as Ovid's Philomel can weave wool, she, like Philomel (whose tongue was cut out to prevent her from identifying her rapist), is unable or unwilling to speak aloud.

Writing thus offers a prosthetic means of communication that bypasses speaking. Consider how Amyotrophic Lateral Sclerosis, or Lou Gehrig's Disease (as in the case of physicist Stephen Hawking), spurred the development of the prosthetic writing device known as the Possum, and

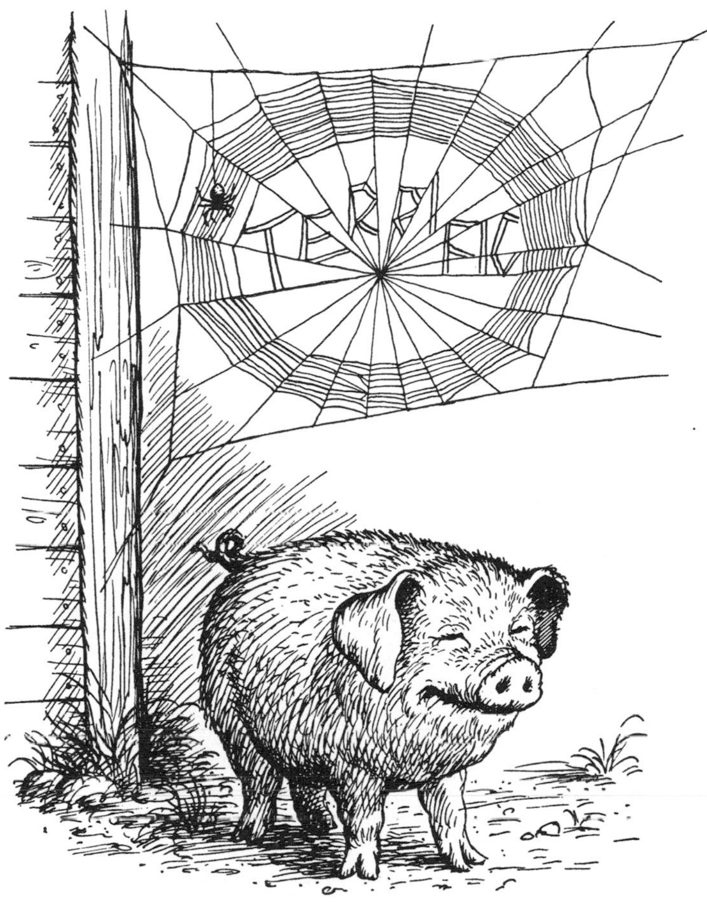

2. Garth Williams, *Terrific,* with Wilbur the pig and Charlotte the spider. From *Charlotte's Web,* by E. B. White (New York: Harper, 1952), p. 95. Copyright © 1952 by E. B. White; text copyright renewed 1980 by E. B. White. Used by permission of HarperCollins. Photo courtesy of the Harvard University Library.

likewise how bulbar polio (as in the case of writer Richard Chaput) sparked the invention of the *tongue stick*. People who suffered from bulbar polio, speechless inside caesura-enforcing iron lungs, wrote the most useful typing manuals—for example, the novelist Ruth Ben'ari at the Roosevelt Institute for Rehabilitation, in Warm Springs, Georgia.[143] If not paralysis of the vocal chords, then paralysis of the breathing muscles in neck and chest made for the breathing stops that the stutterer too knows.

For some people, writing might even present itself as a cure for stuttering rather than as the avoidance of speaking that is symptomatic of stuttering. Thus, Hoagland reports: "At the Ethical Culture School in New York . . . a woman taught me to stick my right hand in my pocket and, with that hidden hand, to write down over and over again the first letter of the word I was stuttering on."[144]

But even if Hoagland is correct in his basic assumption that stuttering is essentially a dysfunction in *speaking* (or if current theorists are right in saying that "stutterers are not aphasics and their word choice and grammar are normal"), it would not follow that stutterers' writing (style) is "normal."[145] In fact, there are several indications that stutterers, even when they are not stuttering, speak 15 percent slower than nonstutterers, which goes some way toward suggesting that stutterers might also write differently from nonstutterers. Consider the case of Porky Pig. In *Porky's Papa* (1938), Porky is unable to say his name. And when he tries writing it out, he does so only by "fits and starts." Porky can write his name only disfluently. Some graphology researchers argue that stutterers' handwriting generally differs from that of nonstutterers.[146] The film *The Court Jester* (1956), which stars Danny Kaye doing tongue-twisters, suggests that it is possible to stutter in sign language.[147]

So how *does* a stutterer in the real world r-r-r-write? One way to begin addressing this question might be to consider whether other types of hesitancy carry over into a writer's style. Walter Scott evidently thought they did, since he claimed to stutter with his pen. (In fact, Scott came from a long line of paralytic "lamisters": his ancestors included John the Lamiter, in the twelfth century, as well as William Boltfoot.)[148] Likewise, some readers of Emily Dickinson link her frequent use of dashes with the theme of psychological paralysis (her own) or physical paralysis (her mother's) that informs so many of her poems.[149]

A further word about the dash: As in Dickinson's work, it is often used "in writing or printing to mark a pause or break in a sentence, a parenthetic clause, an omission of words or letters or of the intermediate terms of a series, to separate distinct portions of matter, or for other purposes sometimes implying the use of strong language; hence as a mild substitute for *devil.*"[150] In this book I often use a dash to indicate a type of parataxis that is different from either parentheses or ellipsis dots. A dash often suggests an unspeakable or at least unspoken "connecting" passage (literally, a "metaphor"). The novelist Anna Nicholas indicates one such when she refers to "a dreadful thought which if put in print would have contained a dash."[151] The Latinist textual editor and translator James Muirhead points to another such use when he reminds his readers, "Passages that are illegible in the manuscript . . . are indicated by dashes."[152] But as we shall see, for the stutterer, the *dreadful thought* or *illegible passage* is initially and always the "unspeakable." It is like a thinker or manuscript caught permanently in oscillations between temporary caesuras. In this sense, *—And the Stutterer Talked,* by Kanter and Kohn, is remarkable for the dash in its title. Likewise, the stutterer

Lewis Carroll's extraordinary *Sylvie and Bruno* (1889), with its variously speech-impeded characters, begins apparently in midsentence with a dash: "—and then all the people cheered again . . ."

Another way to deal with the question, "How does a stutterer r-r-r-write?" would be to reconsider the actual writing styles of writers-who-stutter-when-they-speak. Among these are Lewis Carroll (who identifies himself with the stuttering tutor Balbus in his story "A Tangled Tale"), Margaret Drabble (who has made "a public declaration of public silence"), John Updike (who has written of the "paralysis of stuttering"), and Somerset Maugham.[153]

Henry James presents a telling case of the relationship between the way stutterers write and the way they speak. James's "slow way of speaking," wrote Edith Wharton, "was really the partial victory over a stammer which in his boyhood had been thought incurable." On the one hand, James apparently wrote as if his writing was always supposed to be read aloud. The literary scholar and essayist William Lyon Phelps said that James told him, "I have never in my life written a sentence that I did not mean to be read aloud, that I did not specifically intend to meet that test; you try it and see." On the other hand, James, according to his contemporary George William Erskine Russel, "talked like a book."[154] Yet often what James spoke aloud could not easily be written down, because he so frequently used *er* ("the inarticulate sound or murmur made by a hesitant speaker") and *ah* (like *uh,* a "representation of . . . inarticulate sound").[155] Elizabeth Jordan alludes to James's "habit of hemming and hawing."[156] (In *Lord Jim,* Joseph Conrad represents "stammering" in terms of hawing: "Aw—I am—aw—your new captain, Mister—Mister—aw—Jones.")[157] By way of illustration, Jordan reports

James's response when she asked him whether he thought Arnold Henry Savage Landor's *In the Forbidden Land* was a true account. This is Jordan's transcript of James's reply:

> "Eliminating—ah—" he said, "eliminating, ah-h—eliminating nine-tenths—nine-tenths—nine-*tenths* (slowly)—of-of-of (very fast)—of what he claims—what he claims (slowly) —what he claims (very slow)—there is still (fast)—there—is still—there is still (faster)—enough left (pause) enough left (pause) to make—to make—to make (very fast) a remarkable record (slow)—a remarkable record—ah—ah—(slower)—a re-markable re-cord."[158]

John Updike properly reminds us that "no two cases of dysphemia that I have known are quite alike."[159] I find equally intriguing the fact that there are so many different ways to indicate on the page that a particular speaker is stuttering or to render the particular stutter. Sometimes the difference among methods results in confusion about how a certain person stutters or even *whether* he or she stutters. (One finds the same variance in writers' attempts to present dialect, accents, and interjections.)

Consider, for example, two reports about the stutter of Somerset Maugham. On the one hand, Arthur Marshall represents Somerset Maugham's stuttering as "I felt I h-h-h-had to tell him the t-t-truth."[160] Marshall insists this typographical representation is an "accurate" reproduction of how Maugham "actually spoke." On the other hand, there are those who claim that Maugham did not stutter by repeating sounds (saying "h-h-h-h"); they insist that he got stuck "like a typewriter key." This is how Ted Morgan puts it, even as he claims that Maugham's stutter was "a speech defect that cannot be imitated in type."[161] According to Morgan, Maugham would often fall silent, sometimes for as long as a minute, and then start up again. Maugham would pause, frozen in speech, and "say nothing," in the midst of a paragraph. This is, in some ways, how we might imagine Pyrrhus as reported in the "Player's speech" in *Hamlet:* he would pause and, as if suddenly paralyzed, "do nothing." No wonder Updike and others refer to "the paralysis of stuttering."[162]

In the case of the stutterer Moses, as we shall see in Chapter 4, it is alphabetic writing in particular that becomes the essentially legislative *possum* of language itself.

Rhetorical Terminology and Neurological Nosology

Compensatory verbal substitution has many apparently different rhetorical means. For example, a person who stutters may turn an intended euphemism ("son of a gun") willy-nilly into scatology ("son of a . . . bitch"). Likewise, he may turn an apparently involuntary repetition into an apparently orderly anadiplosis. By way of example, Francis Bacon—the author of an important essay on stuttering—says: "Men in great place are thrice servants: *servants of* the sovereign or state; *servants of* fame; and *servants of* business."[163] Or a stutterer may take a phrase that he is particularly good at pronouncing and employ it as anaphora. Winston Churchill—a stutterer—exemplifies this in one of his speeches: "*We shall* not flag or fail. *We shall* go on to the end. *We shall fight* in France, *we shall fight* on the seas and oceans, *we shall fight* with growing confidence and growing strength in the air, *we shall* defend our island, whatever the cost may be, *we shall fight* on the beaches, *we shall fight* on the landing grounds, *we shall fight* in the fields and in the streets, *we shall fight* in the hills. *We shall* never surrender."[164] By the same token, an individual who stutters might turn a lack of grammatical sequence (typical among stammerers) into anacoluthon.[165] Or he may turn a full stop into the sort of abrupt halt one encounters in real life (as in Somerset Maugham's speech patterns) and in literature (as in the Virgilian "Player's speech" in *Hamlet*). This stop might even appear as the sort of ellipsis called aposiopesis, which in the original Greek suggests silence.[166] In aposiopesis, the speaker comes to a sudden halt as if unable or unwilling to proceed. The traditional literary example comes from Virgil's *Aeneid;* another comes from Shakespeare's *Julius Caesar,* where Antony interrupts his own speech at Caesar's funeral.[167]

The stutterer may turn a speaking block into the condensed, even laconic expression called brachylogy.[168] Or he may terminate his utterance with an instance of synecdoche (as when Porky Pig concludes his statement—"If there's one thing I don't need"—with a word indicating the whole canine species instead of a single breed) or may substitute a part for the whole (as when Eliot's hesitant Prufrock says, "I should have been a pair of ragged claws / Scuttling across the floors of silent seas").[169] Likewise, the stutterer may turn involuntary repetitions into artful paronomasia: "Thou art Peter [Greek: *petros*], and upon this rock [*petra*] I shall build my church."[170] Or he may turn a verbal omission into an artful praeteritio, or prolepsis: "That part of our history which tells of the military achievements which gave us our several possessions, or of the ready valour with which either we or our fathers stemmed the tide of Hellenic or foreign aggression, is a theme too familiar to my hearers for me to dilate on, and I shall therefore pass it by" (Thucydides).[171] Sometimes the stutterer provides an ending unanticipated by either rhyme or reason, in the form of a paraprosdokian: "There but for the grace of God—goes God," said Churchill about Sir Stafford Cripps.[172] Like Hamlet in the quatrain he delivers after the performance of "The Mousetrap," the stutterer does not provide the rhyme expected, because he cannot or will not say it. There results a more or less involuntary expression of something that is contrary to, or different from, the first more or less intended meaning: the words say one thing but mean another. This disjuncture separating sounds from meaning is often called irony or antiphrasis ("Yet Brutus says he was ambitious; / And Brutus is an honourable man").[173] So the stutterer earns a certain compensatory control: in some cases it sounds "diseased," while in other cases it sounds "poetical."[174]

Literary critique is useful in analyzing stuttering partly because the intellectual history of rhetorical terms, like those I use in this book, often matches the scholarly development of concomitant ideas in neurology. The term *palilalia,* for example, derives from *pali* (meaning "again") and *lalia* (meaning "talk"). It designates a speech condition "characterized by repetition of words, phrases, or sentences." Neurologists usually know only what *palilalia* means in the narrow range of present-day medical textbooks. I would suggest, though, that it straddles the line between neurology and rhetoric. For the neurologists who depend on the usual textbooks, "*palilalia* refers to a decrescendo (in the volume of the sound) of whole words and phrases and is most commonly associated with Parkinson's disease." (Contemporary neurologists generally use *palilalia* with reference to Parkinson's disease; it is also used for describing symptoms of schizophrenia and various brain injuries.)[175] Most would argue that it would be a blunder to conflate palilalia with stuttering. Yet the *Oxford English Dictionary* says that *palilology* is "the repetition of a word or phrase, especially in immediate succession, for the sake of emphasis." (The term *emphasis* here retains its strictly rhetorical meaning: "The use of language in such a way as to imply more than is actually said; a meaning not inherent in the words used, but conveyed by implication." In *Mysterie of Rhetorique Unvail'd,* John Smith speaks in the same way of *palilogia.* And in *Ekskubalauron; or, The Discovery of a Most Exquisite Jewel,* Thomas Urquhart refers to *palilogetick elucidations.*)[176] And palilalia, with its various analyses, has an ongoing two-thousand-year history in the very thought on which neurology originally depended and on which it continues to depend, since it is a developing science and stuttering still remains something of a mystery to it. In early neurological history, palilalia was associated with stuttering, partly because both stutter and palilalia disappear when a person "sings." No one has yet been able to determine why this happens.[177]

Older humanist doctors remind us that "those familiar with such symptoms as automatic writing, palilalia, perseveration and verbigeration are inclined to wonder whether or not the literary abnormalities in which [the individual] indulges represent correlated distortions of the intellect."[178] In this way of thinking, the apparently disorderly becomes the apparently orderly, and the apparently involuntary becomes the apparently voluntary. So speech impediment becomes literary art, or vice versa.

2 Testing the Word

> It is not madness
> That I have uttered. Bring me to the test,
> And I the matter will reword.
>
> —SHAKESPEARE, *Hamlet,* 3.4.148–150

The ability to speak language in general is often taken to be a sign of membership in the group of "human beings." Likewise, speaking a particular language properly is an important component of any given "culture"; people cling to the notion of speaking properly as a "necessary sign" of membership in their own "tribe."

In this context, "language tests" really matter. They are a matter of life and death. The guidelines are usually pretty clear.

1. If you can't speak at all, then probably you are not a human being.
2. If you speak a little, then you might be a human being, but just as likely you could be a parrot.
3. If you can't speak my particular language in my particular way, then you probably aren't a member of my tribe.

On the basis of such "guidelines," some "nonspeakers" often lose such "rights" to life as are based on, or derived from, membership in a common humanity or in a particular tribe. By the same token, some humanoid bipeds whom (or that) *we* might actually call "human beings" might never get those rights as conferred by *others.* All too often in human history the motives for *linguicide* (destroying a language)[1] verge on the terrible purposes of *genocide* (destroying all the individuals of a culture). This is, after all, the history of language wars. If you fail the language test, you die.

For a stutterer in this battlefield, the only safe place—would that there were one!—seems to be silence. For him, *all* words are test words, passwords, or catchphrases whereby one gains or loses social acceptance or credibility. For him, the typical word test is not a predictable shibboleth term that he can or cannot learn to pronounce without "accent." Instead, his dreaded "catch" is the verbal trip-up. The concern is not his inability to pronounce some word or phrase fast enough; it is one's inability to say *any* word fluently in *any* language. It is not a "foreign" accent that gives one away as a member of another tribe; it is the fact that one stutters on any and all words *regardless* of "pronunciation." According to the Italian-language tongue-twisting dictum, "Traduttore, traditore" ("[The] translator [is a] traitor"), but it is not interlingual translation that betrays the stutterer; it is, rather, panlingual stuttering.

Regarding the stutterer's seeking refuge in silence, there is a relevant incident in the Icelandic "Foster Brothers' Saga."[2] Thormod is being pursued by an avenging horde. He goes over a cliff and hangs onto a rock to hide. There he clings all day, until his pursuers give up and leave. When his foster brother Thorgeir finally finds him, Thorgeir asks why he didn't call out for help. Thormod replies that he didn't dare: his stutter would have given away his identity. (Thormod is, of course, supposed to be a poet.)

There are many cases of individuals' being caught—caught out—by a stutter. Earle Stanley Gardner's whodunnit *The Case of the Stuttering Bishop* provides a good instance.[3] One might think of the tongue twisters in Gilbert and Sullivan's *Mikado:* here the only solution is "To sit in solemn silence in a dull dark dock / In a pestilential prison with a life-long lock."[4] This is, for a while, the unhappy condition of Papageno in Mozart's opera *The Magic Flute:* when the three ladies padlock his mouth shut, Papageno can "hum" well enough, like any stutterer, but he cannot speak or sing. The relevant history of stuttering in opera would include the extraordinary stutter-singing of Irus in Claudio Monteverdi's seventeenth-century *Il Ritorno d'Ulisse in Patria*. The counterpart history of comic stuttering in European street theater, on which Mozart here relies, has yet to be written.

Tongue Twister

To squeeze a profusion of syllables
past voice box and over lips till
always that torturous tongue
gums the works,
the schoolyard bully
cinches the spigot
clenching thoughts tight,
hoards words piled knotted
and perched in the just past,
a record repeating
half step out of time
stranded on discordant note.

—SHAWN PATRICK DOYLE, "stutter, *v.*" (2002)

A tongue twister per se is, according to the *OED,* "a sequence of words, often alliterative, difficult to articulate

kill. According to the Book of Judges (12:16), the Gideonites (or Gileadites) pronounced the Hebrew *shibboleth* with the "sh" sound; the Ephraimites could not say the "sh" and pronounced it *sibboleth.* Here is the tale, in the 1833 English translation by Noah Webster:

> And the Gileadites took the passages of Jordan before the Ephraimites: and it was so, that when those Ephraimites who had escaped, said, Let me go over; that the men of Gilead said to him, Art thou an Ephraimite? If he said, No; Then said they to him, Say now: and he said Sibboleth: for he could not frame to pronounce it right. Then they took him, and slew him at the passages of Jordan. And there fell at that time of the Ephraimites forty and two thousand.

The two-pronged rule of thumb here is: All members of my tribe are able to pronounce *shibboleth,* and those who are not members of my tribe cannot pronounce *shibboleth* the way I do. The tale is retold often in the literary tradition.[8]

People have often been killed as a consequence of being unable to pronounce a word "properly." (In order to avoid such problems at the international level, spy schools employ foreign-language teachers. One such would be the "Hungarian" in *My Fair Lady*—one of Professor Higgins' two star students.) For example, there is the War of the Sicilian Vespers. This war began with the famous shibboleth massacre that took place outside a church in Palermo on Easter Day, 1282. Frenchmen who could not pronounce "properly" the Italian word *ciceri* were killed.[9] There is likewise the Wat Tyler Rebellion, also known as the Peasant Rebellion, which took place in England in 1381. "They had a Shibboleth to discover them, he who pronounced

quickly." Part of the difficulty stems from the fact that the speaker needs to repeat certain sounds unusually fast. Tongue twisters as such often operate to mark out those who are intralinguistically or interlinguistically different from the speaker. The Greek term for "tongue twister"—*glóssodétes* (from *deno,* meaning "to tie up")—indicates that the *glóssodétes* revolves not only around the interlinguistic detection of an accent or inability to pronounce a "foreign" sound but also around confusion of the native speaker through a need for rapid combination of unusual "mother-tongue" sounds. Consider "Tuphlos ta t' óta, ton te noun, ta t' ómmat ei" ("You are blind in your ears, your mind, and your eyes"), which is what Oedipus says to Tiresias in Sophocles' *Oedipus Tyrannus.* Even native speakers of Greek have trouble pronouncing this sentence.[5]

The same teachers of elocution who help people avoid problems of stuttering and "cluttering" (tachyphemia) likewise try to correct intralinguistic dialectal accents.[6] Eliza Doolittle's Cockney accent in G. B. Shaw's *Pygmalion* and in the musical *My Fair Lady* might make a woman into a flower seller at Covent Garden instead of a successful Cinderella at the ball. It is a social disease. Professor Higgins, her elocutionist, is modeled partly on such language scientists as Alexander Melville Bell (as Shaw points out in his preface). It is no accident that Bell was interested in stuttering—as was his son Alexander Graham Bell, inventor of the telephone, who worked toward an "establishment for the correction of stammering and other defects of utterance."[7] At the beginning of *Pygmalion,* Professor Higgins calls Eliza an "animal" because of her Cockney accent. But by Act 3 he comes to praise her as being "just like a parrot." Eliza is able to play the grand princess thanks to her newly acquired accent. Formerly unable to articulate an as-pirated "aitch" (a lack that is characteristic of Cockney dialect), she eventually masters such tongue twisters as, "In Hertford, Hereford, and Hampshire hurricanes hardly ever happen."

Many similar tongue twisters have ethnic content. They are also designed to root out such "ethnics" as the Cockney, or "East End," Doolittle family. For example, the Catalan *embarbussament* (tongue twister) may be difficult for native speakers of Catalan to pronounce well. "Diu qui, diu jo, diu si, diu tu, diu qui, diu jo, diu no, diu Ah!" ("Says who, says me, says yes, says you, says who, says me, says no, says Ah!") was designed or used to identify nonnative speakers, specifically Castilian speakers, since this twister contains phonemes (*/dz/, /dzh/, /zh/*) that do not occur in close proximity in Castilian. Consider three Serbo-Croatian tongue twisters apparently aimed at Muslims:

> "Ture bure tura, bula bure valja, bolje ture bure tura nego bula bure valja." ("A Turk turns the barrel, a Turk's wife rolls a barrel, the Turk turns the barrel better than the Turk's wife rolls it.")
>
> "Ture bure valja; bolje bure Ture neg Ture bure." ("A Turk rolls the barrel; the barrel pushes the Turk. It is better for the barrel to push the Turk, than for the Turk to roll the barrel [away].")
>
> "Bog te sačuvao Osmana dizdara i kriva kantara, popuzljiva mosta, podrugljiva gosta, prtene vreće i zle sreće." ("God save you from the Ottoman fortress-commander and the crooked scales, from slippery bridge, from mocking guest, from carrying a sack and from bad luck.")

A German *Zungenbrecher* ("tongue breaker") used against Algerians might be: "Allergischer Algerier, alger-

ischer Allergiker" ("Allergic Algerians, Algeri[people]"). An Austrian dialect tongue twister us Gypsies might be: "Zehn zottate Zigeina zahn ze ner Zement zam zau zuwie" ("Ten shaggy gypsies ging ten hundredweights of cement over to the Compare the Kurdish: "Çume çemmî Çeqan çeltûkî eteqan" ("As I came to the Cheqan River, tl was cleaving ears of wheat"). If these tongue twis difficult for native speakers to pronounce, they are all the more difficult for outsiders: those whose nati guage is different.

For the stutterer, though, they are all always impo

Shibboleth

> Oh say can you say?
>
> —Dr. Seuss, *Oh Say Can You Say? Oh My Brothers Oh My Sisters These Are Terrible Tongue Twisters* (1979)

A shibboleth is a test word, or series of test words, wh one group of people can pronounce properly and anotl group cannot, due to a peculiarity of pronunciation or a cent. The English term *shibboleth* is distinct from almost other words, in that its original meaning in Hebrew ("e of corn" or "stream") differs altogether from its meanin in English ("secret test word" or "unconscious social discriminator"). That is to say, speakers of English take *shibboleth* to mean not *what* it means in Hebrew, but the *way* it is used in a particular passage in the Bible (i.e., to detect a mispronunciation). The term describes a linguistic instrument used for the purpose of distinguishing foreign speakers from native speakers and hence figuring out whom to

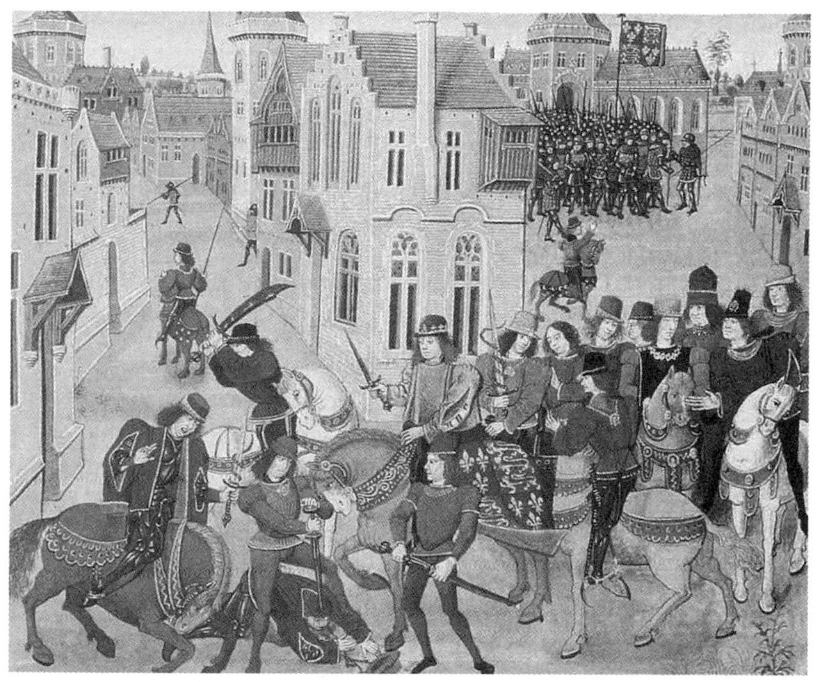

3. Anonymous, *The Death of Wat Tyler.* Illustration from a fifteenth-century Flemish manuscript of Jean Froissart's *Chronicles* (FR2644, fol. 159v). Bibliothèque Nationale, Paris.

Brot and *Cawse* for Bread and Cheese had his head lopt off."[10] And in 1663 James Heath wrote the following about a battle at Worcester: "There were slain in Field and in Town . . . and in pursuit some 3000, and some 8000, taken prisoners in several places, most of the English escaping by their Shiboleth."[11]

The use of shibboleths has been recorded for conflicts in Yemen, Egypt, and the Berber territories.[12] They were also employed during the Peasants' Revolt in Flanders, in the town of Bruges (Brugge), on May 18, 1302. One story has it that Flemish-speaking peasants caught French-speaking nobility by telling them to repeat the Flemish slogan "Schild en Vriend" or "Scilt ende Vrient" ("Shield and friend"). The French-speakers could not pronounce the "sch" in the Flemish word for shield, and so they were "unshielded." (Another version has it that the Flemish catchphrase was "Des Gilden Vriend.")

A similar shibboleth technique was used during World War II by the Dutch resistance and British intelligence to reveal German SS spies pretending to be Dutch civilians. The Germans were unable to pronounce the place-name *Scheveningen,* which is pronounced with a "sk" in Dutch, a sound that the Germans could reproduce only as "sh." In the literature, this Dutch-language shibboleth sometimes has elaborate formulations—for example, "Op scheve schaats naar Scheveningen rijden" ("Riding your oblique ice skates to Scheveningen").

A shibboleth test is the key to the New Testament's story of Peter's denial of Jesus (Luke 22:56–62). Here we must distinguish between the meaning of Peter's words, "I do not know him" (which he says three times), and the accent with which he speaks them. It is his accent that betrays him as a liar to his examiners' ears.

The Dominicans' slaughter of thousands of Haitian immigrants at the Massacre River in 1937 involved the inability of the French-speaking Haitians to pronounce *perejil* ("parsley") in the same way that the Spanish-speaking Dominicans did. This historical event has become the subject of literary novels, such as *The Farming of Bones,* by Edwidge Danticat. Rita Dove, in her poem "Parsley," says of the Dominican leader Trujillo: "He will / order many, this time, to be killed / . . . / for a single, beautiful word."[13]

kill. According to the Book of Judges (12:16), the Gideonites (or Gileadites) pronounced the Hebrew *shibboleth* with the "sh" sound; the Ephraimites could not say the "sh" and pronounced it *sibboleth.* Here is the tale, in the 1833 English translation by Noah Webster:

> And the Gileadites took the passages of Jordan before the Ephraimites: and it was so, that when those Ephraimites who had escaped, said, Let me go over; that the men of Gilead said to him, Art thou an Ephraimite? If he said, No; Then said they to him, Say now: and he said Sibboleth: for he could not frame to pronounce it right. Then they took him, and slew him at the passages of Jordan. And there fell at that time of the Ephraimites forty and two thousand.

The two-pronged rule of thumb here is: All members of my tribe are able to pronounce *shibboleth,* and those who are not members of my tribe cannot pronounce *shibboleth* the way I do. The tale is retold often in the literary tradition.[8]

People have often been killed as a consequence of being unable to pronounce a word "properly." (In order to avoid such problems at the international level, spy schools employ foreign-language teachers. One such would be the "Hungarian" in *My Fair Lady*—one of Professor Higgins' two star students.) For example, there is the War of the Sicilian Vespers. This war began with the famous shibboleth massacre that took place outside a church in Palermo on Easter Day, 1282. Frenchmen who could not pronounce "properly" the Italian word *ciceri* were killed.[9] There is likewise the Wat Tyler Rebellion, also known as the Peasant Rebellion, which took place in England in 1381. "They had a Shibboleth to discover them, he who pronounced

ischer Allergiker" ("Allergic Algerians, Algerian allergic [people]"). An Austrian dialect tongue twister used against Gypsies might be: "Zehn zottate Zigeina zahn zehn Zentner Zement zam zau zuwie" ("Ten shaggy gypsies are dragging ten hundredweights of cement over to the fence"). Compare the Kurdish: "Çume çemmî Çeqan, Çeqel çeltûkî eteqan" ("As I came to the Cheqan River, the jackal was cleaving ears of wheat"). If these tongue twisters are difficult for native speakers to pronounce, they are usually all the more difficult for outsiders: those whose native language is different.

For the stutterer, though, they are all always impossible.

Shibboleth

> Oh say can you say?
>
> —DR. SEUSS, *Oh Say Can You Say? Oh My Brothers Oh My Sisters These Are Terrible Tongue Twisters* (1979)

A shibboleth is a test word, or series of test words, which one group of people can pronounce properly and another group cannot, due to a peculiarity of pronunciation or accent. The English term *shibboleth* is distinct from almost all other words, in that its original meaning in Hebrew ("ear of corn" or "stream") differs altogether from its meaning in English ("secret test word" or "unconscious social discriminator"). That is to say, speakers of English take *shibboleth* to mean not *what* it means in Hebrew, but the *way* it is used in a particular passage in the Bible (i.e., to detect a mispronunciation). The term describes a linguistic instrument used for the purpose of distinguishing foreign speakers from native speakers and hence figuring out whom to

pirated "aitch" (a lack that is characteristic of Cockney dialect), she eventually masters such tongue twisters as, "In Hertford, Hereford, and Hampshire hurricanes hardly ever happen."

Many similar tongue twisters have ethnic content. They are also designed to root out such "ethnics" as the Cockney, or "East End," Doolittle family. For example, the Catalan *embarbussament* (tongue twister) may be difficult for native speakers of Catalan to pronounce well. "Diu qui, diu jo, diu si, diu tu, diu qui, diu jo, diu no, diu Ah!" ("Says who, says me, says yes, says you, says who, says me, says no, says Ah!") was designed or used to identify nonnative speakers, specifically Castilian speakers, since this twister contains phonemes (*/dz/, /dzh/, /zh/*) that do not occur in close proximity in Castilian. Consider three Serbo-Croatian tongue twisters apparently aimed at Muslims:

> "Ture bure tura, bula bure valja, bolje ture bure tura nego bula bure valja." ("A Turk turns the barrel, a Turk's wife rolls a barrel, the Turk turns the barrel better than the Turk's wife rolls it.")
>
> "Ture bure valja; bolje bure Ture neg Ture bure." ("A Turk rolls the barrel; the barrel pushes the Turk. It is better for the barrel to push the Turk, than for the Turk to roll the barrel [away].")
>
> "Bog te sačuvao Osmana dizdara i kriva kantara, popuzljiva mosta, podrugljiva gosta, prtene vreće i zle sreće." ("God save you from the Ottoman fortress-commander and the crooked scales, from slippery bridge, from mocking guest, from carrying a sack and from bad luck.")

A German *Zungenbrecher* ("tongue breaker") used against Algerians might be: "Allergischer Algerier, alger-

quickly." Part of the difficulty stems from the fact that the speaker needs to repeat certain sounds unusually fast. Tongue twisters as such often operate to mark out those who are intralinguistically or interlinguistically different from the speaker. The Greek term for "tongue twister"—*glóssodétes* (from *deno,* meaning "to tie up")—indicates that the *glóssodétes* revolves not only around the interlinguistic detection of an accent or inability to pronounce a "foreign" sound but also around confusion of the native speaker through a need for rapid combination of unusual "mother-tongue" sounds. Consider "Tuphlos ta t' óta, ton te noun, ta t' ómmat ei" ("You are blind in your ears, your mind, and your eyes"), which is what Oedipus says to Tiresias in Sophocles' *Oedipus Tyrannus.* Even native speakers of Greek have trouble pronouncing this sentence.[5]

The same teachers of elocution who help people avoid problems of stuttering and "cluttering" (tachyphemia) likewise try to correct intralinguistic dialectal accents.[6] Eliza Doolittle's Cockney accent in G. B. Shaw's *Pygmalion* and in the musical *My Fair Lady* might make a woman into a flower seller at Covent Garden instead of a successful Cinderella at the ball. It is a social disease. Professor Higgins, her elocutionist, is modeled partly on such language scientists as Alexander Melville Bell (as Shaw points out in his preface). It is no accident that Bell was interested in stuttering—as was his son Alexander Graham Bell, inventor of the telephone, who worked toward an "establishment for the correction of stammering and other defects of utterance."[7] At the beginning of *Pygmalion,* Professor Higgins calls Eliza an "animal" because of her Cockney accent. But by Act 3 he comes to praise her as being "just like a parrot." Eliza is able to play the grand princess thanks to her newly acquired accent. Formerly unable to articulate an as-

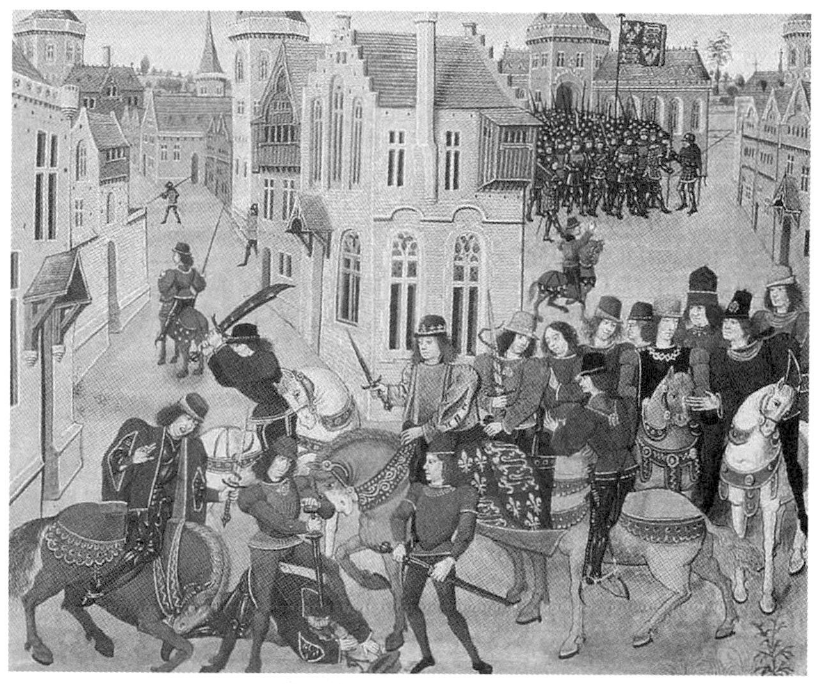

3. Anonymous, *The Death of Wat Tyler.* Illustration from a fifteenth-century Flemish manuscript of Jean Froissart's *Chronicles* (FR2644, fol. 159v). Bibliothèque Nationale, Paris.

Brot and *Cawse* for Bread and Cheese had his head lopt off."[10] And in 1663 James Heath wrote the following about a battle at Worcester: "There were slain in Field and in Town . . . and in pursuit some 3000, and some 8000, taken prisoners in several places, most of the English escaping by their Shiboleth."[11]

The use of shibboleths has been recorded for conflicts in Yemen, Egypt, and the Berber territories.[12] They were also employed during the Peasants' Revolt in Flanders, in the town of Bruges (Brugge), on May 18, 1302. One story has it that Flemish-speaking peasants caught French-speaking nobility by telling them to repeat the Flemish slogan "Schild en Vriend" or "Scilt ende Vrient" ("Shield and friend"). The French-speakers could not pronounce the "sch" in the Flemish word for shield, and so they were "unshielded." (Another version has it that the Flemish catchphrase was "Des Gilden Vriend.")

A similar shibboleth technique was used during World War II by the Dutch resistance and British intelligence to reveal German SS spies pretending to be Dutch civilians. The Germans were unable to pronounce the place-name *Scheveningen,* which is pronounced with a "sk" in Dutch, a sound that the Germans could reproduce only as "sh." In the literature, this Dutch-language shibboleth sometimes has elaborate formulations—for example, "Op scheve schaats naar Scheveningen rijden" ("Riding your oblique ice skates to Scheveningen").

A shibboleth test is the key to the New Testament's story of Peter's denial of Jesus (Luke 22:56–62). Here we must distinguish between the meaning of Peter's words, "I do not know him" (which he says three times), and the accent with which he speaks them. It is his accent that betrays him as a liar to his examiners' ears.

The Dominicans' slaughter of thousands of Haitian immigrants at the Massacre River in 1937 involved the inability of the French-speaking Haitians to pronounce *perejil* ("parsley") in the same way that the Spanish-speaking Dominicans did. This historical event has become the subject of literary novels, such as *The Farming of Bones,* by Edwidge Danticat. Rita Dove, in her poem "Parsley," says of the Dominican leader Trujillo: "He will / order many, this time, to be killed / . . . / for a single, beautiful word."[13]

Americans often claim that they don't have deadly shibboleths. It's widely believed that Americans usually pass off language mistakes as *boners.*[14] A boner, according to *Webster's Third New International,* is a "ridiculous and usually embarrassing or painful mistake or slip often arising from a sudden and fortuitous lapse of understanding, tact, or decorum." In fact, though, Americans have used shibboleth tests in much the same way that other groups have used them: in order to distinguish those people who are "within" a group from those "outside" it, and likewise in order to differentiate those whom one might want to love from those whom one might want to kill. For example, the uniquely American word *lallapaloosa* served U.S. intelligence as a shibboleth for unmasking Japanese prisoners who claimed to be Chinese.[15] During the Civil War, Americans also used the shibboleth test devised by specialists in North-South accent differences in American English. Patricia Beatty's novel *Skedaddle* tells of a man who is all but killed for the *way* he speaks, rather than for the sense of his utterances.[16] (In Canada, according to the *Random House Unabridged Dictionary,* the word *skedaddler* often indicates "a U.S. citizen who fled to Canada rather than serving in the armed forces during the American Civil War").

Intralinguistic dialect difference in the United States often affects romantic comedy and its perception of marriage. One widely influential work in this regard would be the song "Let's Call the Whole Thing Off" (1937) with words by Ira Gershwin and music by his brother George. (The brothers were members of that assimilationist Russian-Jewish American cohort that was influenced by anglophone "elocution schools.") Sung by Fred Astaire and Ginger Rogers in the roller-skating scene in the film *Shall We*

Dance? (1937), "Let's Call the Whole Thing Off" suggests how easily a simple difference in pronunciation can reflect and even trigger conflict.

> You say eether and I say eyether
> You say neether and I say nyther
> Eether, eyether
> Neether, nyther
> Let's call the whole thing off
> . . . . .
> You like potato and I like potahto
> You like tomato and I like tomahto
> Potato, potahto
> Tomato, tomahto
> Let's call the whole thing off
> . . . . .
> You like vanilla and I like vanella
> You sa's'parilla, and I sa's'sparella
> Vanilla, vanella
> Choc'late, strawb'ry
> Let's call the whole thing off
> . . . . .
> So if you like oysters and I like ersters
> I'll take oysters and give up ersters
> For we know we need each other so we
> Better call the calling off off
> Let's call the whole thing off

Sung, with variations, by many artists—among them Billie Holiday, Ella Fitzgerald, Louis Armstrong, and Michael Feinstein—"Let's Call the Whole Thing Off" is a wooer's song of warring against war by way of contrapuntal harmony (calling off the calling off). Sometimes the singer will change the conflict from one of accent to one of dialect: so Harry Connick Jr., in the film *When Harry Met Sally* (1989), changes the conflict from the level of accent (*tomato* versus *tomahto*) to dialect (*tomato* versus *Creole*).

"Let's Call the Whole Thing Off" bears comparison, in this regard, with the American musical stage-play version of Shaw's English stage-play *Pygmalion*. Here the servant-student Eliza, during the course of her intralingual elocution lessons from Professor Higgins, takes on the English accent of her teacher (as in "The Rain in Spain" in *My Fair Lady*). Here, too, elocution lessons generally are much promoted by the professor, as in the song "Why Can't the English Learn to Speak?"

Lisp

> Well no-one's ever seen what I mean
> From the age of n-n-n-n-n-thirteen
> We've all been caught in a m-m-mouth trap
> So join with us and do the st-st-st-st-st-st-st-stutter rap.
>
> —Tony Hawks, "Stutter Rap (No Sleep Till Bedtime),"
> sung by Morris Minor and the Majors (1988)

Lisping (saying "mouth" instead of "mouse") and *stuttering* (saying "st-st-st-st-st-st-st-stutter" instead of "stutter") have similar linguistic and cultural connotations. Indeed, the very word *lisp* refers both to "stammering" and to "lisping." (According to the *OED*, one etymology of *lisping* derives the term from Old High German *lisp* or Middle High German *lispen,* meaning "to trip in speaking.") In fact, many English words mean both "stuttering" and "lisping"—*short-tongued, balbuties, blesiloquent, traulism,* and *maf-*

fling. It is as if the two conditions were essentially one and the same.

In the medical realm, moreover, theorists of lisping and stuttering often conceived both disorders' etiology as lying similarly between the voluntary and involuntary realms and conjoining similarly the psychological and biological realms. Not surprisingly, therefore, the same speech therapies are often used for stutterers as for lispers. Thus, Abraham Tucker would "prevent lisping, stammering, and other such like imperfection," and Raphael Holinshed says that "*aqua vitae* keeps . . . the tongue from lisping, the mouth from maffling."[17] My own Victorian-era elocution school in Montréal had several books on its shelves that treated lisping and stuttering in the same way: Walter K. Fobes, *Elocution Simplified: With an Appendix on Lisping, Stammering, Stuttering, and Other Defects of Speech* (Boston, 1877); Kate Emil Behnke, *On Stammering, Cleft-Palate Speech, Lisping* (London, 1907); and Edward Wheeler Scripture, *Stuttering and Lisping* (New York, 1912).

Poets often do the same. So William Cowper's poem "There Is a Fountain Filled with Blood"—best known as a nineteenth-century American religious hymn—includes the lines, "When this poor, lisping, stammering tongue / Lies silent in the grave."[18]

Both stuttering and lisping are conceived as being sometimes a bad trait and sometimes a good one. For instance, when they are characteristics of "baby-talk"—understood both as the talk *of* young babies and as adult talk *to* babies—they are generally viewed in a positive light. ("A nurse to a child . . . lisps in broken language," says William Beveridge. And Robert Sanderson remarks that "nurses talk half syllables, and lisp out broken language to young children.")[19]

There is also the adult "baby-talk" stuttering by actresses like Marilyn Monroe, whose speech patterns we will consider in Chapter 5.

Lisping sometimes has positive aspects because it softens one's utterances. In the Prologue to *The Canterbury Tales,* Chaucer says that the Friar lisps "to make his English sweete upon his tonge." Lisping can also signify the speaker's thoughtful intelligence or "aristocratic affectation." A common comparison here is to the interjection *haw haw*—an expression of hesitation, like "hemming and hawing," sometimes called *hackering,* which according to the *OED* (s.v. "hacker") is a regular synonym for *stuttering* and often taken to resemble upper-class speech.[20] Sometimes lisping indicates a foreign affectation. For instance, a character in George Etherege's *The Man of Mode* (1676; part 1, ch. 1) remarks: "What a pretty lisp he has!" His interlocutor responds: "Ho, that he affects in imitation of the people of Quality of France." Or lisping "becomes" (i.e., graces or adorns) the speaker, as Jehan Palsgrave wrote in *Lesclarcissement de la langue françoyse.*[21] Thus, many a person affects a pretty lisp, as Richard Steele claimed.[22]

Lisping, like stammering, may be designed to indicate the speaker's genuineness, as when Marlon Brando hesitates in speech while method-acting. Or stuttering implies "honesty," as in the film *The Maltese Falcon* when we hear this exchange:

> *Joel Cairo (Peter Lorre):* You've always got a smooth answer . . .
>
> *Rick (Humphrey Bogart):* Whatta ya want? Learn to stutter?

The Spanish vocal group Estopa has a well-known song, "Vino Tinto," which includes the line, "Si estamos a solas tar-tar-tar-tar-tartamudeo y no son trolas" ("When we are alone I s-s-s-s-stutter and I am not telling lies").

Sometimes, indeed, the tripping tongue is a sort of give-away. "The tripping tongue sometimes tells truth," Thomas Gataker wrote in 1646.[23] One gives oneself away through a "Freudian *slip.*" In certain raw situations, people treat stuttering as an obvious sign that the speaker is a liar: "You lying, cuz you stuttering," says Joe Thomas in the song "Stutter."[24] In *The Golden Notebook,* by Doris Lessing, the fictional novelist Anna Wulf stammers when she speaks in bad faith.[25] The influential German philosopher Johann Georg Hamann, who struggled with a speech impediment of his own, often relies on much the same topos. In a letter to Immanuel Kant, for example, Hamann implies that sincerity would loosen even a dumb person's tongue: "Your silence concerning matters about which sincerity would be enough to loosen a dumb person's tongue is an insult to me."[26] John Updike suggests much the same thing when he confesses (in his essay "Getting the Words Out") "I stutter when I am 'in the wrong.'"[27]

In some cases, God himself is said to be a lisper: He imparts his meaning only to those attuned to hearing Him. In Miles Coverdale's 1535 translation, Isaiah 28:11 reads: "The Lorde also shal speake with lispinge lippes and with a strange language onto this people." (Whether Isaiah's remark means that the Lord speaks esoterically, I shall consider below. In the present context, it at least suggests why lisping is sometimes seen in a more negative light.) In fact, lisping is often decried as an instrument of flattery—as in *Father Hubburds Tales,* by Thomas Middleton.[28] At other times, lisping—like stuttering—is taken as a sign of mental retardation or of the clever "cunning" of children, as Joanna Baillie puts it in her novel *Count Basil.*[29]

Frequently, adults who lisp are often criticized for doing so, as is Lady Charlotte in Fanny Burney's diary.[30] Lispers are sometimes even killed as members of a dangerous tribe. After all, what is the biblical tale of the shibboleth/sibboleth but a simple lisping test?

Lisping, as a socially condemned action, can be "cured" in three general ways.

First, one can change the way that the lispers speak—for instance, they can learn word substitution or hire speech therapists and medical surgeons (techniques that do not always work). One might be killed for saying *sin* instead of *shin*. Many a lisper is unable to pronounce differently *he* and *she*—words that are often unavoidable and that lack synonyms—with what consequences I leave to the imagination. Margaret Drabble, as we have noted, tends to stutter on the word *woman,* and runs into trouble when she is driven to say *lady* instead.[31]

Second, one can turn all nonlispers into lispers so that the telltale quality or discomforting aspect of lisping all but disappears. One storied explanation of the origin of the Castilian lisp has it that a fearful or admiring populace emulated the "interdental fricative" of King Ferdinand II.[32] In similar fashion, followers of Hotspur in Shakespeare's *Henry IV, Part 2,* choose to imitate his talk and walk—his "gait" and his "speaking thick."[33]

Besides turning lispers into nonlispers and nonlispers into lispers, there is a third method for curing human society of the disease that is lisping: removing the lispers from society. Both hospitalization and execution work. For Thomas Fuller, "the Tribual [tribal] Lisping of the Ephramites"—their "lisping accent"—is what does them in.[34] Such tribal speaking characteristics are often associated with barbarism, or "lithping gibberish," as Richard Fanshawe calls it.[35]

Barbarian

> How shall we sing the Lord's song in a strange land?
>
> —Psalms 137:4

The Latin term *balbus,* which means "stammering," is related to the Greek word *barbaros,* a term which has a similar primary reference to speech. In fact, the English *barbarian* often comes down to meaning a person who cannot speak *our* language "properly," or one who cannot speak *any* language without an objectionable accent (see the various definitions in the *OED*).

For the stutterer, as we have seen, every word is potentially a shibboleth. And the stutterer's situation in a multilingual setting is often very different from his situation in a monolingual one. When I was growing up in Québec in the 1950s, for example, we stutterers on both sides of the English-French linguistic fence knew well what Edward Hoagland meant when he described, in "The Threshold of Pain" (1988), how different cultures react differently to stuttering: "I could write a Stutterer's Guide to Europe . . . the titters in old Vienna, the knowing English remembering their King [Henry IV], the raw scorching baitings I met with in Greece."[36] For the stutterer, his individual culture—or his various cultures—really matter. (René Bernard's book *Le Bègue sur la scène française,* or *Stuttering on the French Stage,* is an important study in this regard. So too is Maurice Sand's study of Tartaglia, the stock-character stutterer in Italian Commedia dell'arte.)[37] When an individual is bilingual—speaks two languages equally well—he may speak one language fluently and the other disfluently. (There is relevant research on Puerto Rican stutterers in New York City and on North American Indian stutterers in their particular anglophone context.)[38] Whereas some stutterers find "therapy" for stuttering in their mother tongue when they try speaking another tongue, others discover that the effort to speak another tongue precipitates stuttering in the mother tongue.

Concerning language-switching stutter therapies, I recall my elocution teacher in Westmount (Montréal's anglophone stronghold) telling me about three stutterers who made the transition from using English to using French: the first was Erasmus Darwin, grandfather of the British evolutionary biologist Charles Robert Darwin; the second was Henry James, the American novelist; and the third was Somerset Maugham, the British novelist.

Erasmus Darwin believed that exposure to a non-English language such as French would cure his son Charles's stutter. According to Anna Seward's *Memoirs,* he "sent Charles abroad . . . from a belief, that in the pronunciation of a foreign language, hesitation would be less likely to recur, than in speaking those words and sentences in which he had been accustomed to hesitate." After returning from France, young Darwin no longer stammered, although "his utterance was, from that, somewhat thick and hurried."[39]

Concerning Henry James, who stuttered only in English, Mrs. Humphrey Ward reported that he "spoke French to perfection." Similar testimony came from Edith Wharton: "French people have told me that they had never met an Anglo-Saxon who spoke French like James; not only correctly and *fluently,* but—well, just as they did themselves."[40] So James became fluent thanks to the transition from his native English to another tongue.

Many a stutterer growing up in a sociolinguistically fraught setting feels that he suffers from an almost congenital physical defect—like "puella bilingui," as the eighteenth-century physician Johann Dolaeus called it, or "cleft tongue," which is the usual modern diagnosis.[41] And indeed, some stuttering theorists argue that a major "cause" of stuttering can reside in making the transition from one language or tongue to another. My favorite example of the way in which multilingualism can induce stuttering involves Somerset Maugham. Maugham, who spent his early childhood in France, learned French as his native tongue. He did not stutter at all until he was orphaned at age ten or eleven,[42] at which time he went to live in England. One biographer concludes that "Maugham's stutter was probably the result of [among other things] . . . the sudden demand to speak in a second language."[43] Maugham's masterpiece, the semi-autobiographical English-language novel *Of Human Bondage,* seems to bear this out. Fears of just such multilingualism-induced speech disfluencies bolster that American rhetoric about language and pedagogy which encourages educators not to teach any "foreign languages" until students are thirteen or fourteen years old.

Québécois bilingualism affected my speech in various ways. Even before I was aware that I had any speech "problem," I was sent for weekly two-hour lessons at an elocution school in Lower Westmount. Most of the people who went to this school did so hoping to learn to speak English properly—that is, with the appropriate "Canadian-Anglican" accent for assimilating into the then relatively wealthy anglophone minority in Québec. A single elocution textbook would give instructions for eliminating foreign accents as well as stutters. As Benjamin Humphrey Smart had put it in 1810, elocution lessons were "calculated to assist in removing every objectionable peculiarity of utterance arising from either foreign, provincial, or vulgar habits, or from a defective use of the organs of speech [including] stammer[ing]."[44] For Grace McCullough and Agnes Birmingham, whose 1925 textbook provided my school with its guiding principles, "correcting speech defects and foreign accent" amounted to the same thing.[45]

So I was taught in Lower Westmount that I had *two* sorts of speech impediments and that they were interrelated. The first impediment was *general* disfluency in speaking *all* languages, a problem from which stutterers suffered—or so said the experts. The second impediment was my particular inability to speak a *particular* language with the proper accent.

As I saw it at the time, my speaking with a stutter and speaking with an improper (Yiddish) accent were similar problems. After all, it is not only disfluency in speech but also ignorance of one's interlocutor's language, or inability to speak it without accent, that can disable a person.[46] Concerning this problem, Glen Doman has written: "In no area is man more vulnerable to misunderstanding, criticism and downright abuse from his fellow man than if he should fail to develop speech, or having gained it, should lose it—for when man loses the ability to express himself by speech he is suspect . . . of having lost, also the [faculties to arrive] at the conclusions which he would express in speech. The world feels . . . that if he can't say his name . . . he doesn't know his name."[47]

Elocution and breathing were special interests of Mrs. Trotter, my seventh-grade teacher. A Christian Scientist, she had two pieces of advice for the stutterer.

First, she said I had to have faith. She cited the Gospels to the effect that faith could move mountains: "Have faith in God. In truth I tell you, if anyone says to this mountain, 'Be pulled up and thrown into the sea,' with no doubt in his heart, but believing that what he says will happen, it will be done for him" (Matthew 21:21–22). At the time, I knew about moving mountains only from the Hebrew-language Psalm 114 (verses 1–8 are read at Passover seders every year). It tells how "the mountains skipped like rams" after the stutterer Moses led Israel away from "a people of strange language." The King James Version reads: "When Israel went out of Egypt, the house of Jacob from a people of strange language; / Judah was his sanctuary, and Israel his dominion. / The sea saw it, and fled: Jordan was driven back. / The mountains skipped like rams, and the little hills like lambs. / What ailed thee, O thou sea, that thou fleddest? thou Jordan, that thou wast driven back? / Ye mountains, that ye skipped like rams; and ye little hills, like lambs?" Was it human faith that made the mountains dance? Was it the faith of Moses that made him stutter?

Second, Mrs. Trotter had pulmonary advice for how I might learn to make my words go "trippingly on the tongue." As it happens, breathing and stuttering were the twin subjects of a children's book published about that time: *The Contrary Orphans,* by Elizabeth Stucley.[48] But the more I tried to breathe properly, the worse I stuttered: my involuntary caesuras became longer and longer. Arthur C. Clarke—better known for his breathtakingly influential science fiction writing—felt much the same way as he escaped the iron lung "by the thickness of a nerve fiber."[49] Was *rattling*—a common synonym for *stuttering* in the corner of the British Commonwealth where I grew up—thus related to the *death rattle* that characterizes a person's last breaths?[50]

Mrs. Trotter's advice was that I should believe the right thing and breathe the right way. Yet just as I could not *actively* control my breathing stoppages, so I could not *actively* manage my disbelief that my faith could move mountains.[51] Moreover, I knew well enough from the Book of Exodus that God does not cure Moses' stuttering. He cannot cure Moses—despite His suggestion that He can: "Who has made man's mouth? Who makes him dumb, or deaf, or seeing, or blind? Is it not I, the Lord?" (Exodus 4:11). God has already shown Moses how easy it is for Him to cure such problems as leprosy (Exodus 4:4–7), from which one of Moses' historical antecedents presumably suffered. In any case, Moses does not ask God to cure him of his speech impediment—the implications of which I will discuss later.

Regardless of my skepticism about Mrs. Trotter's views on faith in God, her faith in *me* was a help. (These days I wonder whether Mrs. Trotter ever got into trouble for messing with my stuttering. In the movie *Johnny Rocco,* a teacher's life is threatened when she decides to help a young boy who has begun to stutter after learning that his father is a crime boss.)[52] The fact that my good friends had faith in me was similarly beneficial. When I joined the high school debating club in the town of Mount Royal, my partners Michael Krashinsky and David Caplan put up with me. They suggested that, after all, debating and stuttering both belonged to the province of "rhetoric." (One of the books our debating coach passed along to us was A. M. Drummond's *Studies in Rhetoric,* published in 1962. It contained essays not only about the great speakers of the past and about "the literary criticism of oratory" but also about stuttering. Public speakers had long been interested in stuttering. An example from 1837 is Andrew Comstock's *Remarks on Stammering,* which was part of a lecture on elocution.)[53] Michael is now a professor of economics at the University of Toronto; David is a professor of linguistics at MIT; I teach courses in economics and language at Harvard.

"Could a stutterer like me become a teacher?" As a high school student in the early 1960s, I wondered. In a 1959 *Perry Mason* television episode, *The Case of the Stuttering Bishop,* the main question is the one posed by Mason to the bishop himself: "Is it possible for a stutterer to be a member of the clergy?"[54]

In the novel —*And the Stutterer Talked,* the stutterer figures wrongly that he might be able to become a teacher: "By what reasoning he arrived at the belief that he could teach, with his speech impediment daily growing stronger upon him, only he knew."[55] When a teaching career was denied to the film theorist André Bazin because he stuttered,[56] he seems to have "compensated" by writing his pathbreaking essay "Evolution of the Language of Cinema."[57] Lewis Carroll—who called himself "Dodo"—declined to preach in church, or was prohibited from doing so, because he stuttered. That Johann Georg Hamann never held an academic or ecclesiastical position is sometimes explained in terms of his having had a marked speech impediment. James Hynes's fictional work *Publish and Perish,* with its stuttering English professor, presents something of the same dilemma for stutterers who need to speak publicly in the secular sphere.[58]

A far greater dilemma dogged the trilingual stammerer Moses at age eighty: Can a stutterer deliver his people from bondage? Would Moses need help? Could someone besides Moses speak for Moses?

Alaric's Hexameter

> Teteroromamanunudadatetelalatete.
>
> —Alaric, king of the Visigoths (d. 410)

The terms *stutterer* and *barbarian* both refer to "those people who do not speak our language." It does not matter much whether these people speak a human language other than "ours," such as Macedonian, or whether they make sounds that seem barely human to us—what we might call *gibberish*.[59] *Barbarian,* in fact, often suggests "a people whose language 'we' do not understand"—those who speak mere *gibberish,* say, or those whose languagc is not ours. The Latin *balbus (stammerer)* and its English cognates have much the same double meanings.[60]

The terms *stutterer* and *barbarian* both also refer to "those people who, although they *do* speak our language, do not speak it 'in our way.'" It does not matter much whether these people speak English with a foreign "accent," domestic "dialect," or more general speech "impediment." *Barbarous* often suggests "without good linguistic skills in a particular language" and "a people who are not fluent in 'our' language."[61] To boot, John Ruskin, in his *Political Economy of Art,* writes of "a wholly barbarous use of the word, barbarous in a double sense, for it is not English, and it is bad Greek."[62] Stuttering suggests the same. John Hill Burton tells of a "brave and reckless prince, who could not speak French, and only stuttered German."[63] In *Scourge of Villanie,* by John Marston (a contemporary of Shakespeare), we read of "The vildest stumbling stutterer / That euer hack'd and hew'd our natiue tongue."[64]

Sometimes the double meanings of the terms *stutterer* and *barbarian*—"people who do not speak our language" and also "people who do not speak our language in our way"—are tellingly conjoined by political actors and literary writers. For example, King Alaric—the presumably non-Latin-speaking Visigoth whom the Romans famously called "barbarian"—suggested these meanings of the term through a mightily ironic stutter in a palilogical register. Upholding a tradition extending back as far as the stutterer Moses, this Arian (Christian) pronounced his hexameter as a conqueror outside the gates of Rome on the fateful day of August 24, 410 B.C.E.

Alaric:
Teteroromamanunudadatetelalatete.

Reduplication:
Te—te / ro—ro / ma—ma / nu—nu / da—da / te—te / la—la / te—te.

Latin:
Te tero, Roma, manu nuda. Date tela. Latete!

Translation:
I'll crush you, Rome, with my bare hands! Hand over your spears. Hide![65]

The Gothic-speaking conqueror uttered this hexameter in stuttering Roman Latin (and maybe also bilingually in some sort of impeded Gothic). A good rhetorician, Alaric then acted out his words: he sacked Rome, as the sixth-century writer Procopius of Caesarea (Palestine) reports.

At the time, tongue-tied Saint Jerome wrote: "Roma vale! Haeret vox et singultus intercipiunt verba dictantis" ("Farewell, Rome! My voice sticks in my throat, and sobs interrupt my words as I speak").[66] It was the first time in 797 years that Rome had been conquered.

Moses, the Egyptian prince or Hebrew slave who put down Egypt by speaking through his brother Aaron's mouth and by writing through his father-in-law Jethro's alphabet, was just such a one as Alaric, as we will see in Chapter 4. So too, in his own way, was the slave Aesop: he spoke through animals.

3 Animals That Talk

When I was a child, my favorite stutterer was Aesop. I was sure that Aesop had really existed.[1] My edition of his works made it plain that Aesop was handicapped both in body and in speech: he was born "most deformed" and "coulde not speke."[2] John Vanbrugh wrote in his comedy *Aesop,* "Esop . . . that piece of deformity! that monster! that crump!"[3]

The frankly esoteric quality of Aesop's "animal fables" suggested to me that Aesop had a special need to speak with "forked tongue." Some people told me that Aesop needed to "mask his thoughts" because of his status as a slave (the "Brer Rabbit" tales, they sometimes added, work in much the same way). I thought that this survivor's need to "hold his tongue" was linked with Aesop's speech impediment. The congruence between his political predicament (he was a slave who could not speak his mind) and his linguistic condition (he was a stutterer who could not speak well) must have led Aesop to invent the "talking animal" story.[4] Such congruence is highlighted in the writing of the Haitian-born neurologist Jean Métellus, who lives in Paris. Speaking of his stuttering novel *La Parole prisonnière* (Speech Imprisoned), published just as the dictator Baby Doc Duvalier was removed from power, he said that the book allies censorship at the sociopathological level with stuttering at the psychological level: "Having written *La*

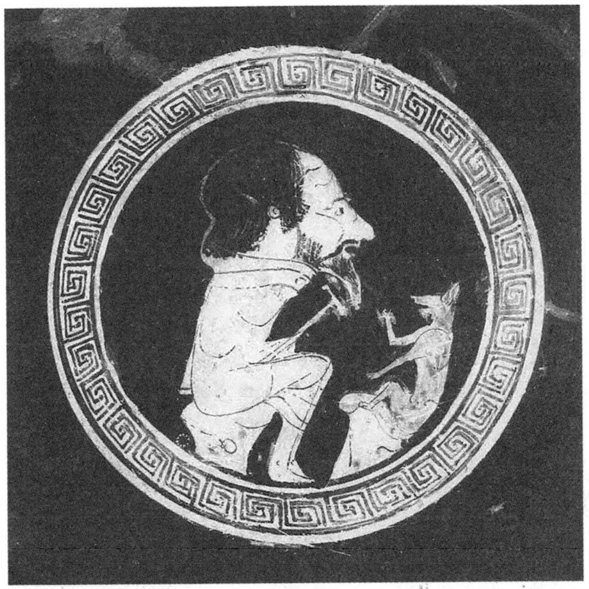

4. Anonymous, *Aesop and the Wolf.* Interior of an Attic cup from Vulci, fifth century B.C.E. Museo Nazionale di Villa Giulia, Rome. Copyright © Alinari / Art Resource, New York.

Parole prisonnière at the level of state concerns and the conditions of Haitian political life, I described the conditions of living that interdict speech."[5]

Isaiah's statement about divine hesitation in speech—"For with stammering lips and another tongue will [God] speak to this people"[6]—operates here as a gloss on the African-American slave writings that Dwight Hopkins and George Cummings gather together in their book *Cut Loose Your Stammering Tongue.*[7] In any case, the "talking animal" genre allows human beings to speak ventriloquistically through dummy animals. Put otherwise, the "talking-animal story" allows dumb animals to speak as if they were human.

In the movies that were so much a part of my growing up, there are many real-seeming animals that seem to talk, as in the film series *Francis the Talking Mule,* which ran in the 1940s and 1950s, and in the follow-up television series *Mister Ed* of the 1960s. There were also many unreal-seeming animals—cartoon animals—that had funny, humanoid speech impediments. But real animals don't talk (or so we're told). It is true, of course, that many human beings talk to animals and also treat their supposedly dumb animals—their pets—as flesh-and-blood ventriloquists' dummies that seem to speak back to them. (Nine-tenths of American pet owners talk to their pets as though the animals were human.[8] Half of these pet owners also put words into the mouths of their animals, just as if they were God opening the mouth of Balaam's mule. Thus, James Russell Lowell endows his dog with the ability to speak.)[9] But human beings who stutter do not stutter when they speak with (or to) real animals. To people who know traditional rhetoric, it comes as no surprise that the presence of dummy animals and dumb animals can help human stutterers. (Hence, pet therapy and hippotherapy are frequent speech treatments.)[10] Nor is it unexpected that children's literature is replete with fictional talking animals who stutter. For example, a stuttering alligator is the main character in Stephen Cosgrove's *Creole.*[11]

Real alligators do not quite talk. But real parrots do talk (or so we're told). Thus, Long John Silver's parrot in Robert Louis Stevenson's *Treasure Island* (1883), and likewise the parrot in John Skelton's mysterious *Speke, Parrot* (1521), seem to have human speech.[12] On the other hand, Polynesia, the parrot in Hugh Lofting's *Doctor Dolittle,* actually speaks human languages—including English. Polynesia also speaks hundreds of animal languages—including parrotese, which uniquely toes the line between the human and the animal. Many old-fashioned scholars used to claim that parrots—and the entire tribe of birds who imitate the human voice—are mere tape recorders without speech of their own. For example, Friedrich Max Müller argues in *Natural Religion* that "the parrot never speaks parrotese."[13] But Müller and his ilk never met the interspecies language-teacher and elocutionist that is Polynesia. Nor, as I shall suggest, did they ever meet the stuttering zebra finch.

The tension between parrots' imitating human speech and their managing parrotese is especially enlightening in the case of stuttering parrots in fiction like Robert Arthur's *Mystery of the Stuttering Parrot* and Leo Edwards' *Poppy Ott and the Stuttering Parrot.*[14] That fictional talking animals should stutter is already suggested by the English language, which has many words that mean both "to stutter" (on the part of a human being) and "to utter a sound" (on the part of an animal). One case in point is the term *tattle,* which means not only "to stutter" and "to produce baby-talk" (according to the *OED*) but also "to sound like a goose."[15]

In the 1950s, questions of human speech impediment and of animal talk often went hand and hand. On the popular stage, for example, Rex Harrison played the technologically and phonetically up-to-date Professor Higgins in the stage-play version of *My Fair Lady* (1956); and he became equally famous for his incarnation of the animal-talk expert Dr. Dolittle, who, in the film of that name (1967), based on the books by Hugh Lofting (first published in the 1920s), talks Solomonically with the animals. Likewise, Julie Andrews played opposite Rex Harrison as Professor Higgins' perfect elocution student Eliza Doolittle in the stage-play version of *My Fair Lady;* and she became equally well known for her title role in the movie *Mary Poppins* (1964), where Andrews specialized in tongue twisters like "supercalifragilisticexpialidocious."

Judging from such works as *My Fair Lady* and *Doctor Dolittle,* the interrelated goals of elocution lessons would seem to be twofold: first, to teach some *human beings* (the stutterers) how to speak fluently and other *human beings* (those with "foreign" accents and "domestic" dialects) how to speak in more recognizably standard fashion; and second, to teach *animals* to talk like human beings. Irene Pepperberg thus taught her parrot Alex to "talk."[16] Similarly, when Professor Higgins, in *My Fair Lady,* first meets Eliza at Covent Garden, he says the impeded sound that she produces—the sound that she herself *is*—is more like an animal's than a human being's.

But what if an animal has a speech impediment? In the popular movie culture of the mid-twentieth century, there was a "feeling that all great cartoon characters had a speech impediment."[17] The humanoid celluloid creatures I remember best from the 1950s are Gerald McBoing Boing (a sort of boy) and Porky Pig (a sort of little pig).

Gerald McBoing Boing, a boy who spoke using non-animate sound-effects, was the brainchild of the tongue-twisting Dr. Seuss. Dr. Seuss's script for the first *Gerald McBoing Boing* animated film (1951) consisted almost entirely of voice-overs and sound effects; Dr. Seuss used polysyllabic sound effects to fill out lines and rhyme. *Gerald McBoing Boing* was immensely popular: the 45-rpm recording (1950), the movie (1951), the book (1952), and the weekly TV show (1956–1957) made the character of Gerald impossible to escape.[18] Like other young stutterers at the time, I recall being especially sensitive to how Dr. Seuss conjoined tongue-twisting "nonsense" with speech im-

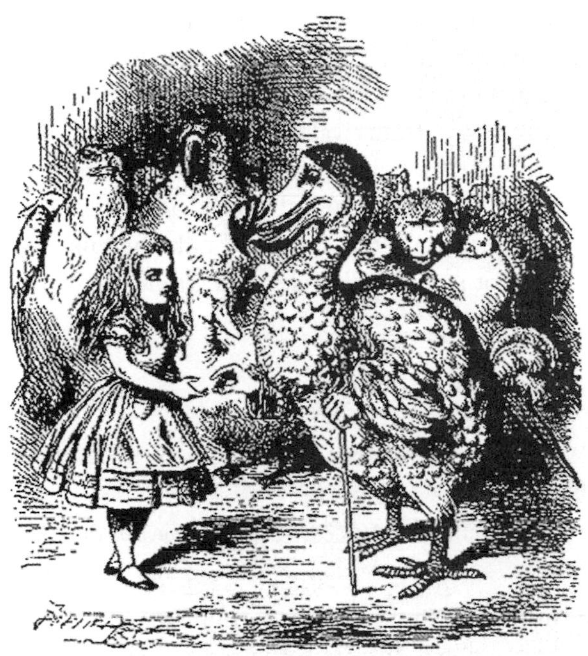

5. John Tenniel, *Alice and the Dodo.* From *Alice's Adventures in Wonderland,* by Lewis Carroll (New York: D. Appleton, 1866; orig. pub. 1865), p. 40. Photo courtesy of the Harvard University Library. "Dodo" was the nickname that Carroll himself adopted.

pediment—almost in imitation, it seemed to me, of the stutterer Lewis Carroll.

Carroll's self-chosen nickname "Dodo" indicates "a stupid person." The flightless dodo was believed to be a dimwitted bird, partly because it had a clumsy body that did not allow it even to *walk* gracefully (as the *OED* tells us). The dodo could neither walk the talk nor talk the walk. Silence became him.

Silent film, which was introduced to world culture

around the time of Lewis Carroll's death (1898), helped to make once-stationary images of animals (including humans) seem perfectly mobile ("animated"). In something like the same way, the arrival on scene of *talking film* ("talkies") in the 1920s helped mobile but still mute images of animals seem to talk fluently. So Dodo in Wonderland could now both walk the walk and talk the talk—like the gigantic parrot in Carroll's *Sylvie and Bruno.*[19]

Talkies

> When you hear your favorite star sing in the talkies, don't be too sure of it.
>
> —"The Truth about Voice Doubling," *Photoplay* (July 1929)

Talkies of the 1920s cured the dumbness, or verbal paralysis, of silent cinema. In much the same way, cinema cured the motionlessness, or bodily paralysis, of still photography. Technically proficient means of synchronizing sound with moving film—including "lip-synching" and "speaking photoplay"—now allowed cinematic drawings and photographs to talk. In fact, many early silent films had already depicted cures for deafness and muteness. In such silent films as *Rimrock Jones* (1919) and *The Big Little Person* (1919), curing muteness and deafness was the essential subject. One finds the same in *The Silent Voice* (1915) and *The Man Who Played God* (1922), both based on Jules Eckert Goodman's play *The Silent Voice,* in which a concert pianist goes deaf. The theme was so long-lived that *Sincerely Yours* (1955), likewise based on Goodman's play, was a popular film when I was coming up the speech ladder.

A concomitant early subject of many talkies was: What should we do now with the old silent picture "stars" who turn out to have no "stage voice"? First, one might cure them of their speech "disability" by means of elocution lessons. The comedy *Once in a Lifetime* (1932) thus thematizes the transition from silent films to talkies.[20] In this movie, three New York vaudevillians working in 1929 are determined to get rich by teaching silent-film stars to speak "properly." They teach acceptable English-language accent and inflection of the sort that nonanglophone immigrants and other nonstandard speakers in America were attempting during the same historical period.

Second, one might turn the screen stars into dummies through whom others speak ventriloquistically or ekphrastically. Dubbing and lip-synching were thus the more or less secret "cures" for many film stars whose speaking or singing voices were "wanting." The advent of the talkies gave rise to an apparently deceptive ekphrasis: Who, really, is talking?

Third, one might fire, or discharge, the voice-disabled star. This is what eventually happens to silent-screen star Lina Lamont (played by Jean Hagen) in *Singing in the Rain* (1952), which drew, in part, on *Once in a Lifetime.* Lina wants people to believe that she talks as well as she walks, so she puts out a bit of news that's duly reported in the press: "Monumental Pictures Wildly Enthusiastic over Her Singing Pipes and Dancing Stems!" But Lina can't make the transition to talkies, despite diction and elocution lessons. Her voice ("singing pipes") does not measure up to her body ("dancing stems"). Lina's lower-class New York accent and squeaky voice—reminiscent of Judy Holliday's characterization of the not-so-"dumb" blond Billie Dawn in George Cukor's *Born Yesterday* (1950)—are not easily retrained. Unlike Eliza Doolittle in *My Fair Lady,* Lina cannot learn to talk right, and she requires a voice-woman ventriloquist: Kathy Selden (played by Debbie Reynolds), who both sings and talks—dubs and doubles—for her.[21] People discover the "dubbing" deception thanks to a performance onstage that might remind us of the exposing of the marvelous professorial Wizard in the *Wizard of Oz* (1939). Kathy then takes over Lina's role both onstage (as the fictional lover of the leading man, Don) and in reality (as Don's "real-life" lover).

There is an irony in these films: the actors who play the "best-spoken" women are themselves often dummies. The real Debbie Reynolds, whom film audiences believed to be the actual voice-woman Kathy Selden in *Singing in the Rain,* does not actually do the singing for Lina; Jean Hagen does.[22] Similarly, the real Audrey Hepburn, who plays Eliza Doolittle in the film version of *My Fair Lady,* does not do her own singing: Marni Nixon sings for her. The "theme" of voice change and illusion in cinematography was often thus reproduced in "production."[23]

In *Singing in the Rain,* the diction coaches and elocution teachers are far more successful with Don Lockwood (Gene Kelly) than with Lina Lamont. Don does really well with the tongue twister "Moses Supposes":

> Moses supposes his toeses are roses
> But Moses supposes erroneously.
> Moses he knowses his toeses aren't roses
> As Moses supposes his toeses to be.

After all, the stutterer Moses also needs a voice-man: his brother, Aaron.[24]

Porky Pig

Just how animation affected our understanding of animals that otherwise could not talk the walk or walk the talk is part of the culture of children's learning about speech. Originally, silent cartoon animation was the study of how animals (including human ones) move. Eadweard Muybridge explored this in his photographic work—for example, in his turn-of-the-century stop-frame depictions of moving horses and human cripples.[25] (Edwin George Lutz's *Animated Cartoons: How They Are Made: Their Origin and Development,* published in 1920, gives more general guidelines for depicting anatomy and motion in cartoons.) The counterpart history of silent cartoon animation in the early 1900s includes many animal characters, such as Winsor McCay's Gertie the Dinosaur (the star of a feature-length film in 1914), Otto Messmer's Felix the Cat (who made his first appearance 1919), and Walt Disney's Mickey Mouse (introduced in 1928).

With the advent of the talkies, photographed animals, including human beings, not only walked—they now also talked. Here, finally, we had "the dumb ass [of Balaam] speaking with man's voice"—as Saint Peter says (2 Peter 2:16). In fact, a fable by Aesop was the basis for the first sound cartoon ever released: an animated talkie by RKO called *Dinner Time* (1928).[26] Soon after the film's success, Warner Brothers inaugurated one of its all-time popular cartoon characters: Porky Pig.

During the 1950s, Porky Pig was the most celebrated of the talking-animal stutterers. His signature line—"Th-th that's all, folks!"—which he struggled to get out at the end of most of his cartoons, was eventually made the subject of a pleasantly official U.S. postage stamp. Many prominent

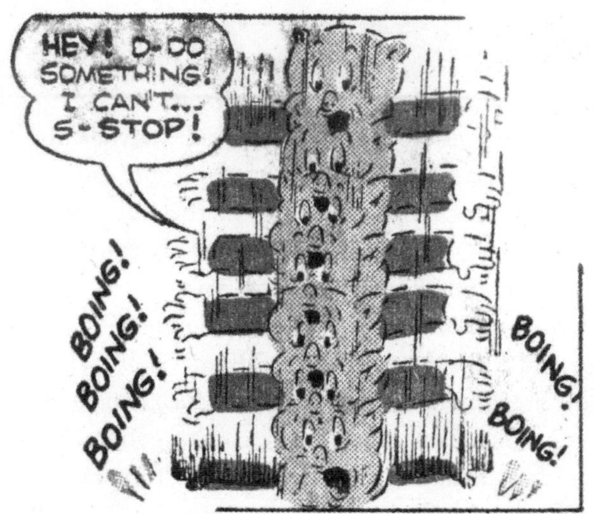

6. Isadore (Fritz) Freleng, *Porky Pig on a Trampoline.* From *Porky Pig,* Dell Comics, vol. 33 (March–April 1954). Collection Selechonek. The original Porky Pig comic book series ran from 1942 to 1962. It was revived by Gold Key Comics in 1965 and continued until 1984.

stutter therapists *still* study Porky's speech patterns—especially his habit of word substitution. It's as if the Porky Pig movies were actually documentaries about human stutterers.[27] (Stutter doctors of the neurological sort are also interested in the ironic Doc—the speech-impeded dwarf in Walt Disney's animated film *Snow White and the Seven Dwarfs,* from 1937.)[28]

The first voice-actor to play Porky was Joe Dougherty, who dubbed for Porky during the early 1930s and who stuttered in real life. His film credits included one of the first talkies, *The Jazz Singer* (1927), in which he was silent. Warner Brothers fired Dougherty, presumably because it was expensive to have an actor who stuttered when he didn't want to.[29] His replacement was Mel Blanc, who would become the most influential voice-man of all time. ("That's all, folks!" is the inscription on his gravestone in the Hollywood Forever Cemetery.)

Mel Blanc sought to re-present in his vocal representation of Porky Pig both an actual human speaker's stutter (Dougherty) and an actual farm pig's sound. English-speaking human beings parrot the sound as *oink oink,* a supposedly echoic term, though humans in general are nowhere near as multilingual in the human languages as the multilingual parrot Polynesia. (Frenchmen imitating pigs say *groin groin,* Vietnamese say *ut ut,* Welsh say *soch soch,* Poles say *chrum chrum,* Albanians say *hunk hunk,* Japanese say *buu buu,* and so on.) In any case, Blanc went out to a pig farm and, in an early bit of method acting, tried to "become" a pig—indeed, he seems to have believed that, in some essential way, he *did* become one. Blanc's first voice-work for Warner Brothers was *Picador Porky* (1937), in which he also played the drunken bull—with a lazy Southern drawl punctuated by hiccups.[30] (Hiccups—those "involuntary spasms of the respiratory organs"—are, as the *OED* says, much like stutters. Blanc picks up on this in Barney Rubble's laughing hiccup in the animated TV series *The Flintstones.* In some languages, in fact, the terms for "hiccup" and "stutter" are the same.)[31]

Mel Blanc, born to a Jewish family named Blank, had grown up in Oregon in the 1910s surrounded by a "medley of foreign accents."[32] Henry James had used the very term "medley" to refer to the animal babbling of immigrant New Yorkers. Blanc turned the barbarian chorus into the voices of a parliament of hundreds of speech-impeded animals. His Tweety Bird sentence "I tawt I taw a puddy tat" became the basis for a best-selling song; his avian

Roadrunner's "Mbeep-mbeep" traveled the world; his Woody Woodpecker was widely celebrated and imitated.[33] Tweety Bird singing "I Tan't Wait till Quithmith Day" and Porky Pig trying unsuccessfully to sing "Blue Christmas" were holiday-time favorites. Sometimes it seemed to me, as I was coming up the speech ladder, that the one dummy persona with a speech impediment that "dub-man" Blanc didn't reduplicate was Moses.

Warner Brothers made a great deal of money from mocking people who did not speak standard English. Mexican immigrants and other Spanish-speaking Americans were outraged by the cartoon mouse Speedy Gonzalez.[34] Blanc's imitations of "Latin-American" speech patterns led to public demonstrations against his voice-acting. French-speaking people in both France and Québec balked at Blanc's Pepe Le Pew, a skunk who stars in such cartoons as *Two Scents Worth* and has a strained French accent.[35] (Cartoons here reflect scientists' claims that some animals have a humanoid ability to differentiate among classes of spoken language on the basis of their rhythmic differences.)[36] Blanc's similarly outrageous imitations of Native American speech patterns (as on the *Jack Benny Show,* December 9, 1951) evoked fewer but equally impassioned complaints. Stutterers were the one group to keep altogether mum—yet Blanc's impersonation of a stutterer in Porky's version of the song "K-K-K-Katy" is, I believe, the most deeply humiliating parody of stuttering ever made in the English language. A close second would be Blanc's performance in *Porky's Poppa* (1938), which also features the unlikely situation in which a stutterer is unable to sing without stuttering. Porky plays a recording he has made to the tune of the song "Old MacDonald Had a Farm," a children's folksong that focuses on reproducing animal sounds. He has a violent, rap-like, percussive reaction to hearing himself stutter; finally, he smashes both the record and the playback machine.[37] Stutterers faced with Porky—Warner Brothers' most popular and long-lived character—did not complain about him until the 1990s, at the time the National Stuttering Project first objected to the stuttering woodpecker Boomer in Walt Disney's animated feature *The Fox and the Hound,* made in 1981.[38]

Stutterers' relative acquiescence about parodies of stuttering as animal speech impediment was the result not only of the difficult and little-studied individual isolation that stuttering entails, but also, as we shall see, of a certain reflexive identification.

Birdsong and Speech

Do birdsong, and the physical and intellectual capacities of some birds to sing, provide a helpful model for understanding human stuttering and human speech in general? Addressing this question, which serves as a reminder that stuttering is a pan-global and pan-cultural human phenomenon,[39] properly depends on our distinguishing carefully between two kinds of musical representation. First there is the representation of stuttering in songs, or in music-with-words. Examples would include popular music like "K-K-K-Katy" and passages in operas such as Francesco Cavalli's *Giasone* and Mozart's *Magic Flute.* As we have seen, one problematic representational aspect of such works is the fact that human stutterers do not stutter when they sing. Second, there is the representation of stuttering in music-without-words. Examples would include Edward Elgar's brilliant "Dorabella Variation."[40] (This is different from the representation of birdsong in music—as in Olivier

Messiaen's *Livre du Saint Sacrement* for organ and Allesandro Poglietti's *Rossignolo* for harpsichord.)

In the most telling instances where music conveys human stuttering, the distinction between music-with-words and music-without-words seems almost to break down. One example occurs at a musical pinnacle in *The Magic Flute.* Mozart had already experimented with dental stuttering in Don Curzio's singing in *The Marriage of Figaro,* with the chattering woodwinds of the overture. In *The Magic Flute,* the Queen of the Night, at the very top of her game, sings out an extraordinarily beautiful schwa-vowel melisma: "ah—ah—ah—ah—ah—ah—ah—ah—ah—." *Melisma* is musicology's term for the "prolongation of one syllable over a number of notes" *(OED)* in such a way that the word halts or repeats, rap-like, in step with the sequence of musical tones. Compare how a speaking human might stutter on the syllable *da,* as does "Loli-ta," or "Aman-da," or "Marilyn Monroe" in Norma Jean Mortenson's performance of "My Heart Belongs to Daddy" in the film *Let's Make Love;* or, appositely, consider how the feather-covered bird-catcher Papageno and his bride-to-be, Papagena, stutter famously on the syllable *pa* in their duet in *The Magic Flute.* (Mozart's librettist Emanuel Schikaneder does something similar in the "Paperl" or "parrot" song in Franz Hoffmeister's opera *The King's Son from Ithaca.*)[41] The stutterers Caracataca and Caracataqué in eighteenth-century French street theater could do no better.[42]

Papageno is, of course, a "bird man." And just as thousands of real-life composers and songwriters imitate birdsong, so many songbirds imitate human speech. For example, there is the *da*—the daw or jackdaw—which we will encounter in Chapter 5.

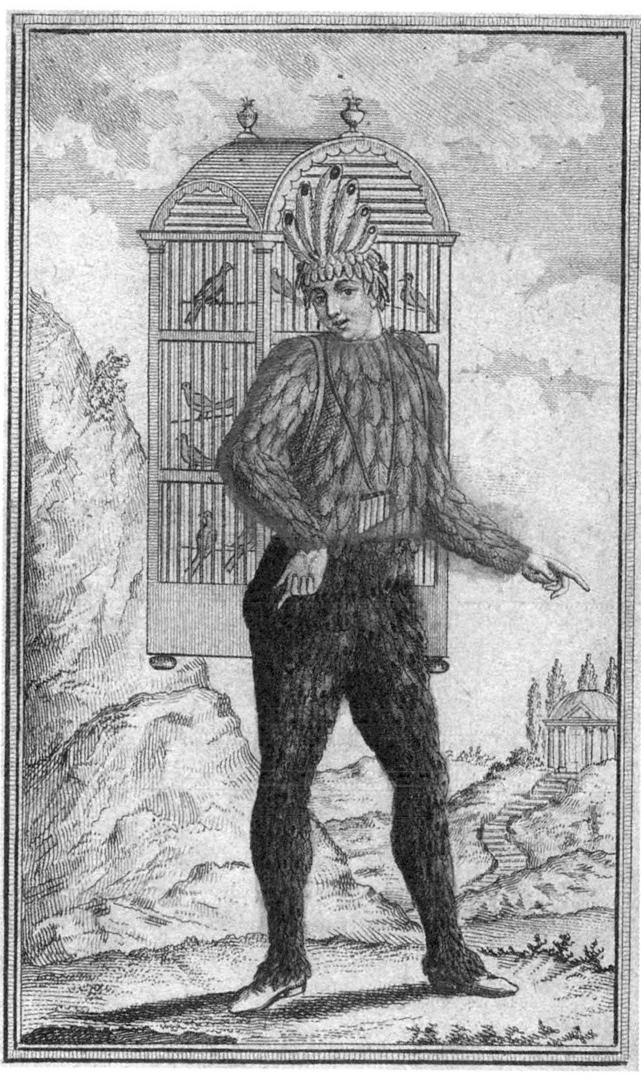

7. Anonymous, *Emanuel Schikaneder in the Role of Papageno.* Engraving from *Die Zauberflöte: Eine grosse Oper in zwey Aufzügen,* libretto by Emanuel Schikaneder, score by Wolfgang Amadeus Mozart (Frankfurt and Leipzig, 1794). Biblioteca Mozartiana Eric Offenbacher of the Eda Kuhn Loeb Music Library, Harvard University.

But if we are to compare humans' musical compositions with the melismatic catches of songbirds, we should probably first seek to dispel three false beliefs about human speech in relation to bird song.

First is the belief that laterality is a reliable distinguishing characteristic of human beings. In fact, just as human speech—stuttering in particular—is related to cerebral laterality (most stutterers are left-handed), so birdsinging is related to the handedness of the bird's syrinx, or lower larynx.[43] Particularized lateralization among human children develops ontogenetically at around the time they are learning to speak. Some researchers think this fact may help to explain why so many children (3–4 percent) "stumble" in speech and then "outgrow" the problem when lateralization is fully developed. Those children who do not fully lateralize are, according to this view, the children who are the "real" stutterers (about 1 percent).[44]

Second is the view that avian soundmaking is usually innate and that, when it is learned, the learning process does not continue past physical maturation. Some bird species do learn their songs in infancy. Like human children, they require tutors. Of these avian song-learners, some are "closed learners," meaning that they keep the same song throughout their lives. Zebra finches are a good example. "Open learners," in contrast, forget old songs and learn new ones as the seasons pass. Examples are canaries and robins.[45] Their ability to forget and learn probably involves the generation of new nerves (neurogenesis). Since most scientists refused for decades to believe that neurogenesis was possible, they did not "us[e] birds [much] in scientific research."[46] (It is worth recalling here that human stuttering is related to gender. On the one hand, 80 percent of human stutterers are male; on the other hand, male canaries—

the open learners—sing and female canaries almost never do.)[47]

Third is the wrongheaded notion that human beings are the only animals that stutter. Individual birds, in some species, stutter. (Hiawatha would have known this: he served the stuttering Iroquois legislator Dekanawida and "learned of every bird its language"—as Longfellow reminds us.) Among zebra finches, for example, about 7 percent stutter. Here, too, there is room for neurological research. Neurological investigation has already determined that when it comes to humans, the brains of stutterers differ from those of nonstutterers. Yet important comparative questions remain: Do the brains of stuttering zebra finches differ from those of nonstuttering zebra finches?[48] In what ways might the brains of stuttering human beings and stuttering zebra finches resemble each other?

Only now are we ready to listen to what the birds say.

The Finch's Stutter

> The finch, the sparrow and the lark,
> The plain-song cuckoo gray,
> Whose note full many a man doth mark,
> And dares not answer nay.
>
> —Shakespeare, *A Midsummer Night's Dream,* 3.1; sung by Bottom the Weaver, transformed into an ass, at the time when Titania the Fairy Queen falls in love with him

> What, billing again?
>
> —Shakespeare, *Troilus and Cressida,* 3.2.60

Many stutterers speak with what some people claim are animal sounds. Thus, the stand-up stuttering comedian Patrick Campbell says that he stammers with a "muted gibbon cry." Gibbons do have a remarkable cry. But it's birds, not apes, that produce sounds the *way* humans do. "Our language has more in common with the singing and calling of birds, than with the vocal signals of apes," argues Jean Aitchison.[49]

Just *how* to study birdsounds is problematic. Some scholars of birdsounds as language focus on birds' apparently weak linguistic conceptualizing ability. That is an error Irene Pepperberg makes when she gives her parrot Alex elocution lessons and then reports on his relatively weak conceptualizing ability compared to that of dolphins and apes, whom researchers regularly provide with prostheses such as pegboards and keyboards.[50] Pepperberg judges Alex's speaking abilities not on his sounds and breathing, but on her own ability to judge Alex's conceptualizing—almost as if her parrot were a human infant trying to speak out or an adult victim of bulbar paralysis. To disassociate soundmaking from language in this way tends to overlook how human language is essentially linked with issues of anticipation in breathing and vocalization. It is also, as we have seen, a prejudice found in much stutter theory.

Another problem concerns the charge that birds engage in mere mindless parroting—or soundmaking without "linguistic meaning." Some may be good at imitating birdsounds of other species. (Mockingbirds—*Mimus polyglottos*—brilliantly mimic the notes of other birds. So do sedge warblers, butcher birds, blackcaps, mocking wrens, lyre birds, parson birds, bhim-rajs, and French mockingbirds, or thrashers.)[51] This capacity has made talking birds, in human guise, frequent targets of put-downs and parodies in literature, film, and everyday speech. On the one hand, we praise a human dialectal elocutionist such as Shaw's Henry Higgins for his ability to parrot the sounds of a wide variety of human beings; on the other, we complain about human beings who merely patter, or "parrot" other peoples' ideas, and we look down on animals, human and otherwise, who "ape" other creatures' gestures or imitate their sounds.[52] Whatever the reason for our denigrating in animals what we often praise in ourselves, we appear anxiety-ridden at any hint of validity in the hypothesis that various animal-like "cries or interjections [like *oink-oink* and *bow-wow*] are . . . the natural and real beginnings of human speech"; this is what the philologist Max Müller called the "Interjectional, or Pooh-Pooh, Theory."[53] Perhaps there is also a long-standing threat in the concomitant view that "human speech originated in the imitation of animal sounds"—the derogatorily named "bow-wow theory" *(OED),* which seems to reduce the essentials of human language to barking instead of conceptualizing. Writes Jonathan Swift in *Traulus* (1730), "And though you hear him stut-tut-tut-ter, / He barks as fast as he can utter."

Do animals *ever* stutter? We should again distinguish here between real animals and fictional animals (say, between a flesh-and-blood pig and Porky Pig), and between real animals that only seem to stutter and real animals that actually do stutter. Real animals that only sound as if they stutter would include the "stuttering frogs" of Australia.[54] And many apes *seem* to stutter like human beings, as when chimpanzees "laugh." (Stuttering, defined narrowly as "the breakdown of the syllable unit, characterized by rapid amplitude fluctuations with the syllable . . . during the production of the combination long call," is a relatively new claim for primate vocal production.[55] Recent evidence from Harvard University suggests that the primate *Saguinus oedipus,* or cotton-top tamarin, when given delayed auditory feedback, occasionally stutters in something like the way that certain birds stutter.)[56] Among humans, however, there is a highly developed thoracic respiratory control that underlies the ability, on a single out-breath, to create multiple strings of vocalizations accurately timed and synchronized with complex vocal-tract movements. This ability, probably absent in chimpanzees, underlies such human singing as stutter rap and melisma, and it partly explains the claim that the evolution of a distinctively human vocal tract is the primary factor in the development of specifically human language.[57]

But although chimps do not quite stutter, some (but not all) zebra finches do. Termed "finches" because their callnotes are represented in English as *spink spink* or *pink pink,*[58] zebra finches—7 percent of them—stutter, in the sense that they repeat syllables of song several times before continuing with their songs, altering syllables, deleting them, or inserting new syllables. Delayed auditory feedback (DA) in zebra finches produces song irregularities resembling human stuttering.[59] These finches, which are otherwise closed learners, do not have parents that stutter, and they have highly individualized avoidance or substitution styles. (Their individual songs are not learned.)[60] That is to say, these particular finches use sound-avoidance techniques which would seem to require reaction if not also "self-consciousness"—techniques of the sort that characterize human speech. Stutterers such as myself immediately underst-underst-underst- . . . barely recognize such strategies when we hear them in the field, the laboratory, and at home (zebra finches make excellent pets).[61] But the sonograms are clear.

In the instant of substitution of one note for another—

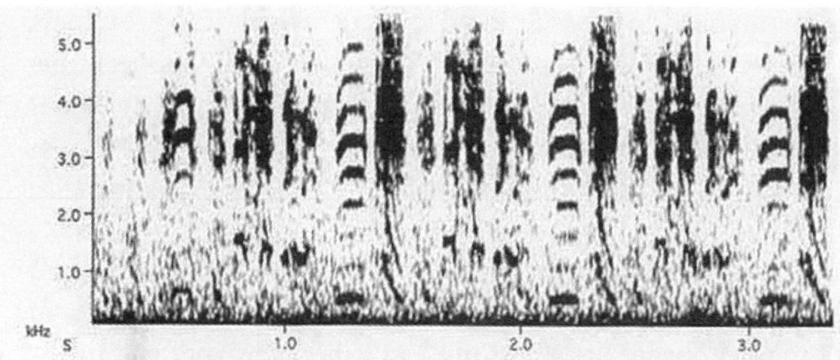

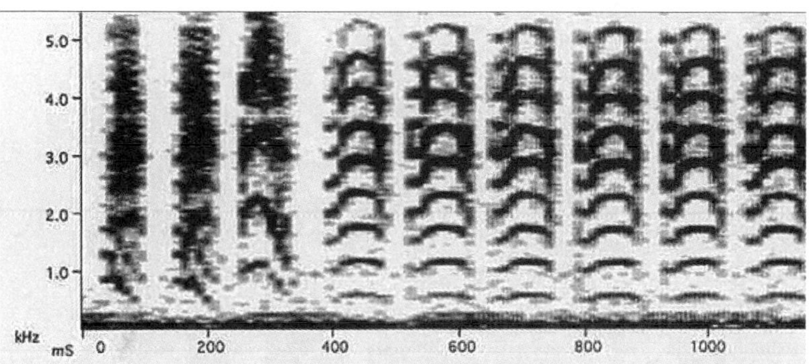

8–9. Sonograms of the songs of zebra finches: normal (top) and stutterer. Courtesy of Dr. David B. Rosenfield and Dr. Santosh S. Helekar, Speech and Language Center, Department of Neurology, Baylor College of Medicine, Houston, Texas.

for example, *re* for *st*—the human stutterer becomes birdlike: he disregards, *almost* completely, the longer-term problems of "meaning" (conceptualization) that his substitution will entail later in his sentence. To all intents and purposes, the stutterer becomes a singer of musical notes. In the case of the bird-man Pa-pa-pa-pa-geno, human speaking is anticipation of the next note, even more than it is production or memory of its supposed conceptual meaning—which, as we have seen, can always come afterward. The example of the zebra finch helps also when we consider stuttering as an impediment involving *anticipation* of faltering in speaking and/or failure in breathing.

Charles Darwin, who came from a stuttering family, argued that "primeval man, or rather some early progenitor of man, probably first used his voice in producing true musical cadences, that is in singing."[62] Indeed, since the eighteenth century, song has been linked to the babbling and hesitant origins of speech.[63] The anatomical characteristics of the human vocal tract are in fact more closely linked to our capacity to sing than to our capacity to speak. The stutterer knows this already, not only because singing increases his subglottalic air pressure in such a way that he can sing without stuttering,[64] but also because, as the work of the ninth-century composer and author Notker Balbulus (Notker the Stutterer) demonstrates, bird-like melisma crosses over into stuttering and usually cancels it out.

Stutterers do not stutter when they singsong melismatically—that is, by prolonging one syllable over a number of notes. Notker long ago located stuttering within the traditions of ornithological melisma when he definitively changed the melismatic sequences of the Gregorian chants.[65] In his day it was customary, where a Hallelujah was chanted in the Mass, to sing on the *schwa*-vowel *ah* a series of long, elaborate melodic passages that prolonged this vowel. Often, what resulted were distinctly bird-like sounds.[66] A good example is the famous aria in *The Magic Flute* sung by the Queen of the Night, Papageno's musicologically opposite number. Her melismatic aria culminates in the representation of speech in music, and music in speech—representation that is a principal formal goal of opera in general and the librettist's art in particular.

Notker claimed (somewhat disingenuously) that in order to better retain in his memory the long wordless melodies of the Gregorian chants, he supplied them with words and notes.[67] He set his new sequences so that each syllable corresponded to a single note.[68] "As many notes as there were in the music, so many words must there be in the text."[69] Notker the Stutterer (in the realm of music), like Moses the Stammerer (in the realm of legislation), introduced a momentous new writing system that changed forever the rules of the language game. One might add that in the tenth century, Abu'l-Faraj ibn al-Muzaffar ibn Sa'id, called al-Lajlaj (the Stammerer), wrote *Kitab mansubat ash-shatranj,* an influential—possibly the first—written work on chess openings.[70]

The Duck's Quack

What makes people laugh? People who talk almost as if they were animals? Animals that talk almost as if they were human? Henri Bergson wrote that what inspires laughter is "the momentary transformation of a person into a thing" —that "we laugh every time a person gives us the impression of being a thing." Sometimes, he says, an animal plays the conceptual role of "a lifeless object," so that when a human being is animalized we laugh. Figaro, in Beaumarchais' play *The Barber of Seville* (the basis for Giovanni Paisiello's opera of the same name) mocks the physician Bartolo as a person who "growls and groans" like an animal.[71] Some scholars, says Bergson, "have defined man as 'an animal which laughs.' They might equally well have defined him as an animal which is laughed at; for if any other animal, or some lifeless object, produces the same effect, it is always because of some resemblance to man, of the stamp he gives it or the use he puts it to." One thinks of the stuttering magistrate Curzio in Mozart's *Marriage of Figaro.*[72]

In the movie *Let's Make Love* (1960), Milton Berle—alias the Thief of Bad Gags—claims that the extinct dodo-bird is the funniest thing in the world. But according to modern research, the talking animal that is universally accepted as the "funniest" is the duck. This was the conclusion reached by Richard Wiseman: "Comparing scores for the same joke with different animals inserted in it, we found that the funniest [talking] animal of all is the duck."[73]

The most famous twentieth-century talking-quacker is Donald Duck. Voice-man Clarence "Duck" Nash's Donald has a special speech impediment. It is not stuttering, as in the case of Lewis Carroll's Dodo; nor does it involve a lisp, like Daffy Duck's *desthpicable,* which voice-man Mel Blanc attributed to Daffy's long mandible, or bill.[74] Rather, Donald Duck has a speech impediment more closely tied with breathing. When he speaks, Donald uses the buccal air-stream mechanism: he makes sounds by forcing out air with the muscles of the mouth.

Human languages, though, rarely use the buccal air-stream mechanism. Most use the *pulmonary* air-stream mechanism, which is either egressive (as in most English today) or ingressive.[75] Languages in which inhalation is important include Tsou, an aboriginal language of Taiwan.[76] Inuit throat games (Katajjait), which are all inhalative, are already a sort of stutter exercise.[77] While stutterers often involuntarily produce ingressive inhalation sounds—whoops, crowing sounds, whimpering noises, and grunts accompanied by long and labored inspirations, together with spasms of the glottis—inhalation therapy for stuttering relies on the observable phenomenon that many stutterers do not stutter on voluntary inhalation.[78] (Charles Darwin observed that cats purr both on inspiration and expiration; many cat owners believe that cats do not purr when their cats are alone, just as people who stutter do not stutter when alone.)[79] Another breathing mechanism common to some human stutterers and cartoon animals involves the *velaric* air stream, which helps to create the following sounds (defined in the *OED*): a partial vacuum resulting in a bilabial *click* ("grandmother's kiss"), a *tchick* for encouraging a horse (a lateral click, also spelled *'ts* and *tut*), and *tisk-tisk* or *tsk-tsk* (an expression of disapproval). An old-fashioned treatment for stuttering combines pulmonary with velaric air-stream breathing. On the one hand, the patient *hums* through the nose by means of the egressive pulmonary method. This entails "making an inarticulate murmur in a pause of speaking, from hesitation, embarrassment, etc." *(OED).* Consider here the stutterer's practice of *hemming and hawing.* On the other hand, the patient simultaneously produces a click by means of the velaric method. This, in short, is the "stutterer's rap."

Animal cartoons of the twentieth century used these and all of the other human breathing mechanisms for speech.[80] A favorite Donald Duck cartoon is *Cured Duck* (1945), which concerns a wise-quacking quack who (or that) cracks us up. A wise-cracking fake doctor, the talking duck makes us laugh. Yet the best theory of stuttering, as a neuronal and motor event linked with problems of breathing and questions of ontogenetic and phylogenetic origin, still remains up in the air—with the birds.

4 Moses' Tongue

As a child I had a habit, frequently ineradicable among young stutterers, of preferring the weak vowel. Instead of saying "da-da-daddy," for example, I would say "duh-duh-daddy." The English-language term *schwa*—sometimes called the *murmur vowel*—names this *uh* sound. My teachers in Hebrew school taught me that *schwa* was related to *sheva,* which in written Hebrew is the sign "placed under a consonant letter to express (what Jewish grammarians regard as) the absence of a following vowel sound," and, they always emphasized, it was "an arbitrary alteration of *shāw',* 'emptiness,' 'vanity.'"[1] As such, the *schwa* recalled for me the Mosaic commandment that we should never speak *lashav* ("vainly") about *adonai* ("God"). "Lo tisa et-shem-*adonai* eloheycha lashav ki lo yenakeh *adonai* et asher-yisa et-shmo *lashav*" ("Thou shalt not take the name of the Lord thy God in vain; for the Lord will not hold him guiltless that taketh his name in vain").[2] Does this commandment mean that one should not use the name of God for any frivolous or malicious purpose, or in magic? Or does it outlaw using God's name to guarantee merely commercial contacts? Or does it only prohibit swear words? In Hebrew school, my friends and I compared this Mosaic commandment with the prophet Ezekiel's complaint about the vanity of false prophets.[3] But as a young stutterer, I took

Moses to mean something like, "Don't use the *schwa* vowel." And for me, that meaning amounted to: "Don't stutter." This was a regulation which, once internalized, all but assured that I *would* stutter.

My most unbearable stuttering experience in Hebrew school was the unavoidable one at the beginning of every class. I would be called upon to announce my presence during the alphabetical roll call. Mr. Teicher—a stern and always disapproving teacher—would begin to read out the roll call in predictable, inexorable sequence. There was plenty of time for me to anticipate my failure. I would tremble fearfully, more and more, until my name, Me-ir, came up. "Me-ir, are you present?"

Every stammering schoolchild rehearses the phrase, "I am present," in his head—over and over and over again—during the hours-long minutes before his turn comes up. (Stutterers who have difficulty saying their own names sometimes resort to changing their names to an easily pronounceable one. Soon afterward, however, they discover that their new names have become difficult to pronounce.) Many stutterers play hooky instead of following through on oral performances.[4] Not a few stutterers—including many Canadians who went on to prominence in the field of stutter therapy—dropped out of school on account of their stuttering.[5] And many young scholars who stutter do not go on to do graduate work, because they fear that they will fail their oral exams—the way I failed fourth grade.[6]

In Hebrew school, I would try to answer, in Hebrew, *Ani poh* ("I [am] present"). But the *schwa,* the *a-a-a-a-ani,* was always too much for me, and my fear of stuttering helped to precipitate the failure I feared. Stuttering at Hebrew school was such a difficult experience—"Except the

Lord build the house, they labour in vain *(shav)* that build it" (Psalms 127:1)—that I often played hooky all day to avoid being there at all.

On such days, I would hide out from Mr. Teicher at the local French-language library. I would identify with Adam, who hid among the trees when God called, "Where are you?" (Genesis 3:8–10). And I would often read over the passage in Exodus, famously authored by Moses himself, where God calls to Moses from out of the burning bush in Midian: "Moses, where are you?"

Moses has a severe speech impediment of his own. Yet somehow he manages to get out a magnificent answer: *"Hineni"*—"I am here!" (Exodus 3:4). I knew that it was even more difficult for Moses to answer *hineni* than it was for Abraham to say it when God and Isaac sought him out.[7] After all, Moses' *hineni* is the great prayer of mediation between the congregation and God that the synagogue cantor recites (both dummy-like and ventriloquist-like) as he takes over leading the crucial services at the beginning of the New Year (Rosh Hashanah).

My colleague Neil Schmitz, at SUNY Buffalo, is right to insist, in his first-person account "To the Speech Clinic," that "at some point in the stutterer's early life there must be a question—a question so powerful that it is forgotten, because all that is remembered is the circumstance. I am obliged to speak. . . . It is not what is to be said that makes the stutterer hesitate, but that it must be said."[8]

At the Burning Bush

At the burning bush, God tells Moses to speak for Him. Why Moses?

On the face of it, God's choice of Moses to be His

dummy spokesperson is odd. Moses is not a person who speaks well. Presumably, an omnipotent God could cure Moses of his speech impediment. ("Who has made man's mouth? Who makes him dumb, or deaf, or seeing, or blind? Is it not I, the Lord?"—Exodus 4:11.) We might presume that God is able to cure stutterers. As Isaiah reminds us, "The tongue of the stutters shal be ready to speake distinctly."[9] God's presumed capacity to cure "tonguelessness" is a principal aspect of the miracle of Pope Leo III's tongue restoration (see Chapter 6). There is also the story reported in Mark 7:33–35: "And they [the disciples] brought to him [Jesus] a man who . . . had an impediment in his speech; and they besought him to lay his hand upon him. And taking him aside from the multitude privately . . . he spat and touched his tongue; and looking up to heaven, he sighed, and said to him, *Eph'phatha,* that is, 'Be opened.' And his . . . tongue was released, and he spoke plainly." Most relevantly for our present purpose, there is Moses' own report about the talking-animal tale concerning Balaam's ass (Numbers 22:28): "And the Lord opened the mouth of the ass." (An ass is a creature which, generally speaking, has not even the faculty for speech. But in Exodus an ass speaks eloquently to the prophet Balaam. During the period of Exodus, God is closer to Balaam than to almost anyone else. And the words that Jews recite every time they enter a synagogue are Balaam's: "How fair are your tents, O Jacob, your dwelling places, O Israel!" (Numbers 24:5). Though some rabbis place Balaam in the same category as Haman and Amalek—presumed evildoers—others say that he is the equal of Moses himself.)

In some religious traditions Moses actually asks to be cured of his stuttering. In the Koran (Sura 20:26–29) Moses says, "Lord, open my breast, and do Thou ease for me my task, / Unloose the knot upon my tongue, that they may understand my words." And Allah cures him. Some Christian interpreters likewise expect that God's presence ought to cure Moses of his speech defect. (The *Easy-To-Read Bible* thus has Moses say, "And now, even after talking to you, I am *still* not a good speaker.") But in Exodus, Moses makes no request to be cured and is not cured. The translation done by Ronald Knox in the 1940s even emphasizes that the appearance of God, while not the cause of the stutter that Moses seems to have had for years, is a factor that "exacerbates" it. Says Knox's Moses, "I am more faltering, more tongue-tied, *than ever.*"

The Stuttering God

Moses is not the only being to hesitate at the burning bush. God does, too. Is that why he seeks out a stutterer? Like a teacher taking roll call, Moses demands that God speak out His name: "What [is] His name?"[10] The stutterer James Malcolm Rymer was right to stress, in his autobiography, God's relevant status as "unspeakable."[11] But God says in Hebrew, "Eheyeh asher ejeyeh" ("I am that I am," King James Version, Exodus 3:14). The prophet Isaiah more strictly recalls this passage in his reduplicative paraphrase, "Anoki anoki hu" ("I, even I, am he," King James Version, Isaiah 51:12, 43:25). The Septuagint's Greek-language translation of Isaiah's paraphrase in 51:12—"Ego eimi ego eimi" ("I am I am")—likewise brings out the divine stutter/repetition or existential doubling. The Vulgate's Latin translation by Saint Jerome—"Ego ego" ("I am I am")—suggests complete doubling.

When I was coming up the speech ladder in the 1950s, my francophone Jesuit teachers interpreted Jerome's "Ego

ego" mainly in terms of Jesus' nominal self-presentation in John 8:58. But I had my doubts, since we all knew the anglophone Protestant doggerel, inspired by Dr. Seuss, that mocked the divine anti-name: "I Am I Am, I Am I Am, / What kind of name is I Am I Am?"[12] At the time, Dr. Seuss had already written books and created animated movies featuring Gerald McBoing Boing, the little boy who spoke only in nonanimate sound effects. Celebrated as a talking-animal poet, Dr. Seuss made puns and fun of "childish" speech defects like mine. (He went on to write about "Sam-I-Am" in *Green Eggs and Ham.*)

God as ventriloquist needed a spokesman because He was unable to speak directly to the people. We will see that the dummy Moses, whom He called on to speak for Him, was both too much and too little like God to do the job. We will also see, though, that the most important aspect of the job seemed to require that the Hebrews' monotheistic legislator and alphabetical scribe be a stutterer.

Heavy and Uncircumcised

> Meine Zunge ist ungelenkt: ich kann denken aber nicht reden. [My tongue is not flexible. Thought is easy; speech is laborious.]
>
> —Arnold Schoenberg, *Moses und Aron,* trans. Allen Forte

> The tongue is not an efficient servant of the intelligence.
>
> —Aristotle, *Problems,* 11.902b

Moses frames his reluctance to call on Pharaoh in terms of two kinds of speech impediment. First, he says that he is "heavy of speech"; second, that he has "uncircumcised lips."

In the former case, the relevant passage (Exodus 4:10) is translated thus by George M. Lamsa, an Assyrian from Kurdistan: "O my Lord, I am not eloquent, neither heretofore nor since thou hast spoken to thy servant; for I am a stutterer and slow [*kaved*] of speech."[13] Lamsa was an expert translator from his native Aramaic (Syriac), often said by certain scholars to be much like ancient Hebrew. But the Hebrew term *kaved* would seem to mean, "literally," something like the English *heavy,* which is how a few translations render it.[14]

The second time Moses brings up his impediment (Exodus 6:10–13), he speaks thus: "The Lord spoke to Moshe, saying: 'Go and tell Pharaoh king of Egypt to let the Israelites depart from his land.' But Moshe appealed to the Lord, saying: 'The Israelites would not listen to me; how then should Pharaoh heed me—a man *of impeded speech!*'"

There are various alternate translations for the phrase "of impeded speech."[15] According to the more literal translators, Moses claims to be "of uncircumcised lips."[16] Indeed, the German Elberfelder version (1871) has the relevant passage as "ich unbeschnittene Lippen habe"—slightly varying the terminology from the great *Bibel* (1545) of Martin Luther. (Luther's momentous "conversion" on July 2, 1505—the day he decided to become an Augustinian monk—took place near the felicitously named town of Stotternheim—sometimes glossed as "Home of Stuttering.") Rashi, or Rabbi Solomon ben Isaac, who lived in the eleventh century in what is now France, says that "uncircumcised" means "closed" or "stopped up," and he gives several examples from other biblical verses to corroborate his view.[17] Some of these verses relate to circumcision events, and a few involve physical "deformity" linked with language disability.[18] But none tell us what it really means to have "closed" lips. Only earlier and later events in Moses' life—and likewise in the concomitant history of monotheism and alphabetical writing—help us to understand what's wrong, or what's right, with Moses' tongue.

Walking the Talk

> Just as when we are children we always have less control over hands and feet, and at a still younger age cannot walk at all, so the young cannot control their tongue.
>
> —Aristotle, *Problems,* 11.902b

We often tend to forget that Moses had trouble walking as well as talking. He really needed that staff of his. Sometimes, in fact, his staff did not suffice. He was sometimes unable to stand on his own legs—or even to lift up his own hands, because they likewise were too "heavy." At the Battle of Adonai-nissi, where the Israelites fought the Amalekites (sometimes associated with Balaam), Moses required a stone chair on which to sit. Human shoulders then propped up his arms and hands. "And it came to pass, when Moses held up his hand, that Israel prevailed: and when he let down his hand, Amalek prevailed. But Moses' hands were heavy [*ki-vae-deem*]; and they took a stone, and put it under him, and he sat thereon; and Aaron and Hur stayed up his hands, the one on the one side, and the other on the other side; and his hands were steady until the going down of the sun" (Exodus 17:11–12).[19]

Had Aaron and Hur not provided Moses with lapidary "wheelchair" and humanoid "crutches," the Israelites would have been destroyed. Instead, they destroyed the Amalekites, who were the descendants of Esau.[20] Esau was, according to one theory, the "stranger" with whom Jacob had had a famous wrestling match.[21] (Other theories say it was God.) On account of that match, Jacob, thereafter known as Israel, became so crippled that he had to use a staff.

The "heaviness" of Moses' hands, to which the Torah refers, was partly the result of his having to stand with arms outstretched for a long period of time without the aid of his usual prosthesis, his staff. Yet the Book of Moses had already identified "heaviness"—which here qualifies his weakness of limb—as the principal factor explaining his stutter. When God commanded Moses to tell Pharaoh to let His people go, Moses was reluctant to take on the mission because, as he insisted, he had a heavy *(kaved)* tongue (Exodus 4:10). The same brother—Aaron, who became Moses' prosthetic mouthpiece at Pharaoh's court—becomes at Adonai-nissi (along with Hur) the prosthetic support of Moses' lame arms. Moses' physical weakness goes hand-in-hand with his oral one. The Knox translation of Exodus brings this out by translating Moses' comment on his "heavy tongue" as follows: "Then Moses said, Lord, have patience with me; but all my life I have been a man of little eloquence, and now that thou, my Master, hast spoken to me, I am more faltering, more tongue-tied than ever." The English term *falter* has long indicated problems both with *walking* and with *talking:* "He felt his legs falter" (late seventeenth century); "Thy tongue falters in thy mouth" (early sixteenth century).[22]

By some accounts, the Egyptian princes whom some scholars have associated and even identified with Moses are likewise lame of leg or arm. Philip Glass, in his opera *Akhnaten,* displays Moses' prototype as lame.[23] Freud, though, gives short shrift to the literal lameness of Akhenaten—presumably Amenophis IV—and likewise to the literal lameness of Moses. Instead, he focuses on the monotheistic aspects of Akhenaten's rule.[24] And following Arthur Weigall, he also looks at an uncannily stuttering likeness: between the sound of the apparently Hebrew term *adonai* ("God"), with its *schwa,* and the sound of the seemingly Egyptian *aten,* or *atum.*[25]

Moses' lameness partly explains why he always has his staff *(matteh)* with him. We first learn about that staff in the section of Exodus where we hear Moses complain about his speech disorder. God responds to Moses' carping about his speaking disability with a question:

> What [is] that in thine hand? And [Moses] said, A rod. And [God] said, Cast it on the ground. And [Moses] cast it on the ground, and it became a serpent; and Moses fled from before it. And the Lord said unto Moses, Put forth thine hand, and take it by the tail. And [Moses] put forth his hand, and caught it, and it became a rod in his hand: That they may believe that the Lord God of their fathers, the God of Abraham, the God of Isaac, and the God of Jacob, hath appeared unto thee.

Whether or not Moses' staff is a Hermetic caduceus like the serpentine staff of cure-all Asclepias,[26] it serves to remind us that Moses' ancestor, Jacob, was lame of hip (as the result of a wrestling match with a "stranger") and carries a staff; that Jews are descendants of Jacob, called Yisrael (Israel), meaning "he who wrestles . . . with God";[27] and that Jacob leans on his staff when he passes on the blessing and when he crosses the Red Sea on his way to Egypt.[28] Not surprisingly, the view is widespread that the staff of the stuttering Moses and the staff of the stumbling Jacob are one and the same. Moses' wife, Tzipporah, apparently said so herself.[29]

Jewish families, descendants of Jacob-Israel, celebrate the holiday called Pesach (Passover) every spring. One etymology of "Pesach" has it that the name comes from the way the Angel of Death "passed over" the Jews at the time of the tenth plague. According to a lesser-known etymology, "Pesach" has the same root as the Hebrew word meaning "to hobble."[30] This term is used with reference to that other lame Jewish prince, Mephibosheth.[31] The English term *hobble,* says the *OED,* is cognate with the Dutch term *hobblen,* meaning "stammer, stutter."

Expelling the Cripples

Ancient Egypt, Moses' native land, is the source of our earliest visual record of the type of crippling caused by polio. The "Polio Stele" in the Carlsberg Glyptotek in Copenhagen provides the first written record of a virus infection. It consists of a hieroglyph from Memphis, the capital of ancient Egypt, and was drawn in approximately 1400 B.C.E. It depicts someone, perhaps a temple priest, who shows the clinical signs of physical paralysis.

The stele recalls the plague mentioned in Egyptian and Hebrew cultural history and mythology. Some writers report that a certain community of people was expelled from Egypt—not because their god caused an epidemic (like the various calamities that Moses instigates among the Egyptians and from which Moses' god safeguards the Hebrews) but because they themselves were the carriers of some "Asiatic illness," an infectious pestilence that may have been leprosy. Pharaoh isolated this people in order to pro-

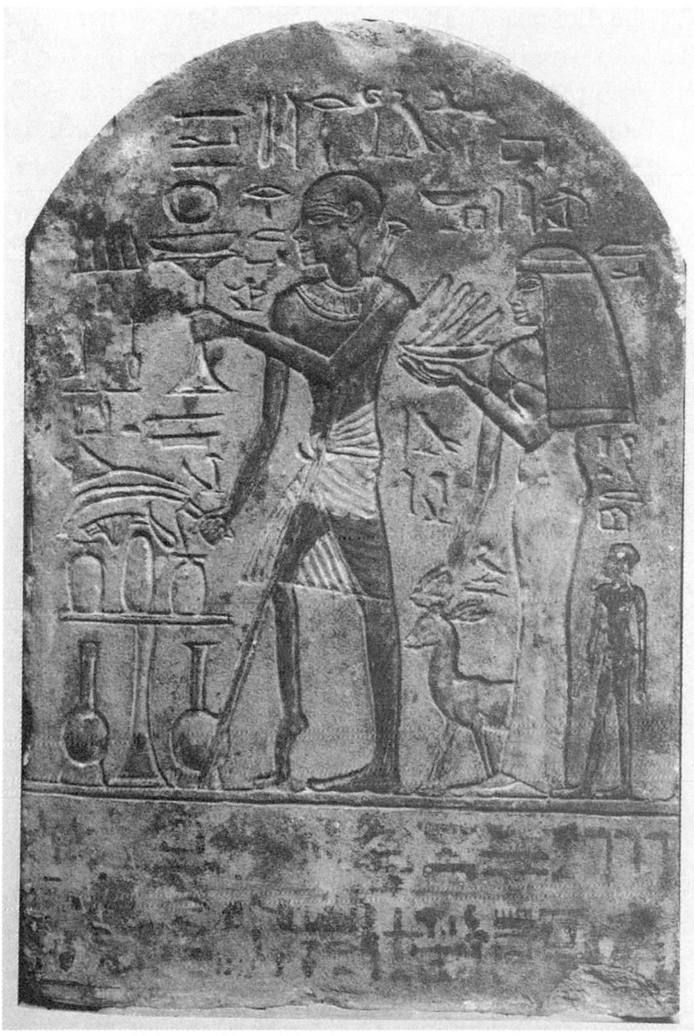

10. The Polio Stele. Limestone with original paintwork. Memphis, Egypt, Middle Kingdom, ca. 1300 B.C.E. Courtesy of the Ny Carlsberg Glyptotek, Copenhagen, Denmark. The man ("Ruma") has a thin, withered leg widely believed to be the earliest evidence of poliomyelitis.

tect the Egyptians from contagion.[32] Many writers take Moses to have been an Egyptian—among them the Egyptian priest Manetho of Sebbenytos (who wrote in Greek), the Roman geographer Strabo (who wrote in Latin), the eighteenth-century English scholar John Toland, and Freud.[33] And many ancient authors claim that the exodus began because Pharaoh (whom the Roman historian Tacitus calls "Bocchorius"),[34] after consulting with the oracle of Hammon, tried to rid Egypt of the portion of his population whose bodies had been deformed: "tabes quae corpora foedaret." (We do not know whether the long-lived historical memory of this *tabes* is to be associated with *tabes dorsalis*—now called "creeping paralysis"—or with syphilis, leprosy, polio, or some other deforming illness.)[35] Only then did a leader (Moses) arise from among those with deformed bodies.[36] Eduard Meyer, who developed this plague thesis for the modern period in his influential *Aegyptische Chronologie* (1904), wrote at around the time that the epidemics, with their deforming effects on both walking and talking, began in the twentieth century.

Burning of the Hand or Tongue

One gloss on Moses' speech impediment has it that the infant Moses was injured in the course of a political hand-to-mouth contest with Pharaoh's counselors (at this time Moses was presumably still without language—literally, *infans*). Moses had worried some of Pharaoh's counselors by sometimes making a grab for Pharaoh's crown. So these counselors offered baby Moses a choice of two plates: one with burning coals upon it, and the other with gold. The infant, directed by the angel Gabriel, chose the coals and burned his tongue, either by placing a live coal in his mouth or by

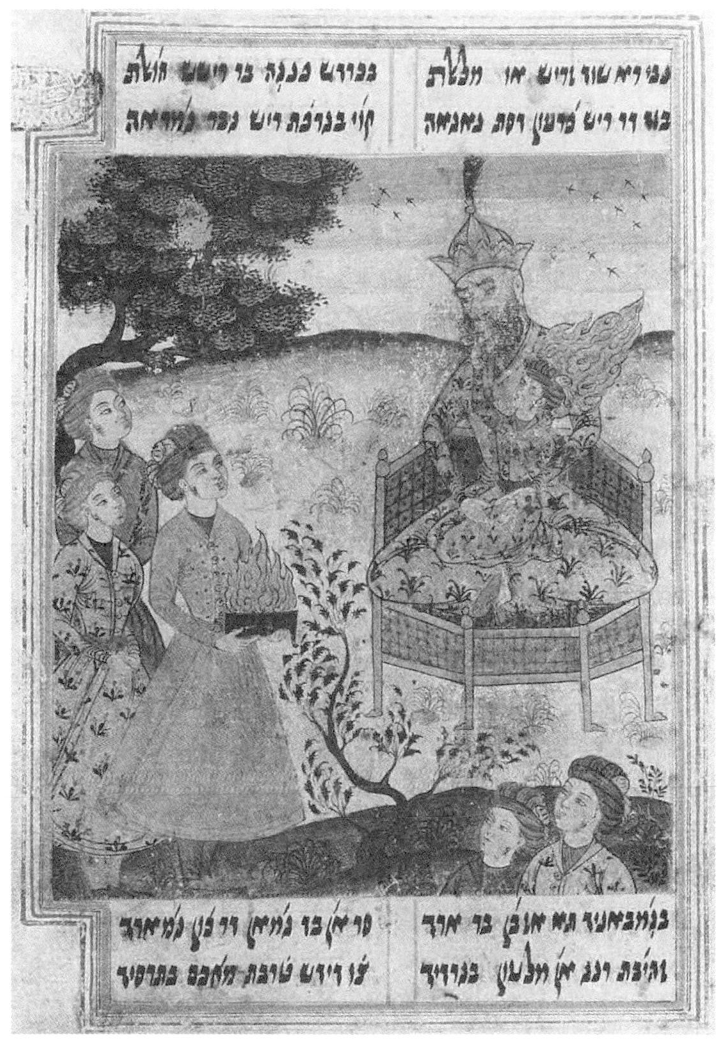

11. Nehemia ben Amshal of Tabriz, *The Infant Moses Challenging Pharaoh and Undergoing an Ordeal by Fire.* From Nawlana Shahin of Shiraz, *Commentary on the Book of Exodus,* Judeo-Persian manuscript (Isfahan, Iran, 1686), fol. 18a. Courtesy of the Israel Museum, Jerusalem.

attempting to cool his hand in his mouth. There is some dispute as to the details—and many different graphic illustrations—in the Jewish and Christian traditions.[37] Still, this ancient story has it that Moses' stuttering is the result of politically necessary physical damage to his tongue during his youth. The damage gives Moses what one stutterer calls a "handicap in the mouth."[38] The tale is silent about any long-term impairment to his hand.

Most Muslims reject the tongue-burning story, just as they insist that Moses was cured of his stutter. Moses, they claim, must have been physically perfect. Many Jews, on the other hand, are willing to entertain the notion that Moses was physically imperfect. In fact, a few medieval Jewish legends have it that Moses had other inferior traits as well:

> A certain king, having heard of Moses' fame, sent a renowned painter to portray Moses' features. On the painter's return with the portrait the king showed it to his sages, who unanimously proclaimed that the features portrayed were those of a degenerate. The astonished king journeyed to the camp of Moses and observed for himself that the portrait did not lie. Moses admitted that the sages were right and that he had been given from birth many evil traits of character but that he had held them under control and succeeded in conquering them. This, the narrative concludes, was Moses' greatness—that in spite of his tremendous handicaps, he managed to become the man of God.[39]

Some rabbis have attempted to ban the further publication of such disparaging legends.[40] But most Jews accept the idea that there was something odd, if not also wrong, with Moses' tongue *(langue)*—and hence also with his various languages.

Moses' Tridental Language

The chronology of Moses' life divides into three forty-year geolinguistic divisions: Egyptian, Midianite, and Hebrew. These periods match Moses' association with three women: Batya, Tzipporah, and Yocheved.

Egyptian. The Egyptian-speaking Batya, a noblewoman, was Moses' "adoptive mother." During his forty-year "sojourn" in Egypt, Moses learned the tongue of Batya—who was Pharaoh's daughter and/or sister. (Presumably, Moses believed that Batya was his biological mother in the same ambiguous way that lame, punning Oedipus believed mistakenly that Corinthian Merope was his biological mother.) If we believe Acts in the New Testament, during this period Moses also learned hieroglyphic writing and Egyptian legal and religious lore.[41] Some people argue that the *only* written language Moses *could* have known, before leaving Egypt, was Egyptian hieroglyphs. In keeping with this view, Freud—who on this point follows historians such as Manetho, Strabo, and Toland—insists that Moses was essentially if not also biologically an Egyptian.[42]

Did Moses also learn to speak a little Hebrew during his first forty years? Perhaps so. As a newborn, before being set adrift on the Nile, Moses had heard Hebrew from his Hebrew-speaking biological mother, Yocheved, and from his siblings, Aaron and Miriam. (It is left unwritten whether this period was long enough for him to have been circumcised.) After being plucked out of the Nile, Moses probably learned a good deal of Hebrew from Yocheved, who then became his nurse-mother. Certainly, Moses knew *some* Hebrew when, at age forty, he killed the overseer of Hebrew-speaking slaves. That incident precipitated his flight to Midian.

Midianite. The flight to Midian marks the beginning of Moses' second geo-linguistic period. In his essay "Israel in the Desert" (1819), Goethe says that when we meet Moses in exile in Midian, he is "barely able to communicate."[43] Presumably, Moses' high-style Egyptian and infantile Hebrew wouldn't do there. But despite his new de facto condition as "infant," the forty-year-old Moses picked up the Midianite tongue, along with the customs and traditions of that people.[44] He also chose a wife, Tzipporah, daughter of the Midianite high priest Jethro (also known as Reuel), and had a son with her.

The notorious passage in the Torah in which Tzipporah flings their son's foreskin at Moses is, as Rashi suggests, not unrelated to the question of Moses' "circumcised tongue." (Circumcision as such is sometimes understood in terms of writing and elision.)[45] Francis Bacon likewise refers to Moses as *linguae praepeditae.*[46] (*Lingua,* according to the *OED,* means "the tongue or a tongue-like organ," as well as "a language," and *praeputium* means "the foreskin, the prepuce." Curiously, Freud does not really pick up on the hint.) Tzipporah has an important role in one of the earliest works on the subject of Moses: the drama *Exagoge,* by the Jewish playwright Ezekielos the Poet.[47]

The Midianites lived near Mount Sinai and held the mountain in awe.[48] Moses was around eighty at the time that God, from the burning bush on Mount Sinai, told him to go back to Egypt. By this time, Moses had been speaking the Midianite tongue, perhaps almost exclusively, for forty years. (The topos is picked up by Zora Neale Hurston in *Moses, Man of the Mountain.*)[49] The Hebrew Torah leaves it unclear what language, if any, God used when he spoke with Moses at the burning bush, or which language Moses used.

Hebrew. We have seen that the Hebrew-speaking Yocheved, Moses' biological mother, became his nurse-mother after his adoptive mother, Batya, hired her. (One legend has it that Moses refused milk from the first nursemaid Batya hired, perhaps because it was unclean, or non-kosher.) In Midian, Moses might well have forgotten a good deal of his Hebrew mother's tongue. (So argued the Tosafot commentator Rashbam, or Rabbi Samuel ben Meir, who lived in France in the twelfth century. Rashbam was Rashi's grandson.)[50] By the same token, in Midian Moses might well have forgotten some of his spoken Egyptian. Moreover, since Midian had a then-strange system of apparently nonrepresentational writing that we would now call "alphabetical," Moses might well have begun to develop a different attitude toward the hieroglyphic writing he had learned in Egypt.

We might here speculate that Moses now "stuttered" because, as a Hebrew who did not know he was a Hebrew, he had "forgotten" who he really was—at least in terms of "ethnic" identity. One consequence of exile and enslavement is the ease with which one's tongue will "cleave to the roof of [one's] mouth." Thus, Psalm 137, in its concern with such forced emigration and forgetfulness of the homeland as often befell slaves, suggests that the consequence of slavery in Babylon is some form of hand-and-mouth disability:

> By the waters of Babylon,
> there we sat down and wept,
> when we remembered Zion.
> On the willows there
> we hung up our lyres.
> For there our captors

required of us songs,
and our tormentors, mirth, saying,
"Sing us one of the songs of Zion!"
How shall we sing the Lord's song
in a foreign land?
If I forget you, O Jerusalem,
let my right hand wither!
Let my tongue cleave to the roof of my mouth.

After the Babylonian exile due to Nevukhadnetsar (Nebuchadnezzar), most of the Israeli people forgot the Hebrew language and were able to say only one Tefilla.[51] If anyone stood in danger of "forgetting" his people, it would have been the infant Moses. This may be one reason for translating Moses' first complaint to God as, "When I get up before a crowd my tongue sticks to the roof of my mouth."[52]

Discoursing with travelers from Egypt, Midianite-speaking Moses may well have noticed that the Egyptian and Hebrew languages had themselves changed during his absence from Egypt. After all, forty years is a long time—enough, as it would turn out, even to build or rebuild a people, its culture, its language.

So Moses, required by Sinai's God to speak to Pharaoh, might have felt heavy of tongue at the burning bush because he had burned his tongue, or did not know Egyptian very well, or had forgotten Jerusalem, or had never known it at all.

Let My People Go: Which Language?

Go down, Moses,
Way down in Egypt-land

Tell old Pharaoh
To let my people go.
—African-American spiritual

It is not clear to us (and maybe was not clear to Moses) which language God wanted Moses to use when he spoke before Pharaoh. When Moses gave his reason for hesitating to take on the job, was he thinking of his inability to speak well in *one* particular language (Egyptian? Hebrew? Midianite?) or in *any and all* languages? The prophet Ezekiel's task is thus apparently much easier than Moses' was, and he knows it. As Ezekiel reports their conversation (3:4–5), "He said unto me, Son of man, go, get thee unto the house of Israel, and speak with my words unto them. For thou art not sent to a people of a strange speech and of an hard language, but to the house of Israel." (As a child playing hooky in Montréal, I used to wonder whether the fact that infants from bilingual homes often "babble" differently in different languages was not itself something to consider when treating the infant Moses' speech impediment. My assumption about multilingual babbling has since become the subject of scientific study.)[53]

Is long-term emigrant Moses prone to stutter in Egyptian, say, because he has lost the diplomatic language of Egypt? That is what the emigrant Rambam, or Rabbi Moshe ben Maimon, suggested in the twelfth century.[54] Or was God requiring Moses to speak Hebrew to Pharaoh, his "father"? That would have been one way for God—through his dummy, Moses—to announce to Pharaoh that the slaves had now become a "nation" in their own right.[55] (J. G. von Herder, centuries later, would say, more simply, that a *Volk,* or *gens,* or nation *is* its language. If Pharaoh had been a late eighteenth-century monarch, he would have understood the *gesture* of such a rebellious Jew as Moses using baby Hebrew in the Egyptian court—even if Pharaoh himself "knew" no Hebrew whatever.) Was Moses worried that, if he spoke Hebrew, Pharaoh would be unable to understand the particular meaning of his words? Or was he more afraid that, if Pharaoh understood the gesture of his using Hebrew, Pharaoh's heart would harden?

The Dummy Brother

When the stutterer Moses hints that God should find another dummy to go to Egypt (Exodus 10:13), the ventriloquist God, himself something of a stutterer, suggests that Moses become a ventriloquist and find himself a dummy of his own. Enter the Hebrew-speaking Aaron, Moses' *elder* brother. (One view has it that Moses hesitated to accept God's mission because Moses thought the honor, such as it was, should go to his older brother.)[56] From now on, Aaron speaks for Moses as if he were Moses' "Lordkeeper." (A Lordkeeper—this was an official title—spoke for the stuttering English king Charles I. Charles was the ostensible author of the strangely iconodule bestseller *Eikon basilike,* and he called himself unfit to speak *in propria persona:* "Now, because I am unfit for much speaking, I mean to bring up the fashion of my predecessors, to have my Lordkeeper speak for me in most things.")[57]

In fact, the Torah often refers to Moses and Aaron as if they were one subject. The grammar of Exodus treats stuttering Moses and his fluent brother Aaron as if they were Siamese twins. The Torah's authors, recognizing the ekphrastic, conjoined personification at work here, often use a singular verb with a double subject: "Moses and Aaron goes." Or they sometimes use a singular subject with a plural verb: "Moses go" or "Aaron go." The Koran is even more explicit on this point.

The issue here relates to the Torah's frequently plural name *(elohim)* for its apparently single God *(adonai),* and it comes out nowhere more clearly than in the need for written Law.

Aleph-Bet

> Moses was the . . . the first man who imparted the alphabet to the Jews.
>
> —EUPOLEMUS (second century B.C.E.), Fragment 1

When the stutterer Moses traveled from Midian to Egypt in order to join up with Aaron, he knew more or less three languages (Egyptian, Hebrew, and Midianite). What language did Moses and Aaron have in common as they started out on their ventriloquist-dummy career? Perhaps it was the "infant Hebrew" that Moses remembered from having played with the son of his Hebrew-speaking nurse-mother Yocheved some eighty years earlier. Or perhaps Aaron knew some Egyptian.[58] Ultimately, it may not matter much which of these two spoken languages—Hebrew or Egyptian—Moses and Aaron used when they spoke with each other. It does not matter, because—in terms of the great intellectual, spiritual, and legislative journey that the variously consanguineous, collactaneous, and conjoint brothers had to make together during the following forty years—*both* the Hebrew language *and* the Egyptian language were seriously defective, insofar as the Jewish God goes. Hebrew was not a written language at that time, and the Jews needed a written language. And Egyptian, though a written language, was also defective: it relied on an image-based, or hieroglyphic, system of representation that was anathema to the Jewish God. (Some scholars understand hieroglyphic script as partly conceptual or nonrepresentational writing, but their overly historical view is, as we shall see, beside the philosophical point. So, too, is the opposite view: that the alphabet is itself partly representational.)[59] As soon as the Jews left Egypt, these dual problems—that Hebrew was not a written language and that Egyptian was an inappropriately written language—became clear. At this point, the writing system of Midianite—a language that fluently speaking Aaron certainly did not know and that stuttering Moses did know—came to the forefront of Jewish spiritual history, where it has remained ever since.

Scholars have long believed that Moses picked up *something* from the Midianites, as well as *something* from the Egyptians. Usually they say that Moses acquired the idea of a violent God (Yahweh) in Midian and the idea of monotheism (in the tradition of Akhenaten) in Egypt.[60] These scholars would do well, though, to focus also on the linguistic factors at work in Moses' variously multicultural backgrounds. After all, the tablets of the Law obtained by Moses on Mount Sinai were written in the North Semitic alphabet, or *aleph-tov,* of Midian.[61] (This speculation is related to the claim in the first fragment attributed to the Greco-Jewish historian Eupolemus in the second century B.C.E., and it is argued by scholars such as Hubert Grimme.)[62] These are the laws that legislator Moses is credited with giving to his people.

So the two brothers need each other: Aaron is able to *speak* properly, like most people, but only the Midianite Moses knows how to *write* properly. The laws that he re-

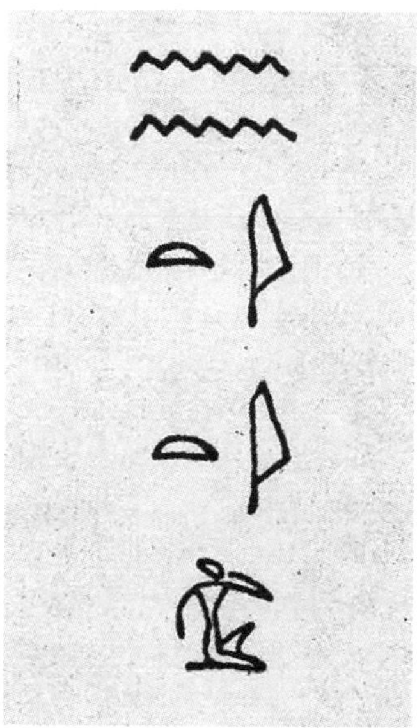

12. The hieroglyph for "stutter." From Vladimir Semenovich Golenishchev, ed., "The Tale of the Shipwrecked Sailor," in *Les Papyrus hiératiques 1115, 1116A, et 1116B de l'Ermitage Impérial à St. Pétersbourg*, facsimile ed. (St. Petersburg, Russia: Manufacture des Papiers de l'Etat, 1913). Courtesy of Widener Library, Harvard University.

trieves from Mount Sinai are written—and must be written—in the generally nonpictographic Midianite alphabet. In order to accomplish God's purpose, Moses needs not only the linguistic help of Aaron (who helps in preparing the geographic exodus from Egypt); he also needs the Midianite alphabet (which helps to complete the spiritual exodus from Egyptian creed and prepare the spiritual entrance to a new religion). The tablets of the Law, which are themselves graven, include the quintessentially important prohibition against "graven images," so it stands to reason that Moses' reproduction of those tablets should not itself be a graven symbol in the same way that the Golden Calf or hieroglyphs were. Hence, the alphabet is crucial in the reformation of the Jewish people as a literate, iconoclastic people.

Even as the new Midianite-Hebrew alphabet was to some extent pictographic, and in this way resembled Egyptian hieroglyphs, so the Decalogue, although it outlawed idolatry, was, to that same (historical) extent, itself idolic, much like the Golden Calf. Reads the commandment: "Thou shalt not make unto thee any graven image." The English word *graven* in the King James translation is not a bad translation of the Hebrew *pesel*. Yet it is all too easy to confuse some letters with some hieroglyphs—that is, to confuse some more or less pictographic or acrophonic, yet still transitionally alphabetic, symbols with the older idolic signs. After all, the same God who *disallows* the graven image *(pesel)* actually *enjoins* Moses to engrave the second set of the stone tablets of the Law (Exodus 34:1): "And the Lord said unto Moses: 'Hew thee [*pisal-licha*] two tablets of stone like unto the first.'" No matter how worried Moses may be that the still-iconodule people will misunderstand the new symbols, God insists that, at the very least, Moses make symbols *like* the ones he smashed.

Nowhere is the inadequacy in Aaron's understanding of the idolic sort of "written language" clearer than when he goes along with the making of the Golden Calf, soon after the exodus from Egypt. This is precisely the moment when Moses is on Mount Sinai receiving the Laws (Exodus 32:2–4): "And [Aaron] received the gold at their hand, and fashioned it with a graving tool, and made a molten calf." In making an Egyptian idol—the graven image of a calf—

Aaron allows for a certain regression to Egyptian quasi-representational symbolization in writing. (Muslim tradition denies Aaron's linguistic "heresy," much the way it denies Moses' stutter: the Koran introduces one "al-Samiri" into the narrative, and it is al-Samiri who makes the idol.)[63]

Moses disliked idols and graven images so much that he angrily smashed the tablets God had given him. (An engraving of Rembrandt's *Moses Smashing the Tables of the Laws* hangs in the Freud Museum in London.)[64] Such anger is often associated with those who stutter, or *happer.* (William Horman, in 1519, wrote of "a foul anger: in which the mouth foams, the nostrils drop, and the tongue happers [i.e., stutters].")[65] The same anger also came to the fore when the *buffer* Moses violently struck the rock in the desert, and some interpreters claim that such anger helps to explain Moses' stuttering. (*Buffing,* according to the *OED,* denotes "speak[ing] with obstructed and explosive utterance, . . . stutter[ing].")

The Golden Calf that so angered Moses was probably a representation of Hathor, an Egyptian cow-deity often shown with a solar disk between her horns.[66] The Theban Hathor was considered a goddess of the dead and wore the interestingly acrophonic hieroglyph for "West" *(amenta)* on her head.[67] From this viewpoint, Moses would have objected to the Golden Calf not merely because it was an idol, or the particular goddess of love, dance, and alcohol, all of which activities recall Hathor. He would have objected to the Golden Calf also because Hathor often bore on her head an exemplar of the very system of quasi-representational writing that Moses was trying to reject. In this sense, the Golden Calf was a linguistic shibboleth-in-reverse. This fact helps to explain the demi-genocide that an acrophone precipitates among the Jewish population after their crossing of the Red Sea.

Arnold Schoenberg, in his great opera *Moses und Aron,* suggests how Aaron, when he allows worship of the Golden Calf, can himself stand for something so presumably *material* as the idol, and how Moses can stand for something so ideally *immaterial* as this alphabetic writing.[68] Moses' words fail in the public sphere, where they are most needed, because the quasi-alphabetic abstraction that people require in order to conceive of the Hebrew God is relatively difficult. Thus, Schoenberg's insightful opera ends with Moses' plaint about how words fail him:

> O Wort, du Wort, das mir fehlt!
> (Moses sinkt verzweifelt zu Boden.)
>
> [O word, thou word, that I lack!
> (Moses sinks to the ground in despair.)][69]

As Michael Gielen says, "[Moses'] Vokabular ist sehr begrenzt. Er gebraucht enorme Konzepte wie 'ewig,' 'allmächtig,' usw., doch Aron ist viel flussiger, redengewandter." ("[Moses'] vocabulary is quite limited. He uses immense concepts like 'eternal,' 'omnipotent,' etc., whereas Aron is much more fluent and more nimble at speaking.")[70]

We have speculated that the "source" of the alphabet was Midian, where Moses spent the middle forty years of his life. But it does not follow that Moses was the only Jew to pick up on it there. It even seems likely that the Jews already had long-standing relations with Midian. First, Jacob's youngest son, Joseph, was sold into slavery (instead of dying in the pit into which his brothers had cast him) thanks precisely to the mediation of Midianite traders.[71] The way to slavery in Egypt was thus by way of Midian, even as the way out of idolatry in Egypt was by way of Midian. Second, Pharaoh's Semitic slaves probably worked the turquoise mine at Serabit el-Khadem, in the Sinai Desert near a spot that scholars say was the historical Mount Sinai.[72] By Midianite trading, the Jews were brought to Egypt as slaves; by Midianite writing, the Jews were freed.

Law Codes

> Also, laws were first written by Moses for the Jews.
>
> —EUPOLEMUS, Fragment 1

Moses' speech impediment indicates a certain kind of legislative capacity. (This is what Martin Luther criticizes about Moses when Luther denigrates stammering in his commentary on Galatians.)[73] By the same token, his stutter suggests the way in which inability to get words out can lead to acting out—and to action. (This is how Goethe sees the matter when, in the great translation scene in *Faust,* he allies the biblical Moses with Faust's transformation of *Wort* into *Tat*—Word into Deed.)[74]

Yet other cultures, too, feature innovative legislators or rulers who stutter. Battus consulted the oracle on account of his stutter, and in this way came to found the Greek colony at Cyrene in Libya (630 B.C.E.).[75] (One legend has it that the name "Battus" means "stutterer.") The stuttering Roman emperor Claudius (41–54 C.E.) made new laws in the area of language, and added three letters to the Roman language. The Iroquois lawgiver Dekanawida (sixteenth century) stuttered, a fact that is sometimes adduced as an explanation for why and how he formed, thanks to his spokesperson Hiawatha, the great alliance with the Iroquois confederation, which Benjamin Franklin suggests was the most sophisticated political entity in North America at the time.[76] (*Dekanawida* likely means something like "two rivers flowing together," as well as "Siamese twin.")[77] There is also the iconoclast Byzantine emperor Michael II the Stutterer (820–829), the French king Louis II, known as Balbus (877–879), the English king George VI (1937–1952), and the above-mentioned King Charles I.[78]

In addition, there is Camille Desmoulins (1760–1794), whose speech impediment has long been an interest of novelists, playwrights, and biographers.[79] Desmoulins was a notary who, on account of his stutter, had no law clients. But in the realm of politics he finally found his persona, or speaking voice. Called "the first republican of France," Desmoulins became fluent on July 12, 1789.[80] On that day, famously, he was the man who called the crowd to arms.[81] That was the beginning of the French Revolution.[82] After that day, Desmoulins' medium of fluency became writing—the Revolutionary press of pamphlets and newspapers.

Do so many legislators stutter because speech dysfunction, and stuttering in particular, might help to create really political language? It is to such enthusiast prophets as Jeremiah and Isaiah that God gives precise instructions about what they should say to the people and to the rulers: "Now therefore go, and I will be with your mouth and teach you what you shall speak" (Exodus 10:12). But in the end, the cure-all was the speech-impeded Moses, whose very *tzit-tzit* memorably reduplicates the stutter. The term *tzit-tzit* ("fringes") refers to the 613 fringe-tassels attached to the corners of the tallith ("prayer shawl") that male adult Jews are commanded to wear; each bit of the fringe signals one of the *mitzvoth* laws that the stuttering legislator Moses passed on.[83] The term *tzit-tzit* already suggests Moses' stutter: it is a "pure" reduplicative, like *murmur* and *barbar.*[84]

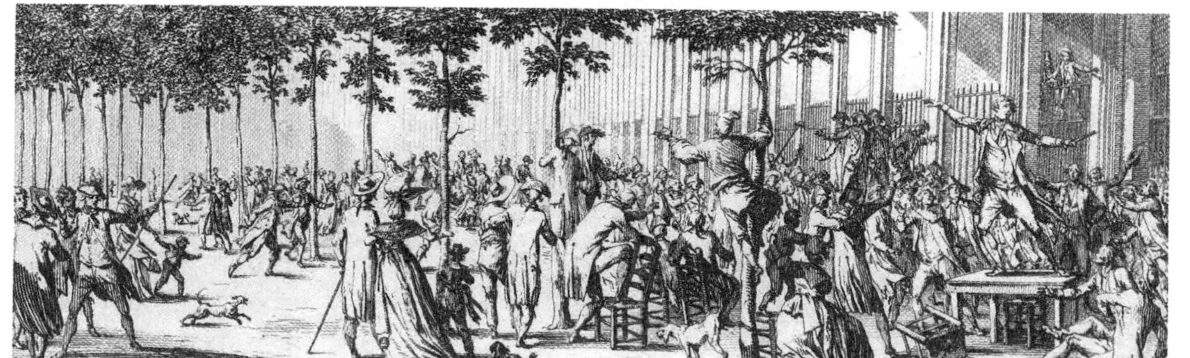

13. Anonymous, after Jean Duplessi-Bertaux, Camille Desmoulins Addressing the People on July 12, 1789, at the Palais Royal (etching). From Claude Fauchet and Sébastien-Roch-Nicolas de Chamfort, eds., *Historical Pictures Representing the Most Remarkable Events Which Occurred during the Early Period of the French Revolution, with a Particular Account of Those Important Transactions, and a Series of Discourses Elucidating the Causes Which Led to That Event; with Portraits and Historical Memoirs of Some of the Principal Persons Engaged; with Vignette Prints Representing the Most Remarkable Event Which Distinguished Each Person's Character*, trans. anonymous (Paris: J. Charles, 1803). Collection Selechonek.

Cure-Alls

The Jewish God would not (or could not?) repair Moses' heavy tongue, so God called upon Aaron to be Moses' spokesperson. But the Christian Jesus cures even mutes. Regarding Isaiah 32:4, "The tongue of mafflers [stutterers] shal speake readily and plain," the Douay Bible (1609) comments: "This prophecy of maffling or imperfect tongues, to speake readily, is fulfilled in the Church of Christ." Not surprisingly, therefore, the Christian apostles did not need the same prosthetic aids that Moses required: spokespersons like Aaron and alphabetic writing like the Midianites'. When Jesus sent forth his apostles and warned them about opposition and persecution, his "enthusiast" dummies were unafraid. Along with His command to spread the gospel was His promise that God would "be their mouth": "When they deliver you up, take no thought of how or what you will speak; for it shall be given you in that same hour, what you shall say . . . For it is not you who speak, but the spirit of your Father which speaks in you" (Matthew 10:19, 20).

God's being "with the mouths of His disciples" is at the very center of Pentecostal Christianity and its definitive endorsement of enthusiast ventriloquism. On the day of Pentecost, it was "given to them what they should speak." For it was not they who spoke, but "the Spirit [who] gave utterance" (Acts 2:4). "The Spirit took full control of their mouths, so that they said not one word except what He wanted spoken. And He wanted only one thing said: '. . . they spoke the wonderful works of God'" (Acts 2:11). In like Christological fashion, the Book of Acts would seem to overcome the issues about multilingualism and language that inform the story of Moses. A few people note inconsistencies here, as when my old neighbor Leonard Cohen sings, "Oh bless thee continuous stutter / Of the word being made into flesh."[85]

We have asked which particular language Moses spoke to Pharaoh. Acts seeks to void this question by "overcoming" (or sublating) the very notion of particular tongues. The familiar may become an "other" one, or the all-fulfilling none:

> And when the day of Pentecost was fully come, they were all with one accord in one place. And suddenly there came a sound from heaven as of a rushing mighty wind, and it filled all the house where they were sitting. And there appeared unto them cloven tongues like as of fire, and it sat upon each of them. And they were all filled with the Holy Ghost, and began to speak with other tongues, as the Spirit gave them utterance. And there were dwelling at Jerusalem Jews, devout men, out of every nation under heaven. Now when this was noised abroad, the multitude came together, and were confounded, because that every man heard them speak in his own language. And they were all amazed, and marvelled, saying one to another, Behold, are not all these which speak Galilaeans? And how hear we every man in our own tongue, wherein we were born? Parthians, and Medes, and Elamites, and the dwellers in Mesopotamia, and in Judaea, and Cappadocia, in Pontus, and Asia, Phrygia, and Pamphylia, in Egypt, and in the parts of Libya about Cyrene, and strangers of Rome, Jews and proselytes, Cretes and Arabians, we do hear them speak in our tongues the wonderful works of God. (Acts 2:1–10)

Acts obscures the various problems posed by the stutterer barbarians of Babel; likewise, Acts shunts aside the various down-to-earth ways of coping with those problems by means of a vastly effective perfect system of absolutely fluent simultaneous translation and murmur. Acts would thus seem to overcome all ordinary and politically needful issues of translation in a post-alphabetical Promised Land.[86]

Moses—as any happerer or buffer might—irascibly struck a desert rock when he was told to talk it into producing water. The failure to speak persuasively to a stone is apparently why this thrice-infanted stutterer was not allowed to enter the Promised Land.[87] He had also smashed the engraved tablets of the law—more stones—when he could not communicate his anger adequately in words. Had Moses, or another of his disabled ilk, not really destroyed the first set of tablets and then really carried down the second, there would have been no Promised Land for anyone to write about as an ideal.

A Glottal Catch

A *glottal stop* is, in Webster's words, "the speech sound produced by momentary complete closure of the glottis, followed by an explosive release." The word for *stutter* in some languages contains the glottal stop, or glottal catch, which is "a complete stoppage of the breath-stream by the vocal cords."[88] In English, speakers make this stop between the two *oh*'s of "Oh-oh!" when it is spoken in surprise or reproof.[89] The feel is very much like a cough—a fact that Henry Sweet, a model for Shaw's Professor Higgins, had pointed out.[90]

In written Hebrew, the first letter, *aleph,* is not, as it is often said to be, "silent." The *aleph* indicates the glottal stop, with which stutterers are so familiar, and the letter is also the alphabetic counterpart of a hieroglyph associated with the ox, or cow, and hence with the Golden Calf.[91] The sound of the sudden opening or shutting of the glottis with an emission of breath encapsulates Moses' difficult role as legislator in a context where the One God is revolted by images, where the divine prophet stutters, where the divine name is unpronounceable as written, and where the system of writing, while alphabetic, remains linked with a polytheistic and still partially pictographic tradition.

The language-stymied Jewish exile Paul Celan ends his great poem "Frankfurt, September" at the point where the glottal stop, or *Kehlkkopfverschlusslaut* (literally, "occlusion of the head of the throat")—all but impossibly manages to break forth into the song that alone would grant fluency.

> Die Simili-
> Dohle
> Frühstückt
>
> Der Kehlkkopfverschlusslaut
> singt.[92]

My teacher John Felstiner translates thus: "The simulate / jackdaw / breakfasts // The glottal stop / Sings."[93] In Mosaic tradition, only the glottal *could* sing. Nikolai Popov and Heather McHugh translate "Die Simili-Dohle" as "The pseudo-jackdaw (cough-caw's double)." They thus seek to recall the Czech word *kavka,* meaning "jackdaw," and the Jewish-Czech author Franz Kafka, who died in silence when an infection utterly stopped up his larynx.

In Celan's "world to be stuttered after," the speech-impeded figure of Moses motivates the poet—as in "Tübingen, Jänner" (Tübingen, January):

> Käme
> käme ein Mensch,
> käme ein Mensch zur Welt, heute, mit
> dem Lichtbart der

Patriarchen: er dürfte,
spräch er von dieser Zeit, er
dürfte
nur lallen und lallen,
immer-, immer-
zuzu.
("Pallaksch. Pallaksch.")

[Should there come
should there come a man
should there come a man to the world, today, with
the lightbeard of the
patriarchs: he would,
if he would speak of this
time, he
would only babble and babble,
ever-, ever-
moremore.
("Pallaksch. Pallaksch.")]

The babbling king *(Lällekönig)* in Basel, the mad poet Friedrich Hölderlin's palilogical "Pallaksch Pallaksch," and Philomel's infantile lullaby in *A Midsummer Night's Dream* —"Lulla, lulla, lullaby, lulla, lulla, lullaby"—have their strong associations here. But the English *lall,* here translated above as "babble," also means "stutter." And the bearded and barbarian Moses, with his *tzit-tzit,* has the last and first say in "Tübingen, Jänner": the reduplicative *zu-zu* that closes the poem also opens it.[94]

5 Marilyn's Duh

> The main exhibition hall [in the Museum of Visible Circumlocutions] boasted a major extravaganza, a hanging of Toon balloons from what the museum grandly titled "The Neo-Comical Era." It proved my own personal rule of thumb—beware the presentations of any art form with more than three syllables in its description. The turning lane of this cultural crossroads consisted of duh . . .
>
> —Gary Wolf, *Who P-P-P-Plugged Roger Rabbit?* (1991)

I saw Marilyn Monroe onscreen when I was thirteen years old. She was acting in the motion picture *Let's Make Love* (1960). At the time, I was still "recovering" from paralysis of the leg—the result of polio some six years earlier. I missed being able to talk and walk well. I had some sense that, in her filmic song-and-dance routines, Monroe was compensating for her own intermittent paralysis of tongue by incorporating a more or less voluntary stutter. I was particularly aware of how smooth walking and fluent talking were both set up as ideals in *Let's Make Love.* Likewise, pedal stumbling and verbal stuttering were both put down as laughable.

In *Let's Make Love,* the richest man in the world (Jean-Marc Clément) learns that he is to be satirized in a new dramatic production. Thanks to his public relations agent, he decides to go see it. Then, incognito, he tries out for the part of himself. Now he must learn how to be funny. The producers hire him, unaware of his real identity. The richest man in the world hires the funniest man in the world (Milton Berle) to teach him how to be funny. "Uncle Miltie" (who plays himself) tries to teach the rich man to stumble and stutter at the same time: to walk *dodo* style and talk *duh-duh* style.[1] Berle was *the* specialist in comedy—even as Gene Kelly was *the* specialist in dancing and Bing Crosby was *the* specialist in singing (both Kelly and Crosby play themselves in the film). So who could argue with Berle's view that nothing could be funnier than making fun of a person intermittently paralyzed in limb and tongue in such a way that he dances and sings like a spastic?[2]

In the 1950s, Milton Berle—like Jerry Lewis and Danny Kaye—was pleased to raise money on behalf of crippled people through various telethons for the Foundation for Infantile Paralysis and the Muscular Dystrophy Association, even as he was satisfied hilariously (and presumably also good-naturedly) to parody cripples' walk and talk in profitable movies and television shows.

So the comedy specialist in *Let's Make Love* tries to teach the money specialist how to do the *dodo* walk and the *duh-duh* talk. Berle splays his feet outward, like a crippled polio survivor; and then, walking in that way, he stutters explosively, "Duh duh duh."[3] In creating this peculiar tapdance-like song-and-dance routine, Berle may have in mind not only animal dances[4]—including the French-American (Cajun) dance called *fais-dodo*—but also the *duh duh duh* refrain of the Fantastic Emanons, the rhythms of popular doo-wop singing, the triple *da* in *The Waste Land* ("Datta, dayadhvam, damyata"), the *duh-duh* stuttering Porky Pig in cartoons like *Dough for the Do-Do* (1949) and *Porky in Wackyland* (1938), and the side-splitting *duh*'s of the wooden dummy Mortimer Snerd in ventriloquist Edgar

Bergen's popular radio and television act.[5] In the 1990s, on the cartoon TV show *The Simpsons,* Homer Simpson's *d'oh* worked the same tradition, in a much diminished way.[6]

When a speaker says "Well, duh!" the implication is that his listener is a da. The term *da* comes from *jackdaw,* denoting the small crow-like bird that is easily taught to parrot human words, and connoting a "simpleton or fool."[7] Unfortunately for the richest man in the world in *Let's Make Love,* he is apparently such a da that he cannot even learn to imitate Milton Berle's *schwa*-vowel *uh* with its consonantal *d* that makes up the sound of *duh.* To begin with, the rich man is francophone, and confusions surrounding the sounds of *d* and *th* are one of American anglophones' favorite ways to mock Frenchmen, or trip them up. "The *th* with its twofold value is one of the most characteristic features of our language, and more than any other [sound it is] the Shibboleth of foreigners," wrote philologist John Earle.[8] Along with Alexander Melville Bell and Henry Sweet, Earle was a model for Shaw's Professor Higgins.

A rich Frenchman might do extremely well with French-language tongue twisters *(virelangues)* involving the letter *d.* I recall one of these from my own elocution classes in Montréal in the late 1950s. "Didon dîna, dit-on, du dos d'un dodu dindon, don dû d'un don, à qui Didon dit: Donne, donc, don, du dos d'un dindon dodu" ("Dido dined, they say, on dorsal meat from a plump turkey, donation due to a Spanish don, to whom Dido said, 'Do, then, Don, donate some dorsal meat from a plump turkey'"). Margaret Drabble has said, "The nice elocution lessons I went to as a child in Sheffield were largely a waste of time, though I did learn some good poetry through them."[9] I, too, learned poetry. But practicing such francophone shibboleths does not help the rich man when it comes to the English *th.*

Uncle Miltie suggests another reason for the rich francophone's laughable inability to say *duh* properly. He has too much *dough*. Says Berle to the rich man, "You sound as if *duh* doesn't mean anything to you."[10] A billionaire has no need for "dough" (meaning "money") and so the rich man has no financial incentive to learn how to pronounce the word *duh*.[11] Bing Crosby, the rich man's singing instructor, later takes up a similar theme when he tries to teach the rich man the "do-re-mi," whose financial aspects (one recalls the musical banks in Samuel Butler's *Erewhon*) the folksinger Woody Guthrie considers in his anticapitalist version of the musical scale (his song "If You Ain't Got the Do Re Mi").[12]

In *Let's Make Love,* the counterpart to the *richest* man in the world is the *most beautiful* woman in the world. Her name is Amanda Dell. She is played by Marilyn Monroe, whose real name was Norma Jean Mortenson. Offstage, Norma Jean was a stutterer. And, as we shall see, the specifically musical poetry of the *duh* in *Let's Make Love* constitutes both Norma Jean's linguistic stumbling block and her greatest performance. At the same time, Marilyn Monroe's performance helps to shed light on originary and motivating links between music and speech.

Singsong

> Noo an' than he mantit [stutters] in his sang.
>
> —PATRICK BUCHAN, *The Guidman o' Inglismill* (1873)

> They . . . go too far in their commandments . . . who enjoin stutters, stammerers and mafflers to sing.
>
> —PLUTARCH, *Morals,* trans. Philemon Holland (1603)

As we have seen, there are practical therapies always working to treat the supposed disorder of stuttering. Among the main "schools" of stuttering therapy in the 1950s were those aimed less at achieving "normal fluency" than at controlling or moderating stuttering.[13] Therapists of the moderating sort aimed at "help[ing] individuals become better adjusted to their 'handicaps.'"[14] Charles Van Riper, for example, aimed at replacing "involuntary stuttering," generally regarded as iatrogenic, with "voluntary stuttering." Other therapists aimed at stutter-free fluency, but Riper aimed at fluent stuttering, by means of voluntary pullouts, cancellations, bounces, and breathy breathing.[15] I myself knew Riper's methods, not only from teachers at elocution school, but also from that first time I heard a stutter from the starlet called Marilyn Monroe.

Norma Jean Mortenson stuttered. Many actors do not stutter onstage but instead speak (almost) normally. (This is a linguistic pattern of *persona,* related to ventriloquism.) But I could hear that Marilyn Monroe, unlike the others, overcame her stutter onstage *not* by speaking normally but instead by breathy singsong. This stutter has been the subject of scattered pseudobiographical and autobiographical speculations often focusing on how that "breathy talking . . . was taught by a singing coach to reduce her stuttering."[16] And even nowadays, people with "spasmodic dysphonia" and caesura-stutters treat their disorder with a technique they call the "Marilyn Monroe voice."[17]

As a young boy with polio, I had heard about Marilyn Monroe from her work with paralyzed children as a March of Dimes celebrity and from her appearance in the polio film *Fireball* with Mickey Rooney (1950), but I first heard her stutter when she was on the radio, singing Irving

Berlin's "Heat Wave," which had been made into a song-and-dance routine in Walter Lang's musical *There's No Business Like Show Business* (1954).[18] Like most persons whose speech was intermittently blocked, I could articulate words fluently only when singing. I was astonished at how Marilyn Monroe singing "Heat Wave" could stutter on the word *can,* in such a way that, working with the chorus on deliberate stoppages and caesuras, they all could sing and dance the *can-can,* both haltingly and fluently.[19] The singers' trips and trip-ups of the tongue are almost arresting:

> *Vicky (Marilyn Monroe):* I certainly can
> [stoppage]
> *Chorus:* Can can
> *Vicky:* Can can

Monroe's "withholding" of the second *can*—a voluntary stutterer's caesura—frustrates the chorus. Who does not want to complete a stutterer's w-w-w-w-w-words? (In the movie *The Man Who Shot Liberty Valance,* a stutterer ordering in a restaurant says "Dee-dee-dee-dee." The waitress finishes his utterance with, "Deep-dish apple pie?" Laughs follow.)[20] In the fashion of many stutterers' interlocutors, the chorus completes Monroe's phrasing—anticipates the metrics and rhyme—as "can can can can can."

"Can can can" is the simplest of *battologisms*—that is, "sentences built by repetition of the same words or sounds." The triple *can* suggests the lexical structure of two then well-known playground tongue twisters:

> Can you can a can as a canner can can a can?

> How many cans can a cannibal nibble
> if a cannibal can nibble cans?

As many cans as a cannibal can nibble
if a cannibal can nibble cans.

The "oil can" in the film *The Wizard of Oz* is the rusted Tin Man's means for curing his verbal and bodily paralysis. The can can cure.

Now, stutterers like Marilyn Monroe don't stutter when they sing or hum.[21] The author of "Psellism" in Charles Dickens' periodical *Household Words* rightly remarks, "Chanting, instead of speaking, or talking in recitative like operatic dialogues, has been tried as a mode of training [for stutterers]."[22] Edith Wharton reported that Henry James chanted poetry, instead of reciting it, with the result that "his stammer ceased as by magic as soon as he began to read."[23] The singer Carly Simon has written, "I felt so strangulated talking that I did the natural thing, which is to write songs, because I could sing without stammering, as all stammerers can."[24] Other such stutterers include the opera singer Robert Merrill, the country singer Mel Tillis, and the Puritan preacher Cotton Mather, who spoke in a "drawling . . . little short of Singing" that enabled him to preach.[25] The perseverating Hamlet ("Words, words, words") is, I believe, nowhere more fluent than when he singsongs, "Why, let the stricken deer go weep."[26]

That stutterers do not stutter when they sing or hum makes the representation of stuttering a test case for serious composers of opera. In *The Magic Flute,* the bird-catcher Papageno hum-sings when the "Three Ladies" lock up his mouth and, jackdaw-like and rap-like, he singsongs "Pa-pa pa-pa" with his Papagena.[27] Benjamin Britten set Melville's brilliant novella *Billy Budd* to music, with a libretto written by Eric Crozier and the stutterer E. M. Forster.

As to why stutterers do not stutter when they sing, there

are many speculations, none definitive. One favorite notion is that singing tends to empty sounds of semantic meaning, to the point where they effectively become music. In a response to a question from Marshall McLuhan about stuttering and music, John Lennon said: "Language and song is to me, apart from being pure vibrations, just like trying to describe a dream. And because we don't have telepathy or whatever it is, we try to describe the dream to each other. And the stuttering [analogy] is right, because we can't say it—it's never how you want to say it." McLuhan added, "The moment you sing, you feel you are communicating much more," and Lennon responded, "Yes, because the words are irrelevant."[28] The stutterer Alvin Lucier's landmark electro-acoustic work *I Am Sitting in a Room* (1970) seems to bring out this semantically empty, musically rhythmic repetition informing all human soundmaking: "I am sitting in a room different from the one you are in now. I am recording the sound of my speaking voice, and I am going to play it back into the room again and again until the resonant frequencies of the room reinforce themselves, so that any s-semblance of my speech, with perhaps the exception of rh-rh-rh-rhythm, is destroyed."[29] Further on, we'll look at the way in which punning can sometimes empty sound of meaning.

Relevant to the specific ontogeny of Marilyn Monroe's stutter and to her compensatory mechanisms for musical ways of dealing with it are the various "stutter songs" popular around the time she was growing up. These would include "Oh, Helen," "Tell Her I Stutter," and "K-K-K-Katy."[30] Such stutter songs follow a superficially lighthearted tradition going back to an eighteenth-century song called "Goody Groaner: The Celebrated Stammering

Glee."[31] During the 1950s, Mel Blanc made a vinyl recording in which Porky Pig *tries* to sing "K-K-K-Katy" but stutters so badly—he substitutes words that *don't* rhyme for words that really *should* rhyme—that the chorus finally orders him to "shut up." Porky's compensatory mechanism for stuttering—he apparently stutters even when singing—is the usual on-the-fly substitution of a synonym for a word on which he stutters or fears he will stutter.[32] This method works better in talk than in song, and better in prose than in poetry, where it upsets the listener's expectations for both rhyme and reason.

Who Is the Rich Man?

> My art belongs to Dada 'cos Dad e' treats me so—well . . .
>
> —Tom Stoppard, *Travesties* (1974)

Let's Make Love is a romantic comedy about the richest man in the world and the human love goddess. The French-accented Wall Street billionaire Jean-Marc Clément (played by Yves Montand). The billionaire falls for Aman-*da* Dell (played by Marilyn Monroe), whose Latinate name, *Aman-da,* seems to mean "loving," or "giving love," as well as "loving *Da.*"

Clément is the last in a line of wealthy tyrants of the sort that Plato describes in his *Republic.* His family's capital derives from the application of agricultural methods involving fertile natural generation from potato seed, or *faenus,* to the "unnatural" monetary realm of *finance.* (The idea is well known from eighteenth-century France. The term *potato* is itself not without its monetary aspect.)[33] Tyrants typically forswear love (natural reproduction) in order to get the power of money (unnatural production). Aristotle complains in his *Politics* that money-making tyrants make metal breed unnaturally. And the tension between "natural" love-making and "unnatural" moneymaking is a topos that ranges from Herodotus' stories about wealthy tyrants like Gyges and Croesus to Richard Wagner's opera *Das Rheingold,* in which the almost unnatural Alberich forswears love and hence fashions a powerful golden ring.[34]

Clément, though, is a degenerate tyrant: he *will* seek love. If ever he is to have love, though, it will not be found "ready to hand." Nor will love be "bought," like so many paintings by Renoir, Matisse, and Van Gogh. ("You don't measure art by money," Clément knows.) Nor is love flattery—the bane of rich men. Rather, Clément and his beloved—whoever she may be—will have to *make* it themselves. Hence the usual title of this movie: *Let's Make Love.* It means the poetry *(poiēsis)* of love: the production of love. You might say, in the words of the comedy's most famous song-and-dance routine, that *Let's Make Love* is about how a loving Aman-da manages to "cook up a fine [amatory] enchila-da" with Clément. (In the United States the movie was sometimes called *The Billionaire,* and in France it is still called *Le Millardaire*—but those titles really get it all wrong.)

The first step in the love recipe is Clément's going to the theater. Clément begins to know himself, as the philosophers say, by means of a mousetrap-like theatrical presentation of himself in a satiric off-Broadway musical revue at a Globe-like stage called "Theater in the Round." Clément, whose financial holdings range the globe over, goes to this little theater on the urging of his hired man, Kaufman—the "salesman" who mediates between the world of business and that of theater. He goes to the theater in order to show others that he's being a good sport about how he himself is depicted in the revue and, as he puts it, "to see what [I'm] like." Once there, Clément falls in love at first sight with Amanda, whom he sees performing a song, "My Heart Belongs to Daddy." Adopting the telling pseudonym Alexander du Monde, he joins the acting troupe incognito, with an assignment to play himself.

As an actor, Alexander (Clément) wants to become a great singer, dancer, and joke teller. *Can* he do that? A tyrant can buy experts in various specialties—the comic Milton Berle, the dancer Gene Kelly, the singer Bing Crosby. The rich man can buy anything by way of "specialized" artist-like prostheses, to put it in Karl Marx's terms.[35] A celebrated Casanova, Clément may feel entitled to "cock his *doo*dle *doo*" any time he likes. Yet there is an old saying that "Caesar can give you money and honor, but he cannot make you an orator."[36] And as it turns out in *Let's Make Love,* the moneyed tyrant cannot really *make* himself an artist. For that matter, although Clément "cocks his doodle doo" in the theater (as his fatherly servant puts it), he cannot so easily make himself into a real *lover.*

So during the course of *Let's Make Love,* Alexander du Monde has to learn to discover and play his true self as Clément.

To Daddy

> How, how, Cordelia! Mend your speech a little,
> Lest it may mar your fortunes.
>
> —SHAKESPEARE, *King Lear,* 1.1

The Frenchman Clément enters the Globe Theater at just the point where Amanda Dell—an aspiring young actor studying French in a high school extension class—is about to rehearse Cole Porter's song "My Heart Belongs to Daddy." The rehearsal takes five minutes (the version below is the one sung by Marilyn Monroe as the character Lolita in the show-within-the-film):

PROLOGUE

Chorus:

["jazzy"]

Lolita:

My name is—Lolita
and uh I'm not—supposed to
play—with boys
moi—uh uh
mon coeur est à papa
you know—le propriétaire

PART ONE

Lolita:

While tearing off a game of golf
I may make a play for the caddy
But when I do, I don't follow through [breath]
Cause my heart belongs to Daddy

If I invite a boy some night
To dine on my fine finan haddie
I just adore, his asking for more
But my heart belongs to Daddy

Yes, my heart belongs to Daddy
So I simply couldn't be bad

Yes, my heart belongs to Daddy
Da, Da, Da, Da, Da, Da, Da, Da, DAAAAD

So I want to warn you laddie
Though I know that you're perfectly swell
That my heart belongs to Daddy
Cause my Daddy he treats it so—

INTERVAL

Chorus:

Badedooo

Lolita:

Dadee dadeedada deeda

PART TWO

Lolita:

While tearing off a game of golf
I may make a play for the caddy
But when I do, I don't follow through
Sugadosugaosugaoado ooooo daddy

If I invite a boy some night
To cook up a fine enchilada
Though Spanish rice is all very nice
Badadadad dada

Chorus:

Yes

Lolita:

Yes, my heart belongs to Daddy
So I simply couldn't be bad

Yes, my heart belongs to my Daddy
Da, Da, Da, Da, Da, Da, Da, Da, DAAAAD

So I want to warn you laddie
Though I know you're perfectly swell
That my heart belongs to Daddy
Cause Daddy, my daddy, my little old daddy
He treats it so—

EPILOGUE

Chorus:

How?

Lolita:

That little old man he just treats it so good.

"My Heart Belongs to Daddy," originally written by Cole Porter for the character Dolly in his musical *Leave It to Me,* was an extraordinarily well-known and popular song.[37] There were dozens of recordings by the early 1940s. Mary Martin, who played Dolly in the first production, made a recording in 1939 with Eddy Duchin; her version made the top-ten list.[38] There were many voice recordings in 1939: Pat Kirkwood with the Jack Hylton Orchestra, Helen Hulmes with Count Basie and His Orchestra, Ella Fitzgerald with Chick Webb, Valaida Snow, and Bea Wain with the Larry Clinton Orchestra.[39] There were all-music versions by the likes of Eddie DeLange and His Orchestra.[40] Since the 1930s, there have been hundreds of recordings—including ones by Rosemary Clooney and Anita O'Day.[41] Della Reese's cha-cha-cha version remarkably syncopates the musical beat with triple-stutter verbal repetitions of specific phrases.[42]

Jack Cole did the original choreography and song direction for the "My Heart Belongs to Daddy" routine in *Let's Make Love.* Cole, whose area was American jazz dance, knew the potential of Marilyn Monroe as a singer and dancer, since he had already done the choreography for her movies *Gentlemen Prefer Blondes* (1953), *River of No Return* (1954), and *There's No Business Like Show Business* (1954).[43] Cole's version of the singsong Prologue to "My Heart Belongs to Daddy," written especially for *Let's Make Love,* distinguishes the role of the chorus.[44] More important, it allows Norma Jean Mortenson *qua* Marilyn Monroe *qua* Aman-da Dell to introduce herself as "Loli-ta." And throughout her performance, Norma Jean emphasizes two habitual strategies of the stutterer. Both tricks are written up in stuttering manuals of the period.

First, Lolita, like her counterpart in *There's No Business Like Show Business,* builds us up to expect a certain word—for example, *well.* Yet she behaves like a stutterer who seeks to avoid a word she fears she cannot say fluently. That is to say, Amanda substitutes an intralingual translation or synonym (*good* instead of *well*).

Amanda *qua* Loli-ta twice builds us up to expect the word *well,* with which she began her prologue ("Well, uh"). The first time she does this, Amanda says, by way of providing us with what we may have anticipated, . . . nothing (line 23). That nothing (which is all that Cordelia is able to say when her father, King Lear, puts her on the spot) is followed by the laddie-chorus' term *Badedooo* (line 24) and by Lolita's own *Dadee dadeedada deeda* (line 25). The second time Amanda builds us up to expect the sound of *well,* she substitutes the babytalk-like adverb *good* for the perhaps more grown-up *well* that we expect (line 44).[45] One might almost think here of the 1950s cinematographer's term

"DA," the well-known acronym for "delayed action"—except that, for the laddie-chorus, the action they expect (or for which they hope) is rather more canceled than postponed.

Amanda's word *well,* as an adverb, means, from one viewpoint, that Lolita's Daddy treats her "in a way appropriate to the facts or circumstances: fittingly, properly."[46] Or it could mean that Daddy treats her "successfully in some material respect; profitably; advantageously."[47] Or perhaps it means, specifically in this case, that Daddy treats her in a way that is "profitable for the seller or buyer; at a high or low price, respectively."[48] There is some feeling, however, that Lolita has not treated the laddies (and us rhyme-and-reason hounds) quite well: she has not finished off her rhymes with the word "swell"; or, if you like, Amanda has not taken off *well*'s poetic tumescence. After all, *well* has a teleological sense: "in a manner, or to an extent, approaching thoroughness or completeness."[49] The laddies are *perfectly swell,* says Amanda, and they are left that way—dangling, like hanging participles, kind of. Well, "That's Amore," which is the famous song from the film *The Caddy* (1953).

Lolita does not "follow through." She does not serve the "main course" to the caddie and/or laddie whom she plies with finan *haddie* and enchila-*da*. The laddies, though elegantly *la-de-da* (a term we hear in the chorus), remain swollen, meaning "increased in bulk by internal pressure."[50] Lolita adores the laddies' asking for more, but she plays "guff"—which means to talk nonsense or to *patter.*[51] (The *Abcedarium anglico latinum* speaks of a "superfluouse *patterer* of words, *battologus*"—which suggests the mouthing of all battologisms such as "can can can.")[52] In this way, Lolita keeps *laddies* at the level of mere *ladies.* Similarly, in the movie *Some Like It Hot,* the character Sugar Kane (played by Marilyn Monroe) does not follow through with the "false 'ladies' of the chorus," Jerry (played by Jack Lemmon) and Joe (Tony Curtis).[53]

Concerning such auditory expectation, one might well think of the stutterer Philip Larkin's poem "Next, Please." Larkin pinpoints stammering as a problem of future anticipation: "Always too eager for the future, we / Pick up bad habits of expectancy."[54]

Aman-*duh*'s second typical stutterer's symptom (other than not following through) is her use of the *schwa*-vowel. It occurs many times in this song: *uh, Lolita, haddie, enchilada, la-de-da, deeda,* and so on. Recall, in this context, that in the 1950s stuttering was defined by how a stutterer might try to "get out" the specific sounds *dad, Dada,* and *daddy.* (These sounds are favorite examples in stutter-therapy manuals of the period.)[55] One well-known example is the Porky Pig talking-animal cartoon *Dough for the Do-Do* (1949), with its Alice-in-Wonderland-like stutters on *dodo.* Taken together, the myriad repetitions and stutters on *da*—*Dadee dadeedada deeda*—are *the* informing element of Aman-da's performance in *Let's Make Love.*

In fact, Cole Porter had long been intrigued with the consonantal *da* version of the *schwa*-vowel. Consider, for example, his song "It's Delovely" (1936). It has "rhyming repetitions" of *duh* or *duhl* at the beginning of many lines: *de*lightful, *de*licious, *de*lovely, *de*lectable, *de*lirious, *de* limit, *di*lemma, and *de*luxe. Similarly, "It's Delovely" has the sounds *duh* or *dub* at the beginnings of other lines: *di*vine, *de* victory, *de* voice. Certain words and lines *double* the *duh: de-du*-ctible is an example, and so is the prologue to the song, with its musical scale "me-re-*do*-so-mi-*do*-la-si."[56]

Well, uh, let's take Monroe's *My Heart Belongs to Daddy* from line 1 of her prologue:

Well, uh

Well is a typical "place-marker" for speakers: it functions something like *er.*[57] "Well, uh" sounds like the English word *wella,* which, according to the *OED,* is a twelve-hundred-year-old interjection with a meaning like "Well, then" or "Ah, alas." (To Ophelia's "How goes your Lord . . .?" the typically thrice-perseverating Hamlet responds, hesitatingly, "Well, well, well.")

Lolita's *uh* is, like the word *well,* one of the typical place-markers for American speakers. Moreover, *uh* is sometimes also thought of as an African-American-derived indefinite article like "a"—a factor that helps to bring out the otherwise verbally unmentioned African-American, jazz-like "components" of *Let's Make Love,* which Cole Porter emphasizes.[58]

In the line 2 of the prologue, Aman*da* introduces her character thus:

My name is—Loli*ta*

Now Loli-ta re-employs *uh* (from line 1) and *ta* (from line 2), and in lines 3–4 delivers them together as a playful statement about expectation:

and *uh* I'm not—supposed—*ta*
play—with boys

Now comes a francophone *schwa*-vowel, followed by a double *uh*. First, there is the French-language *moi,* meaning "me" (Amanda is studying French). Second, there is the apparently English-language *uh uh*. Amanda's interpretation of Lolita's use of the double *uh* suggests the yes-no, will she? won't she? quasi-seductive dialectic that informs the lyrics of Lolita's relationship to the chorus of boys. On the one hand, as *unh-húnh* (with the emphasis on the second syllable), *uh-uh* means "yes."[59] (*Uh-uh,* like the intensifier *hunh,* may also have African-American origins.)[60] On the other hand, as *únh-unh,* with the emphasis on the first syllable, *uh-uh* means "no."[61] Both terms, *unh-húnh* and *únh-unh,* should be distinguished from the interrogative interjection *huh?*

Now, in the fourth line of the prologue, Lolita picks up on the English term *uh-uh* and transforms it into the French triple-*schwa* term *à papa*.

mon coeur est *à papa*

Amanda's French-language sentence translates *literally* as "My heart is to papa"—as when Amanda throws her heartfelt knitting (gives her heart over) to Clément at the end of her song-and-dance routine. Less literally, "mon coeur est à papa" translates loosely as "My heart belongs to daddy."

The ambiguities in Lolita's French-language statement about "belonging" are sharpened in the bilingual last line of the prologue.

you know—le propriétaire

Who *is* the proper landlord *(propriétaire)* of Amanda's heart? Actually, Lolita, as stage *prop*—or as theatrical stage *prop-*

erty—is not quite forthcoming about who is the *proprietor* of her heart. And, as it happens, the ownership even of the Globe Theater changes from time to time. As her song-and-dance routine ends, Aman-da, "she who loves Da," removes her sweater (she's a knitter). She tosses that cabling at the newcomer (Clément) with an aim like Cupid's. Though incognito, tyrant Clément is caught—as surely as Agamemnon in the nets of Clytemnestra, or as Macbeth is caught in the warp and woof of the Fates' weaving.

Lolita's *dada* incantation worked. But it requires the rest of the movie to discover, if at all, to which human being—or to what god or God—the heart of Amanda Dell belongs.

Da-Da-Daddy

> Dah-dah-dah.
>
> —Pharaoh mocking stutterer Moses (Ben Kingsley) after Moses' return from Midian, in *Moses,* TV mini-series (TNT, 1996)

Lolita in *Let's Make Love* is a "babe." By *babe,* I mean *infant* in two senses. First, I mean the literal sense of *infant:* "a human being who cannot talk or cannot talk quite well." (*Infant* is derived from the Latin *infans,* meaning "unable to talk or able to talk only 'baby-talk.'")[62] Second, I refer to the connotative sense of *infant:* "a person who needs someone else to take care of her."

As it happens, Marilyn Monroe first hit the big time by presenting herself as a "big baby." In *Ladies of the Chorus* (1949)—which includes chorus girls holding father-like dolls—she plays Peggy Martin and performs the infantile "daddy stutter-song" entitled "Every Baby Needs a Da-Da-Daddy."[63] (Many Indo-European words mean both *stutter* and *baby-talk*. Among these, according to the *OED*, is *tattle*.) Monroe's baby-like performance in *Ladies of the Chorus* was soon well enough known among soldiers to be "quoted" in the movie *Okinawa* (1952), where the "dame-starved," laddy-like soldiers watch a clip of Monroe doing her "Da-Da-Da" routine.

This is the proper place to remind ourselves that part of the Marilyn Monroe legend focuses on an adult's baby-like need for a father. After all, Norma Jean Mortenson's purported biological father (Edward Mortenson) ran out on her biological mother (Gladys Baker) and never acknowledged Norma Jean as his daughter. For the first few years of Norma Jean's life, her biological mother raised her. But when Gladys was committed to a mental institution, Norma Jean became a ward of the state and was raised in foster homes for four or five years. At the age of seven or eight, she was allegedly raped by a "distinguished" elder man—a sort of Clementine tyrant. Her mother was then released from the mental institution, but had to return within about a year. (Interestingly, one of Norma Jean's early movies—*Don't Bother to Knock,* made in 1952—concerns a woman recently released from a mental institution who takes on a baby-sitting job. Monroe herself chose to do this movie, instead of having it assigned to her by a director or agent.) After her mother's return to the asylum, Norma Jean was sent to a state orphanage. (Again, her later professional career picks up on the experience in good method-actor's style: two of her early movies involve orphans: *Dangerous Years,* made in 1948, and *Fireball,* made in 1950.) At this point, a friend of Norma Jean's mother named Grace McKee Goddard informally adopted the girl.

(Yet again, Marilyn Monroe's later career picks up on the theme: her last film—*Something's Got to Give,* made in 1962—concerns a "lost" woman who returns "home" after an absence of many years in order to "adopt" her own children. This film was never completed.)[64] Grace Goddard now convinced Norma Jean to take the blond bombshell Jean Harlow as a role model. Another such model was Mary Louise Dowell. In 1936, when Marilyn was eight, Dowell was hired as a showgirl by Billy Rose in Fort Worth. Dowell became so popular that Rose took her to star in New York,[65] and pretty soon she was dubbed "Stutterin' Sam," in reference both to the song "Stop Stutterin', Sam" (1924), whose music was written by a friend of Rose,[66] and to the song "I'm Always Stuttering" (1922).[67]

Soon after her "adoption" by Goddard, Norma Jean dropped out of high school (like Amanda in *Let's Make Love*). At sixteen she married a factory worker (Jimmie Dougherty), whom she called "Daddy." Her second marriage was to the baseball player Joe DiMaggio; her third, to the playwright Arthur Miller, who soon thereafter became one of the ghost writers of the screenplay for *Let's Make Love.* As if to underscore the apparently methodical merger between Norma Jean's offstage person and onstage persona, the studio publicity for *Let's Make Love* included rumors about an affair between Marilyn Monroe and her Italian-born francophone costar, Yves Montand. The "studio system" at 20th Century Fox thus used Monroe's celebrity as a stage *propriété;* this time, the publicists included gossip about the impending breakup of the marriage between the "babe" Marilyn Monroe and her "daddy" Arthur Miller.[68] (The rumor mills pointed out that Yves Montand had been the lover of the French nightclub performer Edith Piaf, and also that he had starred in the

French-language stage and film production of Arthur Miller's *The Crucible,* titled *Les Sorcières de Salem,* alongside his wife, the French actress Simone Signoret.)

What a life! By the mid 1950s, Norma Jean was already doing therapeutic method acting with Lee Strasberg. She performed the part of Cordelia in Shakespeare's *King Lear.*[69] Cordelia is the daughter who loves her father according to her bond, "no more, no less," and therefore cannot heave her heart into her mouth.[70] Like a stutterer blocked, all Monroe's Cordelia can say is . . . nothing. Reportedly, Norma Jean cried uncontrollably throughout her drawing-room performance of the scene in which Cordelia tries to measure and to measure up to the love of a daddy.

Now, *daddy* is a word meaning, among other things, "a male lover who supports his paramour in return for her sexual favors." (In *Ladies of the Chorus,* "babes" carry dolls that they call "daddies.")[71] *Sugar daddy,* which means "an elderly man who lavishes gifts on a young woman,"[72] plays a central stutter-role in Aman-da's version of "My Heart Belongs to Daddy." There the line "But my heart belongs to Daddy," from Part 1 of Lolita's song-and-dance routine, becomes more simply "Sugadosugaosugaoado ooooo daddy."

"It's me, Sugar"—Marilyn Monroe's most famous line in *Some Like It Hot*—suggests both that the speaker, Sugar Kane Kowalczyk (played by Monroe), is named "Sugar," and also that the person to whom Sugar Kane speaks is likewise called "Sugar." The line was not easy for Norma Jean to learn to speak properly or fluently: the director, Billy Wilder, made forty-seven takes before Monroe got it right.[73] Biographers suggest many reasons for her difficulties. But they do *not* consider that Marilyn Monroe often had trouble "getting out" the word *sugar*—as suggested by Amanda's singsonging "Sugadosugaosugaoado ooooo" the next year. Various meanings of the term *sugar* are likely relevant. *Sugar* means "money," "drugs," "brothel district," and "sugar-baby."[74] There is also the use of *sugar* as a verb indicating "to flatter." J. Manchon writes bilingually in his French-English dictionary *Le Slang* (1923), "To sugar a person up, *flatter quelqu'un*."[75] Some tyrants like their love "sugar coated," but what Clément—a degenerate tyrant—comes to fear most is flattery. Clément fears that Amanda, if she ever sees him for what he is, will brush him off with *da-da,* a form of *ta-ta.* The term means "good-bye," as in the phrase *tatty-bye.*[76] Consider the baby-talk in *The Waste Land* ("Ta ta goonight") or the "Tata" in Shaw's *Buoyant Billions.*[77]

What is the general relationship here between a male *da* and his female *doll?* Maybe the gift-giving man uses the woman as if she were "his" prostitute.[78] (In her movie *The Cop and the Anthem,* Marilyn Monroe plays a prostitute.)[79] Or maybe the gift-receiving woman uses the man as if he were "her" doll- or puppet-like doormat.[80] For example, there is the episode, in Edgar Bergen's 1950s radio show, in which the "dumb blond" Marilyn Monroe almost marries the wooden dummy Charlie McCarthy: Mortimer Snerd becomes *her* dummy doll. The Marilyn Monroe version of the song "I'm Gonna File My Claim," from the movie *River of No Return* (1954), seems relevant here.[81] One might think also of Marilyn Monroe's singsonging "Happy Birthday, Mr. President" to wealthy John Kennedy, "the most powerful man in the world," who himself did not lack tyrannical qualities.[82]

My use of the possessive pronouns—*his* prostitute and *her* doormat—suggests the potentially proprietary, even violent aspect of any such human relationship. In fact, one version of the song "My Heart Belongs to Daddy" includes the following verse:

> So, I want to warn you, laddie,
> though I simply hate to be frank,
> That I can't be mean to daddy,
> cause my da-da-daddy might spank!
>
> In matters artistic,
> he's not modernistic,
> so da-da-daddy might spank.

George Cukor, who directed *Let's Make Love,* required that Monroe drop the reference to spanking from the song. A concomitant debate about property-in-persons is suggested by the opposition of June Christy's title, "My Heart Belongs to Only You" (1953) to Barbra Streisand's title, "My Heart Belongs to Me" (1977).

In any case, the possessive pronouns *his* and *her* also suggest a husband-wife relationship as *ideally* understood—that is to say, conceived aesthetically as both the essential subject and the teleological goal of romantic comedies. It is not surprising, therefore, that in some versions of the song the line "My heart belongs to Daddy" is followed by "And my daddy belongs to my heart." As we shall see, *Let's Make Love* aims at this narratological equilibrium: "I am my beloved and my beloved is mine" (as the Song of Songs puts it).

What sort of "stage property," then, is the "dumb" blond actor who slides down the stripper's pole at the beginning of Amanda's number? She is not only the iconic face and body that launched *Playboy* magazine on the cover of its first issue (1953); nor is she merely the malapropian blond in *Monkey Business* (1952; costarring Carey Grant) who decides to come to work "punctually" because her boss has complained about her "punctuation." She is the star of *How to Marry a Millionaire* (1953) and the lead in *The Prince and the Showgirl* (1957), where, as an apparently naive showgirl, she manages, with a little German-American lingo, brilliantly to trip up a multilingual Carpathian prince (played by Laurence Olivier) and so saves Europe from war.

She is, like most "naïfs," not to be underestimated.

Pater and Patter

> I say *father,* and you say *pater.*
>
> —George and Ira Gershwin, "Let's Call the Whole Thing Off" (1937)

> Superfluouse patterer of words, *battologus.*
>
> —Richard Huloet, *Abcedarium anglico latinum* (1552)

Dada, a term from French baby-talk, indicates the "international movement . . . characterized by a repudiation of traditional conventions and reason, and intended to outrage and scandalize" *(OED).* From its beginnings, the early twentieth-century Dadaist movement, examined for its social anthropology, took aim at the conventions of the "normal" family kinship system. A journal of 1920 emphasizes "Dadaism as being a 'whole-heartedly aesthetic movement,' in contradistinction to 'papaism' [i.e., daddy-ism] and 'nanaism' [i.e., nurse- or grandmother-ism]."[83] Not only does the term *Dada* sound like an infantile stutter—in the Korean language, in fact, *a-da-da* is actually the word for "stutterer"[84]—but the Dadaist movement's "hobbyhorse proponents" often promulgated a theory of language, dear to some theorists of stuttering and the origin of language, according to which a poem is essentially a collection of potentially always "meaningless" sounds.[85] Gilbert Murray asked in 1927, "Does this [Dadaist theory] mean that the words are only sounds and the poem a collection of sounds? That is clearly nonsense—a form of nonsense that is admired in certain French coteries, and is called 'Dadaism.'"[86] If a pun obtains where one sound, *da,* might stand for two (or more) different meanings, then stuttering perseveration would seem to empty a sound, *da,* of meaning. It would do so in much the same way that the Dadaist movement drains kinship terms of specificity to the point where a *dada* might as well be a *hubby.*

Now many comedies of the *Let's Make Love* sort center on a single being who is both lover *and* father—on a person like, say, Humbert Humbert in Nabokov's *Lolita* (1955). Other such comedies center on a being who is both lover and brother—like A*da*m married to the sister-like Aman*da* in George Cukor's movie *Adam's Rib* (1949). Cukor's *Let's Make Love* focuses on another Amanda, and she serves just this kind of dada-ist love, where one loves a *dada.*

What sort of kin is this *dada?* In 1927, the tellingly named *Journal of Abnormal and Social Psychology* discussed the concomitantly "perverse" or ambiguously incestuous implications of such a phrase as "Come on, daddy, let's have some fun"—where *daddy* clearly means "lover."[87] Yet Cole Porter does use the term *daddy* more explicitly to mean "lover" in songs like "Is It the Girl (or Is It the Gown)?"[88] That *dada* sometimes means "lover," though, does not necessarily imply a sort of paternal incest for *our* Loli-ta, or Aman-da. After all, a *dad* is also a "thump . . . on *any* body" (*OED,* emphasis added)—not only a thump from one's own father. Likewise, *to dad* is "to shake or send a shock through" anyone—not only a daughter.

Yet when Cukor's Aman-da had her Lolita say "Daaad" in *Let's Make Love,* it was only four years after Nabokov had published his scandalously quasi-incestuous *Lolita,* and so the incestuous implication of Amanda's daddyism was clear enough.[89] Ella Fitzgerald, in fact, emphasized the line "Yes, I'm gonna *marry* Daddy" in her brilliant version of the song. Rosemary Clooney also includes this line. But Marilyn Monroe simply dropped the line about marrying her daddy—and did so on the advice of director George Cukor.[90] It is easy to guess why one might want to suppress the line, especially when performing before a largely white audience, for whom the term *daddy* did not always have so wide an array of sexual meanings as for African-Americans.[91] Other singers dropped the line for much the same reason.[92] Yet dropping the line has its aesthetic costs: it tends to bend a little out of shape the sort of pseudosecular, or quasi-religious, romantic comedy that is *Let's Make Love.*

Just how religion in *Let's Make Love* blends here with incestuous romantic love should be clarified. According to conventional kinship rules, a man cannot be both a woman's lover and her father, but on the religious level in Christianity, there are exceptions to these rules. In some Christian doctrine, for example, the Virgin Mary has a wonderful, or mysterious, sort of intercourse with a being who is at once father and lover:[93] the widespread *topos* of the loving spouse-of-Christ (Aman-da) figures both a profane and sacred, or incestuous and chaste, understanding of an incorporated *Pater noster.* The same idea, transposed to the plane where Mary's lover is her brother, informs Cukor's movie *Adam's Rib,* in which the quasi-siblings are the lawyer-lovers *Adam* and Aman*da*. Now, maybe Jean-Marc Clément, up in his heavenly top floors, is no Christ, but, as tyrant, he is by definition a kind of *isothéos*—a would-be "god" or "equal-to-god." After all, the term *Dad* is but a synonym for *God*—as well as the typical punster's and stutterer's asseveration for *God.*[94] (Compare English terms like *adad, bedad,* and *dod.*)

Clément understands his own rivalry with, or identity as, god, both when his secret service reports that Amanda is having an "affair" with someone whom she meets regularly in church, and also when he sees Amanda kissing that ecclesiastic in the church. Most of us theatergoers have guessed wrongly that this someone is Amanda's biological father, so that the kiss is a "chaste" kiss. But in *Let's Make Love,* we always know as *little* about moneyless Amanda's consanguineous family background as we know *much* about moneyed Clément's consanguineous family background. And it turns out—surprise!—that Aman*da* Dell has been mysteriously meeting her wonderful priestly *Father* at the Church of Saint Timothy. One might think here of the bestselling song of 1953, "O my Pa-pa / To me he is so wonderful."[95] The Holy Ghost—the wonderful "ghost behind the ghost"[96] in *Let's Make Love*—has sent Amanda out into the world to convert and marry a rich tyrant.[97] Timothy was warned by Saint Paul, though, that "the love of money is the root of all evils."[98]

"Sister" Amanda is also a sort of pagan goddess of love and luck. When sliding down the stripper's pole at the beginning of her "My Heart Belongs to Daddy" song-and-dance routine, for example, Amanda's Lolita is a love-goddess playing Jacks—a gambling game with a globe-like bouncing ball and multidimensional crosses that suggest the universally high stakes for corporate world tyranny and financial power in relationship to love.[99] Marilyn Monroe plays for *jacks* (which can mean "money")[100] even as she uses the *duh* against the *jackdaw* Clément.

At the penultimate moment of *Let's Make Love,* Amanda is again on her way down from the heavenly "top floor" of the Clément Building in an elevator. The fluently accented voice of Clément announces from "on high" to Amanda that *he* is going to lift her back up to him: "I am up here on top of the world." Amanda finally takes pleasure in anticipating her sorority pals' surprise when they learn of her upcoming marital *Aufhebung.*[101]

Let's Make Love "gets over" *(aufhebt)* the always potentially troubling aspect of the *pater,* or Daddy, and likewise our concomitant issues of intermittent paralysis in walk and talk. It does so on an ideal linguistic plane, at least, by means of an assortment of variations on the *duh* in Uncle Miltie's talk and the *dodo* in his "patter walk." *To patter* means "to make a rapid succession of . . . slight sounding strokes" *(OED),* as in the tradition of Aman-Da's stuttering Dadaist "patter-talk." In the end, the semantic content of words is useless. Clément speaks many languages but remains a *da.*[102] "Words, words, words—I'm so sick of words," sings Eliza Doolittle in "Show Me" from the Lerner and Loewe Broadway musical *My Fair Lady.* Quoting the perseverating Hamlet, Eliza seems to encourage Freddie—whom she calls a *dud*—to stop talking to her and instead make love to her.[103] (The names of the two women, Elizabeth and Amanda, are practically synonymous: *Elizabeth* means "consecrated to God"; *Amanda* can mean "loving Dad.") In the title song of *Let's Make Love,* Amanda comes likewise to the same position. She wants to cut out the "patter," the mere "tatter"—a term associated both with stuttering and with animal talk—and get down to the real business of life.

Here we sit and we *chatter.*
What are we thinking of?
Let's not make with the *patter.*
Baby, let's make love!

In the "patter song" genre of the 1950s, a "large number of words are fitted [rap-like] to a few notes sung rapidly,"[104] in a curious reversion to the traditional melisma. The genre is at once the bane and salvation of stutterers: we fear to chatter, yet want music in order to patter.

In the 1950s, Danny Kaye was master of the tongue-twister patter. He was the lead in movies like *The Five Pennies* (1959), which depicts grown-ups raising money for crippled polio children, and he was the celebrated chanter of patter songs with hilarious accents, made-up words, and counterfeit languages, as in *The Court Jester* (1956). Yet the best-known patter song of the 1950s was probably "Moses Supposes." This ditty was composed, according to the plot, especially for dance specialist Gene Kelly, who plays Jean-Marc Clément's movement instructor in *Let's Make Love.* Likewise, "Moses Supposes" was composed, in actuality, especially for the film *Singing in the Rain* (1952), a song-and-dance movie that addresses brilliantly the various problems of da-da-da-dubbing that Marilyn Monroe actually resolves in *Let's Make Love.*

The term *patter* implies tiresome *parroting* of the *Pater noster* even as it recalls the seeming repetitions of stammerers' speech. ("His lips moved in a paroxysm of prayer helpless, parrot-learnt, Latin prayer.")[105] In the line "Let's not make with the patter," the singer's plea to cut out the patter comes as an inducement to make real love. Amanda Dell sings,

Just a tiny section of your affection
In my direction will *do oooh*
. . . .Come to grips with me,
Lips to lips with me, *do ooh ohh ooh*
You'll just love my embraces
Cause they'll fit like a glove.
We could get down to cases, maybe.
Kiss me baby, let's make love.

So works like *Let's Make Love* and *My Fair Lady* are anti-patter pieces. They inveigh against the intra- and inter-linguistic patters and patterns of male talkativeness. Amanda, like Eliza, requires that the male "do something" instead of talk; she wants to "coo like a dove": "lips to lips with me, *do ooh ohh ooh.*" In the song "Let's Make Love," Lolita's dialectical *uh-uh* and stutterer Norma Jean's *dada,* taken together, thus become the sounds of lovemaking. In the 1950s, Kathleen Ferrier's brilliant version of the old folksong "The Stuttering Lovers" was a bestseller.[106]

In the second century C.E., Saint Clement of Alexandria asked, "Who is the rich one that shall be saved?"[107] Jean-Marc Clément, alias Alexander du Monde, is the one whom Aman-duh saves.

6 Hamlet's Pause

Between the acting of a dreadful thing
And the first motion, all the interim is.

—Shakespeare, *Julius Caesar,* 2.1

Hamlet: The interim is mine.

—Shakespeare, *Hamlet,* 5.2

When I first read *Hamlet,* as a high school student in 1963, I was also studying Suetonius' *Life of Claudius,* the biography of the Roman emperor Tiberius Claudius Drusus. As it seemed to me, Claudius' family had dismissed him as "dim-witted" or "brutish" *(brutus).* I was certain, in those days, that Shakespeare's character Hamlet was based on Suetonius' Claudius. That is to say, I believed that Shakespeare based the character as much on Claudius as on the other individuals who, according to my edition of the play, served as sources for Hamlet: the legendary Danish prince Ambleth (or Amleth), the Roman patrician Lucius Junius Brutus (nephew and nemesis of the sixth-century B.C.E. king Tarquin), the legendary Greek king Oedipus, the fabled Greek hero Orestes, and the Roman emperor Nero. The latter analogues were obvious. For example, Hamlet is ostensibly "stupid" like Ambleth (whose name means "mad" or "daft" in the "original" Scandinavian epic) and like Brutus (in accord with the meaning of *brutus* in Latin).[1]

Hamlet himself compares and contrasts himself with Nero, who killed his father-uncle, Claudius, and committed incest with his mother, Agrippina.[2]

As it seemed to me, Claudius was apparently both a victim of polio and a stutterer. But the analogy between the hamstrung, tongue-tied Danish prince Hamlet and the polio Roman emperor Claudius was not evident to my classmates. So I set myself the double task of understanding why they could not see what I saw and of convincing them that what I saw in the play was actually there. This was my first attempt at literary criticism.

In my various attempts to convince my colleagues that Hamlet was partly modeled on Claudius, I stressed four superficial factors. The first was the nominal identity between the Roman emperor and the Danish king, Hamlet's uncle: both are called Claudius. The second was the identity between Emperor Claudius and King Claudius as uncle-fathers who are killed by their nephew-sons, the Roman Claudius by Nero and the Danish Claudius by Young Hamlet. The third was the identity of Emperor Claudius and King Claudius as oppressors of Britain: the Roman emperor was "the first Roman to make British heads bow" (in 43 C.E.) and the Danish king himself reminds us in *Hamlet* of his oppression of Britain (the Danegeld).[3] Fourth, I emphasized the structure of the story's plot: "Hamlet the Dane" is meant to displace King Claudius and essentially *become* King Claudius by means of intrafamilial regicide and incest. But Shakespeare's Hamlet resists committing Neronian regicide and incest, and this very resistance defines both his familial and political position and his character.

As it seemed to me, moreover, Shakespeare had brilliantly done two things at once in constructing his plot. On the one hand, he *clearly* attributed to King Claudius the murderous and incestuous characteristics of Emperor Nero. On the other hand, he *obscured* the ways in which the Danish Hamlet and the Roman Claudius, who were both endangered prisoners of their respective courts, used their considerable "disabilities" in order to make themselves relatively "safe" and "able" agents or actors. Those "enabling disabilities," I would argue with my high school buddies, were the real key to understanding *The Tragedy of Hamlet*.

To show all this, I had my work cut out for me. After all, there was no clear suggestion in the play that Hamlet was disabled physically, at least not in quite the way that the *stumbling* Emperor Claudius actually had "weak hams." And there was no clear suggestion that Hamlet was linguistically disabled, at least not in quite the way that the *stuttering* Emperor Claudius was.

At a crucial moment in the play, though, Hamlet requests of the Players: "Speak the speech, I pray you, as I pronounced it to you, trippingly on the tongue." The meaning of the term *tripping* has an internal dialectic that relates to walking and talking. On the one hand, it means "stumbling," "erring." Thus, one might speak of a *tripper* as "someone or something that causes stumbling," often with reference to the mouth or tongue. (The sixteenth-century Swiss clergyman Heinrich Bullinger thus touches on Moses' situation as stutterer: "The Lord beginneth . . . with the bridle to checke the mouth of his tripping Church.")[4] On the other hand, *to trip* means, "to dance"; hence, *trippingly* means "moving quickly and lightly; light-footed; nimble" *(OED)*. In Shakespeare's *Hamlet,* the word *trip* has both of these polar-opposite meanings. Hamlet instructs the players to speak *trippingly* (nimbly or smoothly—he specifies his terms carefully here), so that Claudius will *trip up* (stumble). He would *trip* Claudius.[5]

Let us look more closely at what Hamlet's stumbling and stuttering have to do with each other.

Weak Hams

> . . . they have a plentiful lack of wit,
> together with most weak hams.
>
> —SHAKESPEARE, *Hamlet,* 2.2

In my high school researches into *Hamlet,* I began by looking through the play for ambiguous references to something like physical disabilities. I speculated first that the word *Ambleth,* as Hamlet's Danish namesake was known in the Latin and French-language sources, not only refers to how Hamlet talks—his intermittent perseveration and dumbness—but also indicates, for the multilingual punster Shakespeare, how horses walk, ambulate, *amble.*[6] It was thought that horses moved like crabs, lifting the two feet on one side together, then the two feet on the other.[7] In *Hamlet,* Shakespeare glances frequently at tricky equine "amblers"—ones that contain human beings (such as the wooden horse in which Pyrrhus hid at Troy), that are partly human (such as the centaur-like knight Lamord, sometimes called Lamond, to whom Claudius refers), or that are forgotten (the hobbyhorse)—almost to the point where Hamlet himself has an "Antick amble," in the sense that Cyril Tourneur used the term.[8] As a polio survivor, I knew well the term "crab walk" (a "doctor's term" for the way many polio survivors move), and wondered at its usage in *Hamlet* (2.2): "Slanders, sir: for the satirical rogue says here that old men have grey beards, that their faces are wrinkled, their eyes purging thick amber and plum-tree gum and that they have a plentiful lack of wit, together with most *weak hams:* all which, sir, though I most powerfully and potently believe, yet I hold it not honesty to have it thus set down, for yourself, sir, should be old as I am, if like a *crab* you could go backward."

The crab walk, with which Hamlet here taunts Polonius, recalled for me the term used to describe the "gait" of the polio-detective Calvin Kane, a character in the 1940s pulp novels by Bruno Fischer (a.k.a. Russell Gray). More to the historical point, it also recalled Masaccio's fresco *Saint Peter Healing the Sick with His Shadow* (1425–1426), a work that casts doubt on the notion that the Renaissance had no polio.[9] Masaccio's painting thematizes Peter's miraculous cure of the sick that takes place in the Book of Acts.[10] Its historically packed figures include Masolini da Panicale, or Maso di Cristofano (who also did a painting of Peter curing the sick), and may also include Donatello and Saint John.

Second, in my adolescent *Hamlet* musings I speculated that Emperor Claudius was a *claudicant*—a term found in the English dictionaries as early as Henry Cockeram's *English Dictionarie* (1623). That is to say, Claudius was "lame," "halting," "limping."

Third, I speculated that Hamlet—Emperor Claudius' counterpart—has "weak hams," as the very name Ham-let suggests. Hamlet himself used the term "weak hams," and in this context Fortinbras' "strong arm"—*fort bras*—is their counterpart (*Hamlet,* 1.1). Might one present Hamlet onstage "gigging," or "jigging"—that is, as the *OED* defines it, "moving up and down or to and fro with a rapid jerky motion"? (The "jig" dance often signaled an empty-headed person. Hamlet accuses Polonius of liking only jigs; and to Ophelia, Hamlet says, "O God, your only jig-maker." "Limping up and down" is often called *jigging.*)

Fourth, I wondered at Queen Gertrude's saying of Hamlet, "He's fat." I understood the term *fat* as meaning not so much (if at all) "obese." (That is a largely modern sense; moreover, it did not seem applicable to Hamlet, who has told Horatio that he has been practicing his dueler's swordplay and is physically able, meaning "in shape.") I understood the term *fat* to mean mainly "fed up for slaughter," "ready to be killed." (Isaiah 6:10, for example, says, "Make the heart of this people fat, and make their ears heavy, and shut their eyes.") But when I looked up *fat* in the *OED,* I learned that *fat* also means "displaying the characteristics of a fat animal; slow-witted, indolent, self-complacent." The obtuse slowness that Gertrude attributes to her son suggests either physical disability or the intellectual "brutishness" which gave Hamlet his name in the first place (the Danish word for *ambleth* translates into Latin as *brutus*).

I am not arguing now that Shakespeare's Prince Hamlet has a physical disability in the sense that, say, Shakespeare's Richard III supposedly has a "hunchback."[11] The reference to a crab may merely suggest aspects of Hamlet's melancholic language or apparently impolitic spirit. (In *The Faerie Queene,* 3.ix, Edmund Spenser writes of "a cancred crabbed carle . . . / That has no skill of court nor courtesie.") And in Shakespeare's romance *Pericles of Tyre,* it is not a Masaccio-like polio but instead Monsieur Veroles who "cowers i' the hams" (4.2). Yet the problem of paralysis, both physical and verbal, remains inescapable in *Hamlet.*

Hamlet's Stops

Several astute productions of *Hamlet* depict the Danish prince, whom his mother calls "scant of breath," as a stutterer. Such productions as that of Mark Rylance catch, on the *verbal* level, those problems of *actional* hesitations—those "hems and haws"—in terms of which most audience members usually understand the plot of *Hamlet*.[12] These verbal catches remind us that Hamlet was modeled partly on the stuttering Roman emperor Claudius, as he is depicted by the historian Suetonius and others. In this context, Shakespeare has in mind two things in constructing his plot. On the one hand, he clearly attributes to his Danish King Claudius the murderous and incestuous characteristics of Emperor Nero, who was Emperor Claudius' nephew. On the other hand, Shakespeare obscures the ways in which the Danish Hamlet and the Roman Claudius, who were both endangered prisoners of their respective courts, used their considerable "disabilities"—they stumble and stutter—to makes themselves "safe" and "able" agents. These "enabling disabilities" are key to understanding the tragedy of *Hamlet* and its variously reduplicative verbal styles.

Although "the primary symptoms of stuttering can be difficult to differentiate from those of normal developmental disfluency,"[13] many of the linguistic "trips of the tongue" we hear in *Hamlet* are common "devices" of stutterers. Indeed, stutterers' instruments pervade not only *Hamlet* but Shakespeare's entire oeuvre, to the point where they are all but "uncontrolled" and hence constitute, like perseverated punning,[14] a principal characteristic of the Shakespearean writing style. (Francis Bacon's almost contemporary essay, "Experiment Solitary Touching Stutting," is relevant here to understanding *all* the works usually attributed to Shakespeare.)[15] Hamlet's wonderfully *dexterous* verbal tricks or tics, which constitute part of his ambiguously feigned "antic disposition," include the following apparently sinister and involuntary behaviors or effects.

1. *Seemingly perseverating palilalia.* Examples include such phrases as "well, well, well" (*Hamlet,* 3.1); "words, words, words" (3.2); and "except my life, except my life, except my life" (3.1). Hamlet's repetitions seem to mimic those of the ghostly Old Hamlet: "List, list, O, list!"; "O horrible! O, horrible! Most horrible"; and the thrice-repeated command to Horatio and Marcellus, "Swear!" (1.5). Hamlet's palilalia here is like a me-mo in the brain.

The term *memo,* like its Greek etymon *mermeros,* is a stutter whose second part remembers the first: *mo* recalls *me.* The echo recalls linguistic and conceptual repetitions in *Hamlet.* On the one hand, Hamlet might seem disinclined to remember: "Must I remember?" The ghost then requires him to remember: "Adieu adieu! Remember me." On the other hand, Hamlet seems determined to remember: "Remember thee! / Ay thou poor ghost, while memory holds a seat / In this distracted globe." Immediately, Hamlet recalls this potentially devastating determination: "Remember thee! / Yea, from the table of my memory / I'll wipe away all trivial fond records" (*Hamlet,* 1.2). Ablaut reduplication *(me mo)* suggests the stutterer's dramatic struggle not to stutter.

"If only I were as eloquent as [the stutterer] Demosthenes," wrote the philosopher J. G. Hamann, "I would have to do no more than repeat a single word three times."[16]

2. *Punning and synonymy.* These entail the use of *one*

sound to mean *two* (or more) things, a device which is often linked with perseveration, and also the use of *two* (or more) different sounds meaning the same *one* thing, a device which is a standard avoidance technique employed by stutterers.[17] Stuttering *diction* thus expresses amatory *addiction,* or recurring obsession with the beloved, in the Canadian group Simple Plan's stutter-song "Addict": "I'm addic—, I'm addicted to you"—or "I'm a dick, I'm addicted to you."

3. *Singsong, rhyming, playacting, and substitution.* By way of example, let us look at the odd quatrain, rhyming *a-b-a-c,* that Hamlet singsongs for Horatio after the players perform "The Mousetrap" (*Hamlet,* 3.2):

> For thou dost know, O Damon deere,
> This Realme dismantled was
> Of Iove himself; and now reigns here
> A very very—Paiocke.

Hamlet, who wrote part of "The Mousetrap," preens himself on his dramatic abilities, and plays on dramatic impersonation and hypocrisy. Here he uses the theater, as do so many stutterers, to speak (and also, for once, to act) relatively fluently. (Just how the theater allows for such fluency among stutterers is suggested in Marc Norman and Tom Stoppard's script for John Madden's film *Shakespeare in Love* (1998). We are not told until the end that the stuttering tailor Wabash is to speak the prologue in the play-within-the-film, *Romeo and Juliet.* Wabash turns out to be perfectly fluent onstage.) In *Hamlet,* the hero's fluid singsong verse (with the expected rhyme of *a-b-a-b*) would obtain at just the moment when Hamlet senses he will overcome his Pyrrhus-like, actional paralysis and get on with killing the tyrant. Yet in the quatrain above, Hamlet ("little ham") adopts the classic strategy associated in the twentieth century with the "little ham" Porky Pig. Instead of saying *ass*—the word we might have anticipated, both semantically and aurally (it provides a near-rhyme with *was*)—he blocks temporarily, like a Pyrrhic stutterer. Then he supplies the extraordinarily unusual, not to say uniquely odd term *Paiocke.* (The *OED* reminds us that the word is known only from this one instance.) Horatio says, "You might haue Rim'd." Indeed, Hamlet does rhyme in the other quatrains he seems to compose off the cuff. There are, for example, the lines that he—or his persona—sends to Ophelia and that rhyme *a-b-a-b:*

> Doubt that the stars are fire
> Doubt that the run doth move
> Doubt truth to be a liar
> But never doubt that I love.[18]

But in the "Damon deere" quatrain, his asinine *Paiocke* hams it up. He might also have ended—echoing the sometimes speech-impeded Hotspur, dying in *Henry IV*—with a stutter bordering on silence: "food for w-w-w . . . for worms."

One may have the sense that although most people find it difficult to pun, Shakespeare—called the "Swan of Avon"—found it relatively difficult *not* to pun. An infant hears a sea of sounds, which then needs discrimination into language and words, but Shakespeare never fully outgrew this stage of language development. Marshall McLuhan once said: "Language is a form of organized stutter. Literally, you chop your sounds up into bits in order to talk. Now, when you sing, you don't stutter. . . . Singing is a way of stretching language into long, harmonious patterns and cycles."[19]

4. *Silence.* This is the *pause,* or breathing-stop *caesura,* between sounds. The effort of speech, thus understood, resides in "the interval silences between sounds" and not in "the interval sounds between silences." The pause in speech is cousin to the musician's *rest* (the technical musical term)[20]—or, as Hamlet calls rests' physical counterparts in the flute, "stops" (3.2):

> . . . govern these ventages with
> your fingers and thumb, give it breath with your
> mouth, and it will discourse most eloquent music.
> Look you, these are the stops.

As the stops become longer and longer, increasing toward infinity, silence rules out breathing and signals death.

Throughout the play, therefore, *breath* and *speech* are all but synonymous.[21] Hamlet is always concerned with "windy suspiration of forced breath" (1.2); and at the end, he would leave Horatio to "draw thy breath in pain / To tell my story" (5.2). The hero's penultimate statement in the play, "The rest is silence," though linked with vows of monastic silence,[22] is best understood in terms of "rest is the only real cure for stuttering." Hamlet's caesura is thus an in-between that defines "Pyrrhic" tragedy: it comes between the conception of a dreadful thing and its enactment.

> But as we often see against some storm,
> A *silence* in the heavens, the rack stand *still,*
> The bold winds *speechless,* and the orb below
> As hush as *death* . . . (*Hamlet,* 2.2)

At the end, Hamlet will be paralyzed (dead) in both movement and speech, before those who are "but *mutes* or audience to this act."

Pyrrhus' Paralysis

> So, after Pyrrhus' pause,
> Aroused vengeance sets him new awork.
>
> —Shakespeare, *Hamlet,* 2.2

> Hector rose, recover'd from the trance.
>
> —Homer, *Iliad,* 11.462, trans. Alexander Pope

Paralysis. This is not a sixteenth-century term, but speakers of English during the Renaissance had many words of similar meaning. According to the *OED, astonishing* meant "deprivation of sensation; paralysis, benumbment"; likewise, *amazement* meant "the condition of being mentally paralyzed, mental stupefaction, frenzy." Horatio says that Hamlet would have been "much *amazed*" to see the ghost (1.2). Rosencrantz reports Gertrude's claim that Hamlet's behavior has *amazed* her (3.2). Old Hamlet, appearing to Hamlet in his mother's bedroom, says that Gertrude is *amazed* (3.4). Hamlet, imagining himself as a professional actor, sees himself as *amazing* and *appalling* his spectators and auditors (2.2). He meditates on how one might overcome by means of "indiscretion" those moments when "our deep plots do *pall*" (5.2), thus seeking to transcend the ghostly *amazement* about which Horatio had warned him from the beginning.

Trance. The word *trance* does not occur in any of the extant versions of *Hamlet,* but we would do well here to think of Pyrrhus' temporary paralytic trance in the player's speech as part of such vertiginous madness, melancholia, and "over"-pensiveness that we usually associate with Hamlet's relative "inaction." Jehan Palsgrave, in fact, defines *paralysis* as "traunce, a sickenesse, trance."[23] Walter Montague used it in this sense in the mid-seventeenth century: "[They] cannot imagine pensivenesse to be any thing but such a trans, as mad men or sick persons are in."[24] In *Romeo and Juliet,* the physician seems to induce a death-like or statue-like trance in Juliet, who is all but buried alive; and in *The Winter's Tale,* Hermione is astonished into a marble statue with something like Locked-In Syndrome.[25] In *Othello,* after Iago poisons Othello (through the ears) and Othello "falls in a trance," Cassio, seeing Othello in a "lethargy," believes that Othello has "fall'n into an epilepsy."[26] Even Christ's condition after crucifixion and before resurrection is sometimes called a trance.[27]

Trance toes the ghostly line between life and death. "She fell downe in a transe, more lyke to be deed than alyve," reads a sixteenth-century translation of Huon de Bordeaux.[28] The notion of trance marks the passage between death and life as surely as the "dead-sowne" (death-swoon) into which the afflicted Francis Bacon—sometimes compared with Shakespeare and even said to have written some Shakespearean plays—was wont to fall.[29] Finally, trance involves the transition between sleep and waking. "And as I so lay half in a traunse, / Twene slepyng and wakyng he bad me aryse," wrote John Lydgate in the fifteenth century.[30] What dreams may come?

Apoplexy. This has been defined as "a malady which arrests the powers of sense and motion." In the bedroom scene (3.4), Hamlet suggests that Gertrude suffers from "apoplexy": "Sense, sure, you have, / Else could you not have motion; but sure that sense / Is apoplex'd." Yet Hamlet, whose uncle has "popped in between the election and my hopes" (5.2), might almost as well be speaking about his own sickly paralysis. In his best-known soliloquy (3.1), sometimes anthologized as "To Be or Not To Be," Hamlet refers to the *pause* between life and death: "For in that sleep of death what dreams may come / When we have shuffled off this mortal coil, / Must give us *pause.*" This is the pause that explains how "resolution" to act "lose[s] the name of action," and likewise why it becomes "*sicklied* o'er." Hence, too, the "deliberate" pause that a desperately diseased King Claudius wants others to see, as Claudius seeks to liberate himself from the disease that he projects onto Hamlet (4.3):

> To bear all smooth and even,
> This sudden sending him away must seem
> Deliberate *pause.* Diseases desperate grown
> By desperate appliance are reliev'd,
> Or not at all.

Claudius, the Danish king, stands in pause even as to his beginning: "I stand in *pause* where I shall first begin" (3.3).

Hamlet depicts paralysis not only in terms of its hero's bodily action or inaction, but also in terms of his speech action or inaction. Ambling Ambleth *stambers,* meaning he stutters *(OED).* Hamlet thus says that he *must* "hold" his "tongue" (1.2). In Act 1, scene 3, he excoriated hypocrisy as a vice ("I know not seems"), but as the action unfolds, he needs to keep his words inadequate to his wants: he prays that "his tongue and soul be hypocrite," so that he will not behave like Nero.[31] No wonder Hamlet stutters. Physically, Hamlet must become, like Pyrrhus at the moment of para-

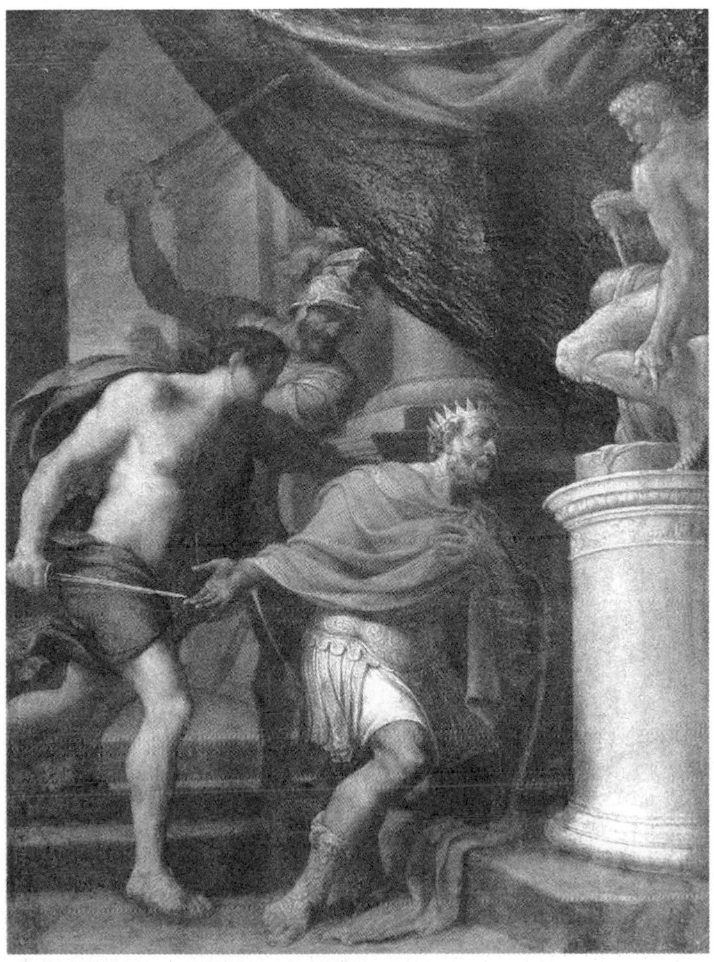

14. Attribution uncertain, *The Death of Priam at the Altar of Zeus.* France, seventeenth century. Photo copyright © Maicar Förlag GML.

lytic pause, "a neutral to his will and matter" (2.2.468). Hamlet becomes still—the way Pyrrhus is depicted "frozen" on some Greek vases and European canvases.[32] Like Pyrrhus, Hamlet is stoppered up when it comes to action.

> So as a painted tyrant Pyrrhus stood,
> And like a neutral to his will and matter
> Did nothing.[33]

The up-to-date term for *painting* here might be the cinematographic term *freeze-frame.* Frame-freezing in this context is not only a matter of "suspended animation"—as when one might "stop . . . a film or videotape in order to view a single motionless frame"; it is, more importantly, "a shot in which the movement is arrested by printing or transmitting the same frame many times" *(OED).* In the latter sense, frame-freezing is a near-perfect analogue, at the level of action, of what stuttering is at the level of words: what Hamlet calls "words, words, words."

Saying or doing nothing, instead of becoming hypocritical or murderous/incestuous, is the basis for the famous "hesitating" (*OED:* "stammering in *speech*") in *Hamlet.* The counterpart, in action, to the speaker's pause or *caesura* (literally, "a cut"), in speech, is Pyrrhus' temporary motor paralysis—as reported in the player's speech.[34] Pyrrhus, also called Neoptolemus or Neptolonius,[35] was, according to John Lydgate, a stutterer: "Neptolonius in speche stamered whan he spak."[36] During the events narrated in the player's speech, "The Fall of Troy," both Pyrrhus and Priam become paralyzed, as if by some strange "poison in the ear." Priam succumbs first (2.2, Quarto 1):

> Anon he [Pyrrhus] finds him [Priam] striking too short at
> Greeks,
> His antike sword rebellious to his Arme,
> Lies where it falls, unable to resist,
> Repugnant to command.

Priam has no strong arm (*bras fort;* cf. "Fortinbras"). His sword is *antike* in its results, much the way Hamlet's disposition is *antick* (1.5). He is "unnerved." Motionless Priam is "the unnerved father"—"senseless Ilium" (2.2, Folio). ("Sense, sure, you have," says Hamlet to Gertrude, "Else could you not have motion.") But then, following Priam, Pyrrhus—though he has strong arms ("The rugged Pyrrhus, he whose Sable Armes . . .")—is likewise paralyzed of sword.

> . . . for lo! His sword
> Which was declining on the milky head
> Of reverent Priam, seem'd i'th air to stick,
> So as a painted tyrant Pyrrhus stood
> Like a neutral to his will and matter,
> Did nothing.

No action. And no speech. The rest is silence. *Hesitation* derives, after all, from the Latin, *haesitare,* meaning "to stick fast" *(OED),* like Pyrrhus' sword, yet something is pent up and pending. It is as when Hamlet decides not to kill Claudius: "Up, sword; and know thou a more horrid hent" (3.3).

Hamlet is, of course, at least as much about the kinesis following stasis as about the stasis. Paralysis ends; action begins. Change happens. Child players, whose vocal "success" onstage depends upon their *not* changing, *will* change by virtue of maturation. In the same way, the unripe fruit to which Hamlet compares Queen Gertrude eventually ripens.

> But what we do determine oft we break.
> Purpose is but the slave to memory,
> Of violent birth, but poor validity;
> Which now, like fruit unripe, sticks on the tree;
> But fall, unshaken, when they mellow be.

Pyrrhus' sword *sticks*—has "become fixed or stationary on account of some obstruction, to be arrested or intercepted" *(OED)*—yet that sword will eventually fall on Priam as surely as children become adults and fruit ripens.

The temporal interim before Pyrrhus' sword falls is a dumb "painting"—like a still photograph—in which the action of him who will be killed and of him who will kill is frozen. Pyrrhus' "pause," is, in this sense, a "frozen frame" —the cinematic term that helps to explain the role of film-editing as an explicit theme in Michael Almereyda's movie version of *Hamlet* (2000). On the political level, the extended interregnum moment in *Hamlet* is the frozen superimposition of the phrase "Long live the king" (and the famous password with which *Hamlet* all but begins) on the phrase "The king is dead"—statements normally spoken without any pause, or caesura, between. In *Hamlet,* the action takes place in an interregnum of only apparent "truce."[37] The Danish kingdom is contested always.

Claudius' Claudication

> *Claudication:* the action of limping or halting.
>
> —*Oxford English Dictionary*

> . . . I wonder in my soul,
> What you would ask me, that I should deny,
> Or stand so mammering [stammering] on.
>
> —SHAKESPEARE, *Othello,* 3.2

"Those that stutter . . . will be soonest melancholy," wrote Robert Burton.[38] Shakespeare's famously hesitant and perseverating Hamlet does not "stutter" in quite the way that Burton attributes to melancholics, but several of the fictional and historical personages to whom he refers did. Among these would be Pyrrhus, the Greek whose namesake stutters in Lydgate's chronicle of Troy, and Virgil, author of the *Aeneid,* which inspired the verbal pause in the player's speech about Pyrrhus in *Hamlet* (2.2.470). Dante noticed bilingual Virgil's legendary Latin-language speech impediment and reproduced it in his Virgil's *parola tronca* ("truncated phrasing") in the *Inferno* (9.1019).[39] But it is the Roman melancholic Emperor Claudius whom we are really investigating here.

Claudius was well known to the British as "the first Roman to make British heads bow," and he figured in Shakespeare's *Cymbeline* (in which the Trojan Brutus, who founded England, has a part). He was a brutish stumbler-stutterer who rose to imperial power when his nephew Caligula was murdered; he fell from power when his nephew and adoptive son Nero poisoned him.

When I was in high school, the prevailing scholarly view of Emperor Claudius' physical lameness—his *claudication*—was that he had had polio. (Just as the word *ambleth* means "daft" and *brutus* means "stupid," so the word *claudius,* from the Latin term *claudus,* means "lame.") A few modern biographers look to other diseases—cerebral palsy, spasticity, and the effects of prenatal and postnatal infections.[40] There can be no certainty about Claudius' illness: medical historians are usually unable to perform autopsies.[41] But the most influential view remains that of Robert Graves: Claudius was a polio survivor.

Graves associated his own shell-shock from the First World War with some of Claudius' paralytic symptoms.[42] He had been badly injured in 1916 during the Somme offensive, in which many soldiers contracted hysterical paralysis—often conflated with such other conditions as "neurasthenia," "battle neurosis," and "hysteria."[43] His colleagues Siegfried Sassoon and Wilfred Owen were officially diagnosed with shell-shock and sent to Craiglockhart Hospital.[44]

In Josef von Sternberg's unfinished movie *I, Claudius*—a work based largely on Graves's novel *Claudius the God and His Wife Messalina* and his first-person "polio-narrative" *I, Claudius*—Claudius is brilliantly portrayed by Charles Laughton as both stutterer and stumbler.[45] Laughton's portrayal of Claudius includes a distinct alliance of stumbling with stuttering: "I l-l-limp with my tongue and st-st-stutter with my leg! Nature never quite finished me."[46] Claudius was *brutus,* or daft, or so people thought. His mother, Antonia, used to call him "a half-formed monster," Suetonius reports (*Claudius,* 3.2). She set him up as *the* standard for brutishness, berating fools publicly by calling them "more stupid than my son Claudius." Some members of the Roman court, however, thought that the stumbler-stutterer was faking symptoms of madness so as to seem no threat to Emperor Caligula. ("Nor what he spake, though it lack'd form a little / Was not like madness," says the Danish King Claudius about Prince Hamlet in Act 3, scene 4.) According to Suetonius, the Roman Claudius himself said that he had only "feigned" imbecility in order to stay alive.

In this respect, he was like Lucius Junius Brutus, who pretended to be stupid as part of a strategy for staying alive and for eventually overthrowing his tyrannical uncle, Tarquin. It was a famous debate: some doubted Claudius' "indifference" and "unconcern"; yet Suetonius reports slyly that a lampoon entitled "The Elevation of Fools" propounded the thesis that "nobody *ever* counterfeited folly."[47]

In the British television series *I, Claudius,* the question of just how cloddish stuttering Claudius is informs episode 4, "What Shall We Do about Claudius?" In scene 2, which takes place in a library, Claudius is doing research for a biography of his father, Nero Claudius Drusus Germanicus, and conversing with the Roman historian Pollio. Pollio tells Claudius how Emperor Nero had poisoned Claudius' father and emphasizes that, in order for Claudius to survive, he must exaggerate his limp and stammer in such a way as to seem harmless: "If you want to survive, exaggerate your stammer and twitch. No one will think you're worth killing." Claudius takes this advice and adopts what Hamlet calls an "antic disposition."[48]

The emperor Claudius, much like the Danish prince Hamlet, was a gifted man of letters. His works, composed mostly in Greek and Latin, included forty-three books on Roman history, twenty-one on Etruscan history,[49] and eight on Carthaginian history; a book on philology; a rhetorical defense of Cicero; and an autobiography in eight books, one of which concerned the murder of his father. (Claudius' nephew Nero supposedly destroyed all these books.)

As scholar and emperor, Claudius went some way toward conjoining two generally opposed views of politics and language: the rhetoricians' view that "Caesar non est supra grammaticos" ("The emperor is not superior to the grammarians"),[50] and the rulers' "political" view (espoused by Holy Roman Emperor Sigismund at the Council of Constance in 1414) that "Ego sum rex romanus et supra grammaticam" ("I am the Roman king and above the grammarian"). Claudius' own custom of reading silently is often cited; unusual at the time, when people read aloud even when in solitude, it eventually became common. More important is the fact that Claudius added at least three new letters to the standard Roman alphabet.[51]

Why should it take a lame and stuttering ruler to begin to realign these two views of politics and language? Such a question returns us to Prince Hamlet, to Moses the great legislator, and to Marilyn Monroe.

Speaking for Another

Soon after the performance of the "dumb show" and "The Mousetrap" in the middle of *Hamlet,* Hamlet speaks his unrhymed quatrain ("A very very—Paiocke") and is chided by Horatio. "The Mousetrap" is the small play that Hamlet has partly written himself and in which a nephew like himself (Lucianus) kills his uncle (Duke Gonzago) much the way Hamlet both wants and fears to kill his uncle Claudius. Thanks to Claudius' reaction to "The Mousetrap," the prince now believes that Claudius, "frighted with false fire," has given himself away as the murderer of Old Hamlet. He congratulates himself on being so expert at drama as to "get me a fellowship in a cry of players." He seems overcome with *ecstasy*—a term that, according to the *OED,* suggests removal of the soul from the body, as well as swoon, trance, or catalepsy. Almost beside himself, Hamlet recites the quatrain, but when he comes to the last line he hesitates or pauses at the word "very": "A very, very— . . ."

The pause is signaled by the same sort of dash—"a horizontal stroke of varying length (-, —, ——) used in writing or printing to mark a pause or break in a sentence" *(OED)*—that I use passim throughout this book. Was Hamlet about to say some such word as *ass?* The word *ass* would denigrate Claudius. And the sound of *ass* might suggest attack by way of the ears. (Bernardo *assails* Horatio's ears at the ramparts.) Or it might recall a disagreement about whether the ghost is believable. The ghost *assumed* "my noble father's person," says Hamlet; but Horatio wisely suggested that the ghost might also *assume* "some other horrible form." (That disagreement, claims Hamlet, has now been resolved by "The Mousetrap": "I'll take the ghost's word for a thousand pound.")

In any case, Hamlet cannot bring himself to utter the word *ass.* He says instead that the being who now reigns is a *Paiocke.* Some poets and scholars, including Alexander Pope, say this term means "peacock"; others, that it means "patchcock" (which may recall Hamlet's denunciation of Claudius as a "king of shreds and patches"). All we really know is that Hamlet, in pronouncing *Paiocke,* appears to choose a sound over the meaning and rhyme he apparently once intended. Whatever mechanism of *ekstasis* allowed him to speak so freely in the first three lines of the quatrain is now gone. Yet, for a moment, perseverant Hamlet's play-writing, acting, and ventriloquism freed up his otherwise ongoing inability to speak straight out. What's *that* freedom about?

The term *ventriloquism,* according to the *OED,* means "the art or practice of speaking or producing sounds in such a manner that the voice appears to proceed from some person or object other than the speaker, and usually at some distance from him." As such, ventriloquism is related to ekphrasis, the poetic mode which "giv[es] voice to a mute art object." Ekphrasis thus often refers to "a human or divine being's speaking for someone (or something) else who (or which) may or may not have, for whatever reason, a voice of his (or its) own."[52]

Human beings without a voice of their own are often figured literally, like those who are without tongues. The same is true for persons whose tongues have been removed (amputated by state-sanctioned glossotomy) for political reasons. For example, there are the "Turkish mutes" referenced in Shakespeare's *Henry IV.*[53] The practice of punishing prisoners by removing their tongues has been widespread throughout history, and has been used recently by Turks against Kurds.[54] In literary works, slave-owners threaten to cut out their slaves' tongues and then seem to regret it, as in Charles Chesnutt's short story "The Dumb Witness."[55] Literature has many scenes in which tongues are removed in order to prevent people from "tattle-telling" ("to tattle," says the *OED,* means to "stutter"). Likewise, many deposed Roman emperors and other nobles had their tongues removed, as Gibbon tells us.[56]

Tongue removal is inflicted on Lavinia in Shakespeare's *Titus Andronicus,* and on Philomel in Ovid's *Metamorphoses.* In these literary cases, the desire to give speech to the "dummy" is explicit: many people want to speak for Lavinia, and Philomel weaves a telltale cloth to report her own plight.[57] Ovid tells the story of Philomel along with that of the statue Galatea, whose creator, Pygmalion, manages to animate his artwork and make her speak.

In the Christian tradition of bodily resurrection, linguistic "animation" often borders on "tongue replacement." Thus, Pope Leo III (elected in the year 795) had his

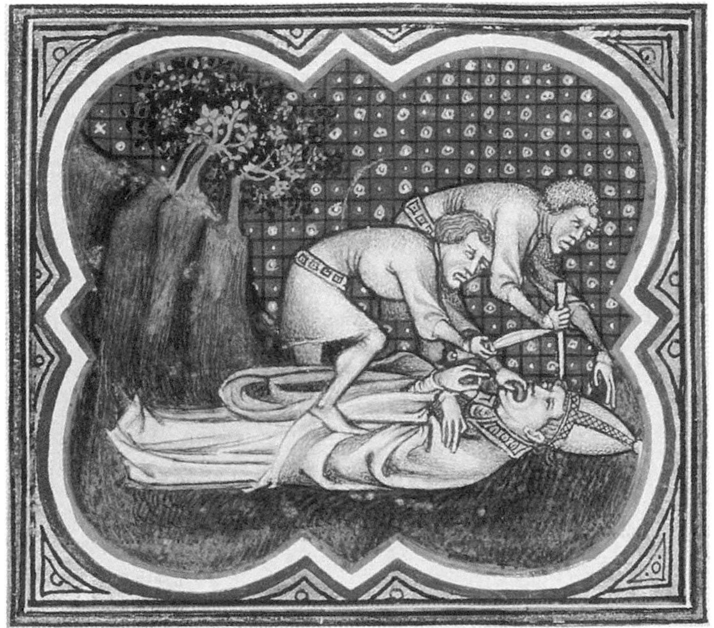

15. Anonymous, *Tongue Amputation (Glossotomy) of Pope Leo III.* Illustration from a fourteenth-century French manuscript entitled *Grandes Chroniques de France* (FR2813, fol. 95v). Bibliothèque Nationale, Paris.

tongue amputated and then restored.[58] The mystery of that tongue restoration smacks of tricks well known from the annals of magic and harks back to the tale about the manuals of ancient Egyptian magicians who tried to outdo Moses at Pharaoh's court.[59]

The typically Ovidian topos of animating a static—hence also mute—statue is an especially popular theme in the first-person polio literature. In such works, the paralyzed persons cannot speak for themselves, and they are often called "statues" or "statue-like."[60] Sculptures like

Stanislav Szukalski's *Stuttering Philosopher* suggest the figural linkage—the most common sort—between bodily stasis and verbal paralysis (see Figure 17 in Chapter 7).[61]

More often than not, though, the popular focus is on situations where a would-be magician such as a ventriloquist, who remains mute, takes up a "dummy"—a statuette, doll, animal, or infant—and seems to allow the dumb dummy to speak for itself. To put it otherwise, the dummy seems mysteriously to become the apparently silent ventriloquist's persona. Sometimes, in fact, the ventriloquist seems able to speak—to overcome his own dumbness—*only* through his dummy. The best ventriloquist-dummy dialogues define an addictive dialectic where the ventriloquist and dummy are as mutually interdependent as Siamese twins where one twin has the will to speak and the other twin speaks for him.

In the 1950s, as any polio survivor knows, the ventriloquist Edgar Bergen and his wooden dummy Charlie McCarthy used to visit bulbar polio patients at the Rancho los Amigos hospital in California.[62] Unable to speak, these polio survivors were locked in iron lungs. They well understood the polar dialectic between dummy and ventriloquist. The Rancho patients, who sometimes thought of themselves as being buried alive, understood stuttering as two beings locked in a single body. For them, the central event in the talking-animal cartoon *The Daffy Doc* (1938)—lisping Daffy Duck tumbles into an iron lung with stuttering Porky Pig—was an ever-present condition.

The topos of living inhumation has long been a focus for terrifying tales about inability to move and to speak. Relevant Gothic tales abound. Edgar Alan Poe's narrator in "The Premature Burial" (1844) describes the grave pressure on the chest and lungs that makes breathing and speaking impossible: "I endeavored to shriek—and my lips and my parched tongue moved convulsively together in the attempt—but no voice issued from the cavernous lungs, which, oppressed as if by the weight of some incumbent mountain, gasped and palpitated, with the heart, at every elaborate and struggling inspiration."[63]

Elizabeth Needham, in her first-person bulbar polio narrative about life in the steel cocoon that is the iron lung, opposes the swishing sound of the iron lung to the shriek she cannot make:

> Swish . . . swish . . . swish. The pines making their lovely song. What a strange and horrible nightmare. I wouldn't wait for morning to tell Jim. I stretched out my hand to wake him. But I couldn't move my hand! It had been no dream! Deep in my throat a scream started but then something sucked away my breath.
>
> A hand was placed on my head. A voice, muffled and compassionate, said, "You're in an iron lung, Mrs. Needham. It's helping you breathe."[64]

Ekphrasis finds its place in the interstices between animate and inanimate, between animal and human, and finally between voluntary and involuntary.

Stutterers often wonder, "Is stuttering something that I do (voluntarily) or that happens to me (involuntarily)?" Does ventriloquist Bergen allow dummy Charlie to speak, in the way that some actors do with their "characters"? Or does Charlie—or the social/psychological condition that this pet doll apparently confers on Bergen—allow Bergen to speak, in the way that personas do with actors who cease to stutter when they play-act someone other than themselves.

An actor views his body as a persona, which he "sounds through" *(per sonare).* The stutterer Gummo Marx—the fourth of the Marx brothers—famously played the part of a pet wooden dummy *through* which his uncle *sounded.*[65] The stuttering ventriloquist in Woody Allen's movie *Broadway Danny Rose* becomes fluent when he uses his dummy. James Earl Jones, in his autobiography *Voices and Silences,* writes that he was "virtually mute" as a child. With the help of his high school English teacher, Jones says, he overcame stuttering by reading Shakespeare "aloud in the fields to myself," and then, pretending to be a ventriloquist, by acting before audiences.

Many stutterers cease to stutter when they take up a dummy or a persona; just so, many people cease to stutter when they play-act at being a "dummy persona." (As J. G. Hamann suggests in his correspondence with Immanuel Kant, they also often give up stuttering when they are inebriated.)[66] For example, young Norma Jean Mortenson stuttered *in propria persona,* but not when she took up her persona: the "dumb blond" known as Marilyn Monroe. Other stutterers who became fluent as actors include Peggy Lipton, Bob Love, and Peter Bonerz.[67] The most revealing such stutterer is probably the French actor and director Louis Jouvet. Sometimes stutterers play roles closely linked to the topic of stuttering: Bruce Willis plays a stutterer's psychotherapist in *Color of Night* (1994); James Earl Jones portrays a stutterer in *A Family Thing* (1996); Michael Palin, whose father stuttered, plays a stutterer in *A Fish Called Wanda* (1988).[68]

In the movie *Shakespeare in Love,* the stuttering Wabash is transformed when he walks onstage: suddenly, he is able to speak Shakespeare's lines fluently. As the stutterer John Updike puts it, "The captive tongue is released into

Maskenfreiheit, freedom conferred by masks."[69] The essay "Psellism" in Dickens' *Household Words* states outright, "It is not rare for stammerers who have assumed a mask, to cease to stammer under their disguise."[70] "Gummo" (Milton) Marx, of the early Marx Brothers, was one of those persons whose stutter did not disappear onstage. And when, in the 1910s, his family's vaudeville routines became less song-and-dance than verbal comedy, Milton quit. He could no longer play the ventriloquist's dummy, as he had done with his uncle. Nor could he play a dumb ventriloquist, as his maternal grandfather "Lafe" (Louis) Schoenberg had done in Germany. And he did not consider seriously that he might actually play a permanent mute, as brother "Harpo" (Adolph) was eventually to do—according to brother "Groucho" (Julius) in "Why Harpo Doesn't Talk." Yet Gummo had a certain advantage: a storehouse of needful synonyms (a synonym being two sounds with one meaning). His son Robert thus reported that Gummo "was very nervous onstage, and stammered, to the point that he made himself a student of the dictionary as a result of that." Gummo therefore "had every innuendo of every word that he could possibly do, because he needed other words to get out, to get the lines out, so the show would go on, in normal timing." Gummo set his hand to writing poems and vaudeville sketches. His *Adam's Apple* (1919), which includes an excursion to Adam's Heaven and Hell and an oblique meditation on the laryngeal "Adam's apple," is of certain interest to stutterers, who have special problems with breath-holding and voice-making. Most people in Gummo's audience might suppose that the term *Adam's apple*—which names the protuberance on the human male's throat commonly understood as the "breath-holding, whisper-, and voice-making instrument"—comes "from a superstitious notion that a piece of the forbidden fruit stuck in Adam's throat, and occasioned this prominence." But punster Gummo, who had played a "Hebrew Boy" in vaudeville, knew otherwise: an influential early French translator had understood too narrowly the Hebrew-language *tappuah ha-adham* ("swelling on the man") to mean only *pomme d'Adam* (Adam's apple). In any case, Gummo's departure from the fraternal world of fast-talking puns (a pun being one sound with two meanings) turned out to be a turning-point in the trajectory of the Marx Brothers. Their journey ended cinematically in musical Harpo's apparently elective, or hysterical, vocal mutism. And by the time of the TV show "Silent Panic" (1960), the jig was up: Harpo plays a robotic, mechanical man who witnesses a murder; but as a deaf-mute without his usual interpreter—namely, "Chico" (Leo) Marx—Harpo is, Cassandra-like, utterly unable to tell anyone about the murder.[71]

Whether donning a mask is similar to other, more markedly auditory techniques for treating stuttering is a subject for another time. Often, when a stutterer is in the act of speaking and his own voice is played back to him with a delay of a fraction of a second, he speaks fluently.[72] As is perhaps the case with vaudeville's little ham.

Hamlet as Porky

> The thinking and reflecting of the hero is not Apollonian insight into his true essence, but rather an illusionary stammering: the hero errs.
>
> —NIETZSCHE, Preliminary study for *The Birth of Tragedy,* trans. Carol Jacobs

> But break my heart
> For I must hold my tongue.
>
> —SHAKESPEARE, *Hamlet,* 1.2

The most famous speech-impeded personage of the 1950s was that "little ham" Porky Pig. So it seemed to me, as I was trying to convince my high school buddies that Shakespeare's Hamlet suffered intermittent and involuntary silent "rests" and "stops," that Porky Pig cartoons might constitute a good gloss on Shakespearean language.[73]

I did not want to argue that the solution to the problem in the animated whodunnit cartoon *The Case of the Stuttering Pig* (1937) was Shakespeare's Hamlet. Rather, I wanted to show that Shakespeare's Hamlet was some kind of stuttering punster and perseverating stutterer. (Shakespeare was the "literary" ventriloquist to his dummy character Hamlet. He wrote *Hamlet* in 1600–1608, after the death of his son Hamnet around 1596.) My classmates were further convinced of the link between stuttering and *Hamlet* when I showed them such cartoons as *Ham on Wry* (1937), *Hamateur Night* (1939), and *A Ham in a Role* (1949) —some starring Porky and some not, but most, like *Hamateur Night,* containing explicit references to *Hamlet*.[74]

Finally, I would point out in class that the very first time Porky Pig appeared on the big screen, he was already associated with perseverative puns on *ham*. In *I Haven't Got a Hat* (1935), there were several cartoon animals named after paired food items. Among these were "Ham and Ex" (two puppies) and "Porky and Beans" (a pig and a cat). Dr. Seuss's *Green Eggs and Ham* (1960), published just as I was entering high school, also springs to mind.

The only character from these films to appear in post-

1935 cartoons was the "little ham" himself, Porky Pig. The voice of the original Porky was supplied by Joe Dougherty. Dougherty had had a part in *The Jazz Singer* (1927), one of the films that mark the transition from silents to talkies. Had he been given the chance, Dougherty, who stuttered in real life and pretended to stutter onstage—would have made a fine Hamlet. Instead, his rest was silence.

7 Last Stop

Stop (noun, 2): A pause or breaking-off made by one speaking.

—*Oxford English Dictionary*

The mystery of this stays with me.

—Kenneth Koch, "To Stammering," *New Addresses* (2000)

The Unspeakable

Ever since the publication of James Rymer's autobiography *The Unspeakable; or, The Life and Adventures of a Stammerer* (1855), the shifting meaning of the term *unspeakable* has played many roles in stutter narratives and quasi-scientific studies of stuttering. Some things or feelings may be unspeakable in the sense of being "ineffable," "indescribable," or "inexpressible": an experience may be "too great" for words, or there are "no words" for it.[1] And even when there are words, a person may want or need to leave them unspoken. For example, there may even be a religious rule against enunciation; thus, God's sacred name, Yahweh, may be termed "unutterable" or "unpronounceable."[2] (Some German theorists linked this unspeakableness with Moses' stuttering.) Or, to take another example, there may be a taboo against using profane swear-words, like those "four-letter" words often represented in writing by dashes.[3] Or a person may clam up before judge and jury: in American English, *unspeakable* means "unwilling . . . to speak—as when a court witness refuses to testify" *(OED)*. But even where there are words to say *and* the will to say them, words may be *unspeakable* if the individual is physically unable to speak. That would be the case for victims of ALS (Lou Gehrig's Disease), Locked-In Syndrome, full-tongue amputation, and certain breathing impairments. It is also the case for speakers of extraneous languages in utterly strange lands.

Most of the fiction writers, autobiographers, and therapists we have considered in this book associate stuttering with one or another of the above-mentioned conditions. They do so partly in order to construct an easily comprehensible literary work, upbeat scientific study, or new therapy that promises a solution to the "riddle of stuttering" or an end to the "stuttering syndrome."[4] So many millions of people have suffered from speech impediments for so many millennia that the rhetoric seems laudable. Many are still waiting for "sweet relief," as Jason Gay calls it on his CD *The Singer and the Song:*

my tongue is tied and the cat's got it, too
my mind is on fire
i'm trapped under the block of gibraltar
and i just want to tell you
that i'm still waiting
i'm still praying for sweet relief
oh yes i'm still waiting
i'm still praying for our sweet relief.[5]

Daffy Docs

HUSH YO MOUF

—Placard in the animated talking-animal movie *The Daffy Doc,* starring Daffy Duck (Warner Brothers, 1938)

In 1895, the French physician Arthur Chervin gave a detailed account of verbal phobias—fears of being unable to pronounce certain sounds and words: "Such phobias appear most often in adults, especially in those who view their stammer as a true tragedy, whether because it interferes with their professional work and social relations, or because they have an innate tendency to exaggerate their ailments. . . . The verbal phobic is afraid of certain letters, usually consonants, . . . and once he becomes convinced that a particular letter is difficult to speak, he feels real anxiety every time this letter shows up in the course of his conversations."[6]

It is difficult to make sense of "disease," as Robert Aronowitz says.[7] Stuttering is an especially mysterious condition, since it straddles the hypothetical line between physiology and psychology and between voluntariness and involuntariness. Ask ten doctors about it and you'll get ten answers; ask ten rhetoricians and you'll get ten more. "For various reasons pertaining to the development of nosology of disease," David Rosenfield remarks, speech disruption is "among the few conditions where the symptom equals the sign equals the disease." The symptom (stuttering) is the sign; the sign (stuttering) is the disease. To say that "stuttering is the response to the problem in speech output, not the problem itself," as Rosenfield does, does not solve the nosological difficulties and literary tribulations, nor does it aid us in understanding just how a condition like stuttering is "socially constructed."[8] Each disease, after all, has its own profile: biological characteristics, socially felt conditions, even moral qualities which shape the actual and eventual, as well as the visible and invisible, responses to it.

In 1936, Dr. S. Loew wrote: "The stutterer's way of thinking about his language (and in general, we would add, the way anyone affected by defects in pronunciation thinks about his language) differs remarkably from that of a healthy person. While the latter has no interest in his speech, the stutterer accords to his own speech an extraordinary and morbid degree of attention. He prepares himself in advance for every conversation; he dreads the pronunciation of certain words. He feels obsessed by these words, by these letters, even in his dreams."[9] That uncured and perhaps properly incurable condition is, after all, what makes stuttering a fit subject for students of language and literature.

Almost all stutterers "list to speak" (want to talk fluently), as tongue-tied Hamlet puts it. Therapists promise hope to such individuals, who account for 4 percent of all children and 1 percent of all adults in a pan-global and pan-cultural context. Yet therapists and theorists, with their monocular and undialectical focus on health (Loew's *santé*) and morbidity, usually sidestep the cultural phenomenology of stuttering—as a conditional event involving sound and silence, spirit and body, and voluntary and involuntary realms. For the stutterer, after all, his condition of comparative or relative speechlessness is highly conditional, unnervingly contingent, and permanently anticipatory. Thus, Jean Métellus' voodoo-informed novel *La Parole prisonnière* focuses on the stutterer's conflict between the will *(volonté)* and the absence of automatism *(absence d'automatisme).*[10] For the most part, however, therapy—like much literary theory—tends to tiptoe around relations of human language to speech and the arts (links such as the ones we've examined here) or ignore them altogether. Like much fiction, speech therapies tend to play covertly the iatrogenic role in the stutterer's tribulations that political correctness —and often the profit motive—force therapists to eschew overtly. It is little wonder that many speech therapists are buoyed by their own well-intentioned attempts to help the stutterer and "cure" him of stuttering—to make him speak out at last.

There are myriad fictional and scientific accounts of how to cure stuttering. I knew many of them even as a young boy. Kanter and Kohn's didactic novel —*And the Stutterer Talked* found its way into our home; the pamphlet "Stammering and Its Extirpation," by Ernest Tompkins, found its way to the bookshelves of Montréal's Elocution Centre, where I was a pupil.[11] Kanter and Kohn told numerous tales of charlatan cures—one of them involved learning to speak "out of tongue"—even as they themselves aimed at the complete annihilation of stuttering.[12] Tompkins aimed likewise at its eradication. In reading such books, I always felt like the buccal-talking Donald Duck in *Cured Duck* (1945): if they could not eliminate my stutter by means of a quack cure, then they would do it by annihilating me.

The Elocution Centre had received the book collection of an eminent Scottish speech therapist, and on its library shelves were many books promising cures by nonsurgical means. Listen to the list: James Sonnett Greene, *The Cause and Cure of Speech Disorders: A Text Book for Students and Teachers on Stuttering, Stammering and Voice Conditions* (New York, 1927); James Wright, *A Treatise on the Cause and Cure of Stuttering, with Reference to Certain Modern Theories* (London, 1835); William Wahab Cazalet, *Stammering: The Cause and Cure* (London, 1858); Andrew Comstock, *Comstock's Elocution and Model Speaker: Intended for the Use of Schools, Colleges, and for Private Study; for the Promotion of Health, Cure of Stammering, and Defective Articulation* (Philadelphia, 1871); L. Klindworth, *Stuttering, and How to Cure It: A Practical and Systematical Handbook for Self-Instruction, Containing an Approved Method of Respiration and the Gymnastic of Voice and Speech* (London, 1896); S. Clesson Pratt, *Hydrokonion; or, Catarrh and Its Complications: Comprising the Causes, Symptoms, and Treatment, by Medical Hydrokonia; with Notes on Diseases and Treatment of the Eye and Ear; the Cause and Cure of Stammering; the Atmisterian Treatment of Deafness; New Theory of the Electrical Relations of Mind and Body, in Health and Disease etc.* (Boston, 1865); Alfred George Farquhar-Bernard, *On the Causes, Treatment, and Cure of Stammering* (London, 1899); *The Philadelphia Institute for the Permanent Cure of Stammering, Stuttering and All Other Defects in Articulation* (Philadelphia, 1902); George Andrew Lewis, ed., *Home Cure for Stammerers,* containing advice by forty experts (Detroit, 1907); Samuel Dowse Robbins, *How to Stop Stammering: A Discussion of Stammering, Its Causes, Effects, and Cure, as Embodied in the Courses . . . Offered by the Boston Stammerers' Institute* (Boston, 1918); and Louis J. Orton, *The Cure of Stammering, Stuttering, and Other Functional Speech Disorders* (London, 1941). There were books in foreign languages as well—for example: Friedrich Wilhelm Kreuels, *Das Wesen des Stotterns und der Weg zur Heilung* (Cologne, 1934). The same promise of successful therapy continues today unabated, as evidenced in Oliver Bloodstein, *Stuttering: The Search for a Cause and Cure* (Boston, 1993). There are also such volumes as Martin F. Schwartz, *Stuttering Solved: Stutter No More* (New York, 1977), with its heavily promoted airflow therapy, as well as David Guy Compton, *Stammering: Its Nature, History, Causes and Cures* (London, 1993).

Elocutionists and speech therapists also promise *correction*—a term recalling orthopedic "correctives" of the first part of the twentieth century. "List, list, O, list!" says Old Hamlet's ghost, and the list continues: Boston Stammerers' Institute, *Course of Private Lessons for the Correction of Stammering* (Boston, 1916); Benjamin Nathaniel Bogue, *Stammering: Its Cause and Cure* (Indianapolis, 1926), reissued in 1939 as *Stammering: Its Cause and Correction* (Bogue was editor of *The Emancipator,* a magazine devoted to the "Interests of Perfect Speech"); Charles Van Riper, *Speech Correction: Principles and Methods* (New York, 1939); Mabel Farrington Gifford, *Correcting Nervous Speech Disorders* (New York, 1940) and *How to Overcome Stammering* (New York, 1940); Edwin Burket Twitmyer and Yale Samuel Nathanson, *Correction of Defective Speech: A Complete Manual of Psycho-Physiological Technique for the Treatment and Correction of the Defects of Speech* (Philadelphia, 1932); William D. Dennison, *The Correction of Stammering* (Toronto, 1941); Frederick Martin, *Stammering Can Be Corrected* (Bristol, R.I., 1936); and Paul J. Wolfe, *A Home Study Course in the Correction of Stuttering and Stammering* (n.p., 1932). The term *correction* is still used in major textbooks, as in the latest edition of Charles Van Riper's book, now titled *Speech Correction: An Introduction to Speech Pathology and Audiology* (Englewood Cliffs, N.J., 1990).

A third therapeutic trope, *remediation*, has had the same staying power over the centuries. Relevant publications include C. P. Bronson, *Stammering: Its Effects, Causes and Remedies; Involving Other Nervous Diseases, Such as Hysterics, St. Vitus' Dance, Spasmodic Asthma, Croup, Trembling Palsy, Epileptic Fits, Hypochondria, Misanthropy, Depression of Spirits, Pe-*

culiar Weaknesses, &c. &c. (Boston, 1855); William Ludwig Rosenberg, *Stuttering: Its Cause and Remedy* (Cleveland, 1930); and Edward G. Conture, *Remediation: Young Children Who Stutter* (Englewood Cliffs, N.J., 1982).

Psychoanalysis, the "talking cure," makes special promises to the stutterer.[13] Alfred Appelt's book *The Real Cause of Stammering and Its Permanent Cure: A Treatise on Psycho-Analytical Lines* (London, 1911) was influential in its day, and was followed by Isador Coriat's prominent *Stammering: A Psychoanalytic Interpretation* (New York, 1928). Smiley Blanton founded the Speech and Mental Hygiene Clinic at the University of Wisconsin in 1914, and underwent psychoanalysis in the 1930s. Blanton's *Diary of My Analysis with Sigmund Freud* (New York, 1971) followed such earlier works as *For Stutterers* (New York, 1936) and *The Hygiene of Speech* (New York, 1919), which he co-wrote with Margaret Gray Blanton. By the 1950s, American psychoanalytic literature on stuttering was flourishing.[14] Its special animus against mothers is one theme of the still-popular stuttering song "Ma Ma Ma My Sharona," written by Doug Fieger and Berton Averre (The Knack, 1979). In P. G. Wodehouse's hilarious story "The Truth about George," the stuttering of the hero is cured when he falls in love: "Her sweet sympathy effected the cure for which he had been seeking so long."[15] Yet George's stuttering poses an obvious problem for his psychoanalyst: no cure without talk. So the analyst tells him to sing everything he wishes to say—which George continues to do throughout his brief course of therapy.[16]

Nowadays, stutterers are offered hundreds of new cures. These range from highly touted medications like Zyprexa to widely distributed mechanical devices like SpeechEasy for providing delayed auditory feedback—devices that are often shunned by stutterers as a "crutch."[17] Recent cures promise simple solutions to complex conditions. One advertisement for a device called the Fluency Master reads, "Giving the Fluency Master to a stuttering person is like giving eyeglasses to a person with a vision problem."[18]

Elementary research and honestly interim make-do technologies are almost always better than daffy promises of cures. In stuttering research, the ideal best is the enemy of the realistic good. It's no accident that in *The Daffy Doc,* the buccal-speaker Daffy Duck holds up a sign reading HUSH YO MOUF. In stuttering therapy, the daft drives out the deft.

In their novel —*And the Stutterer Talked,* Kanter and Kohn describe their hero's search for a cure: "The promises and guarantees of a quick cure have hypnotized him. He goes blindly until he reaches a precipice. And the distance he falls is a long one; the bump terrific. He will try again and again."[19] One day my cure will come.

Stutter Culture

> And besides, the last word is not said—probably shall never be said. Are not our lives too short for that full utterance which through all our stammerings is of course our only and abiding intention? I have given up expecting those last words, whose ring, if they could only be pronounced, would shake both heaven and earth. There is never time to say our last word—the last word of our love, of our desire, faith, remorse, submission, revolt.
>
> —Joseph Conrad, *Lord Jim* (1900), ch. 21

In fictional works, stutterers often try to commit suicide—which is what Jeremy Zorn does in David Shields's autobiographical novel *Dead Languages* (1989). In "Stuttering Blues," the Five Scamps sing: "Sometimes I wanta cry cry / Sometimes I wanta die."[20] "What pen can depict the woefulness, the intensified suffering of the inveterate stammerer, confirmed, stereotyped in a malady seemingly worse than death?" asked the stutterer David Newton in 1920.[21] Real-life stutterers frequently make such suicide attempts.[22]

The main cause of stutterers' distress is neither the terrible stereotyping of stutterers—"bad characters," "low intelligence," and so forth—nor the deplorable discrimination that keeps stutterers from reaching their potential in school and workplace.[23] What is all but unique about the stutterer's world is the individual loneliness and noncommunal aspects of his contingent, unpredictable, and anxiety-producing inability to talk fluently. Some people conclude, from the fact that stutterers are often loners, that they like to be alone: "Usually stutterers like to stay by themselves, because they are more or less accustomed to it," says one fictional stutterer.[24] But that outlook misses the mark.

"Stutter Culture"—if there were one—would be informed by awareness of isolation as an inescapable condition. The isolation of the stutterer is a commonplace and a common experience of stutterers, although it is often denied.[25] Long ago, stutterers hoped that this isolation would end with the historical advent of writing, then of the printing press, then of widespread literacy. Marty Jezer hopes still that it will end with the development of the World Wide Web, with its many virtual "stuttering communities" bearing such names as Speak Easy and the National Stuttering Association. Of course, writing is not speaking, any more than reading is hearing. But the contrast with Deaf Culture is instructive.

Proponents of Deaf Culture say that deaf people have "a voice of their own."[26] To show this, they present studies of talkies (cinema), education, family structure, technological innovation, discrimination, and various written and visual arts, and they point to several deaf-institutions of learning dedicated to deafness and deaf people, including a major university (Gallaudet).[27] Above all, they emphasize that deaf people have a fluent if silent language of their own: American Sign Language (ASL).[28] ASL is a communal *binding* agent: it gathers its individual speakers into a cohesive group partly governed by common syntax and lexis. By the same token, ASL is a political *separating* agent: it demarcates the boundary dividing the "deaf nation" from other linguistically defined groups.

With regard to the issue of separateness and aloneness, there are two significant differences between the deaf community and the individual stutterer. First, stutterers do not claim to have a language of their own—and perhaps essentially, they *cannot* have one—so that, while deaf people do not need to use spoken language in order to "speak out," stutterers do. Second, while the deaf frequently use assistive or prosthetic devices such as teletype and telecommunication instruments when they communicate with hearing speakers, stutterers usually do not use such devices when they communicate with fluent speakers. Stutterers are stuck at the periphery of expressivity. Without a special or national community defined in terms of linguistic bonding and separating, individual stutterers are willy-nilly isolated both from groups who do *not* stutter and from individuals who *do* stutter.

Hundreds of stutter jokes say as much. They often begin with the question, "What happens when two stutterers meet?" and they all imply it is best for the two *not* to meet.

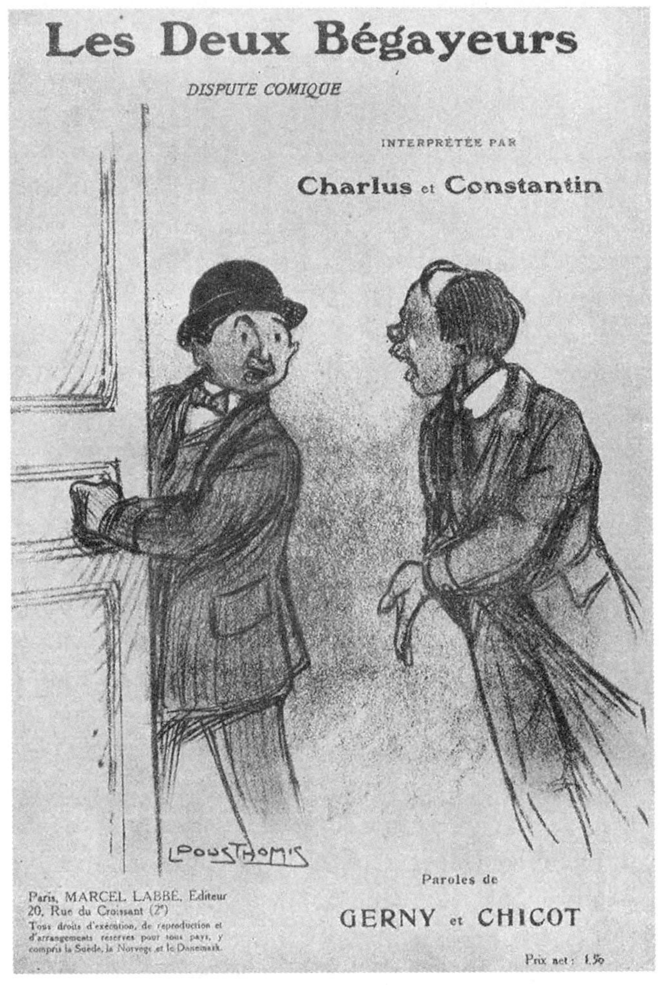

16. Poster, with drawing by L. Pousthom's, for *Les Deux Bégayeurs: Dispute Comique* (The Two Stutterers: Comic Dispute), words by Gerny and Chicot, interpreted by Charlus and Constantin Le Rieur, 1920s. From René Bernard, *Le Bègue sur la scène française* (Paris: Droz, 1945), frontispiece. Bernard's caption, taken from *Les Deux Bégayeurs,* reads: "'A-alors, vous pen-pen vous pensez que je vais man-man manger le po-po—, le pognon que j'ai eu tant de mal à ga— . . . de male ga— . . .' / 'J'en j'en prendrai bien un verre.' / 'Tant de mal à ga-a-gner . . .'" ("'S-so you th-th—, you think I'm going to f-f-fritter away the do-do—, the dough that was so hard for me to g-g— . . . so hard for me to g-g— . . .' / 'I-I-I'd love to have a drink.' / 'So hard f'me to g-g-get . . .'").

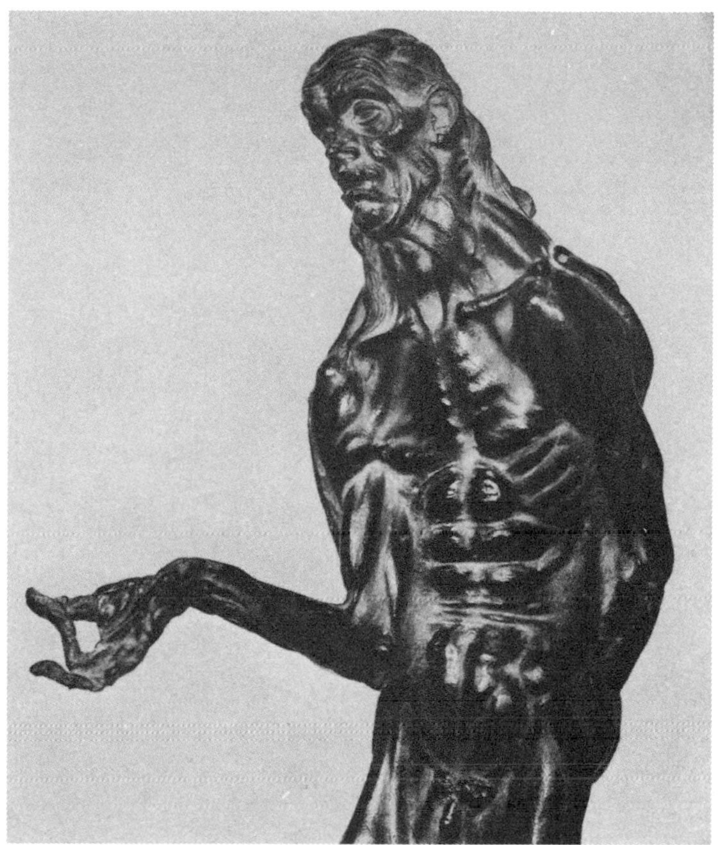

17. Stanislav Szukalski, *A Stuttering Philosopher* (1915). Bronze, 12 inches high. Photo copyright © Archives Szukalski, Sylmar, California. "Stuttering philosopher, while talking, assists his argument with hand and foot. He squeezes his stomach to get a last breath for his impatient words and thereby causes his neck to swell apoplectically." *The Work of Szukalski* (Chicago: Covici-McGee, 1923), unpaginated.

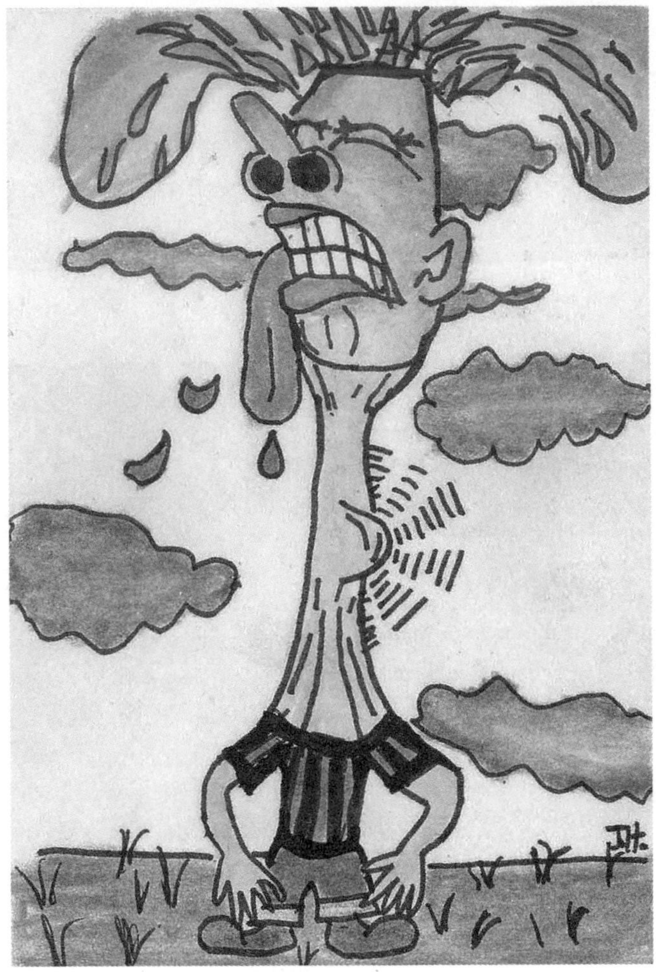

18. Jeremy Hill, *Self-Portrait as a Child Stutterer* (1988). Drawing produced in a grade-school class taught by Adriana DiGrande, Department of Communication Disorders, Sargent College of Health and Rehabilitation Services, Boston University.

That is the gist of many anecdotes in Benjamin Constant's *Memoir of the Hundred Days.*[29] "The Biter Bit: A Tale of Two Stutterers" was a "children's story" I came across at age nine.[30] The meeting of two stutterers on a train is the comic situation that motivates one of the scenes in Wodehouse's "Truth about George."[31] Two stutterers meeting up is an oft-repeated comic situation in French theater. Thus, Florent Carton Dancout's *Le Galant Jardinier* (1704) brings together two characters named Bavardin and Caton; Nicolas de Malezieu's *Tarentole* (1705) includes a conversation between Pincemaille and Rhubarbarin; and in *La Cloyère d'huîtres* (1820), by Pierre Frédéric Adolphe Carmouche, Frédéric de Courcy, and Jean Toussaint Merle, there is a scene between two characters named Begotin and Double-Langue.[32]

Many first-person stuttering narratives seem to end happily. Some conclude that "adversity makes a person better." Others say, "Whatever does not kill a person makes him stronger." The authors of such triumphant accounts tend to resemble Renard the fox in stuttering Aesop's fable: he fruitlessly tries to reach the grapes on the trellised vine and then, famished, he slinks off, muttering to himself that they must have been sour anyway. Yet for many people, stuttering is not without certain real "compensations."

For example, experience with breathing *seizures* might help one become a sensitive scholar of pulmonology or of the literary *caesuras* that inform oral poetry, versification, music, and religion.[33] Familiarity with verbal substitution —use of the same sound to express different meanings (puns) and of different sounds to express the same meaning (synonyms)—might motivate one to publish a synonymicon or a new theory of puns. My own difficulty in pronouncing the word *stutter* helps to explain my hardly cavil-proof acquaintance with many (by no means all) of its synonyms: *abbob, balbutiate, barbarian, block, buff, clutter, drote, dyslalia, faffle, falter, famble, fribble, hack, hacker, hammer, happer, hem, hesitate, hiccup, lisp, maffle, mammer, mant, psellism, rattle, shamble, shrench, stacker, stagger, stamber, stammer, stumble, tattle, titubate, totter, traulism,* and *wlaffe*—each of which has played a distinct role in this book. A "fully bilingual" stutterer—fluent only in his imagination—becomes expert in translation (*argent/money*), word-doublets (*Porky/Pig*), accent (*tomato/tomahto*), and perseveration *(da da da)*. When playmates and doctors labeled me *ambleth,* or daft, because I stuttered, this may have spurred me to offer a novel interpretation of *Hamlet.*

Fluent speakers have the gift of *gab,* or *gob*—meaning "fluency of speech" *(OED).* They take for granted their easy *patter* or *chatter,* as Amanda Dell (or is she Lolita? or Marilyn Monroe? or Norma Jean Mortenson?) calls it in *Let's Make Love.* Like someone who breathes the air without even knowing that there *is* air, speakers with the gift of gab hardly know the involuntary caesura of the poet and singer. From the stutterer's lifelong *gob-gobbling* and *goblobling,*[34] however, comes an almost unconscious avian understanding. He understands why Hamlet—even as "the potent poison quite o'er-crows [his] spirit" (5.2), and though he is a "croaking raven [that] doth bellow for revenge" (3.2)—says to his real friend Horatio, "The rest is silence." Hamlet has already warned Rosencrantz and Guildenstern, who seek shallow therapy and merely politic ends, not to mistake the delicate link between music and human speech—between the recorder's stops and the windpipe's glottal stops. They only seem to know what blocks him, whom only fell death will arrest: "You would seem to know my stops" (3.2).

Writes the stutterer Philip Larkin in his poem "Next, Please": "Always too eager for the future, we / Pick up bad habits of expectancy."[35] Lack of closure and the concomitant desire or need for conclusion are exacerbated by prosaic rhythm, semantic meaning, and logical argument. These wants are the stutterer's burden—and, as we have seen, also sometimes his peculiar boon. In the end, however, the stutterer's stops are closely bound up with the phylogenetic development of humankind and the ontogeny of human individuals. For the time being, stuttering is the mystery where language and culture meet—that *chassé-croisé* where acting, music, song, speech, writing, legislation, and talking cinema take on and put off a common humanity.

Notes

Prologue

1. André Malraux, *Les Noyers de l'Altenburg* (Paris: Gallimard, 1948; orig. pub. 1945)—a novel. "Venice" refers to the poem "Venedig," in Nietzsche, *Ecce Homo,* ed. Raoul Richter (Leipzig: Insel-Verlag, 1908), ch. 7: "Warum ich so klug bin."

2. There are 6.3 billion people in the world, according to the latest estimate by the International Programs Center of the United States Census Bureau. I use .8 as an estimate for the percentage that stutters. As we shall see, figuring the percentage of people who stutter is difficult for a number of reasons: the predisposition of clinicians, the consequential differences among cultures, the importance of variance in the age of stutterers, and the many disagreements about how to define stuttering for the purpose of collecting data. Most authorities agree, however, that .8 percent is a relatively low estimate.

3. The term *gag* "sounds" like the choking that it "means." According to some traditional scholars, this onomatopoeia is the "historical origin" of the term.

4. See the drawings by children stutterers in classes taught by Adriana DiGrande (Department of Communication Disorders, Sargent College of Health and Rehabilitation Services, Boston University), *Boston Globe,* October 22, 2000. Adriana DiGrande and Diane Parris discussed such work in their paper "Monsters, Chains, and Cages: Images of Stuttering," presented at the Convention of the American Speech-Language-Hearing Association (ASHA), Anaheim, California (1993).

5. Thomas Wilson, *The Arte of Rhetorique: For the Use of All Suche as Are Studious of Eloquence* (London, 1553), Book 3, 117b, under the heading "The Parts of Pronunciation": "Musicians in

England have used to put gags in children's mouths that they might pronounce distinctly" (spelling modernized).

6. For the use of the term *gag* to mean "an apparatus for distending the jaws during an operation," see John Eric Erichsen, *The Science and Art of Surgery: A Treatise on Surgical Injuries, Diseases, and Operations,* 10th ed., rev. Marcus Beck and Raymond Johnson, 2 vols. (London: Longmans, Green, 1895), vol. 2, p. 691: "If the patient be efficiently gagged."

7. It is often thought that branks were instruments used only on women; they were sometimes called "scolds' bridles." But they were also often used for men who blasphemed or railed. For drawings of many branks—some gruesome—see William Andrews, *Old-Time Punishments* (Hull: W. Andrews, 1890). See also Edmund F. du Cane, *The Punishment and Prevention of Crime* (London: Macmillan, 1855), p. 14: "For women scolds the branks or gag . . . were authorized punishments."

8. Jon Bee [John Badcock], *Sportsman's Slang: A New Dictionary of Terms Used in the Affairs of the Turf, the Ring, the Chase, and the Cock-Pit* (London, 1823): "*Gag,* a grand imposition upon the public; as a mountebank's professions, his cures, and his lottery-bags, are so many broad gags."

9. Walter Winchell, the Broadway columnist, was the first to dub Berle the "Thief of Bad Gags"; he was referring to the famous movie *The Thief of Baghdad* (1920). Berle had a predilection for stealing other performers' gags. See Milton Berle and Haskel Frankel, *Milton Berle: An Autobiography* (New York: Delacorte, 1974).

10. Hugh Lofting, *The Voyages of Dr. Doolittle* (1922), part 6, ch. 3: "The Red Man's Science."

11. Walter Benjamin, *Goethes Wahlverwandtschaften* [1924–1925; *Goethe's Elective Affinities*] (Frankfurt: Insel-Verlag, 1964).

12. Ralph Waldo Emerson, *Representative Men: Seven Lectures* (London: H. G. Bohn, 1850).

13. The term *parataxis* refers to "the placing of propositions or clauses one after another, without indicating by connecting

words the relation (of co-ordination or subordination) between them" (*OED,* 3rd ed., s.v. "parataxis").

14. *OED,* s.v. "elide," 2.

15. Friedrich Nietzsche, *Thus Spake Zarathustra,* trans. Thomas Common (London: William Reeves, 1898), section titled "Joys and Sorrows." In German, *Also sprach Zarathustra: Ein Buch für Alle und Keinen* (1883–1884; Thus Spake Zarathustra: A Book for All and None), section titled "Von den Freuden- und Leidenschaften": "Deine Tugend sei zu hoch für die Vertraulichkeit der Namen: und musst du von ihr reden, so schäme dich nicht, von ihr zu stammeln."

16. Victoria Nelson, *On Writer's Block: A New Approach to Creativity* (Boston: Houghton Mifflin, 1993).

17. Walkiria Toledo de Araújo, Humberto Vicente de Araújo, and Juliana Toledo de A. Rocha, "Algumas reflexões sobre ansiedade de publicar" (Reflections on Anxiety about Publishing), *Informação e Sociedade* (Brazil), 12, no. 1 (2002).

18. Henry Charlton Bastian, *The Brain as an Organ of Mind,* International Scientific Series (London: Kegan Paul, 1880), pp. xxix, 658.

19. "In less extensive lesions," wrote the Russian neurologist A. R. Luria, who viewed stuttering as a key problem, "the disintegration of writing takes the form of dysgraphia, and examination of the writing of such patients reveals a disturbance of the clear distinction of the sounds of words, confusion between closely related phonemes, and other signs of a defect of acoustic analysis." Aleksandr Romanovich Luria, *Restoration of Function after Brain Injury,* trans. Basil Haigh, ed. O. L. Zangwill (New York: Macmillan, 1963), p. 183. On Luria's general interest in stuttering, see C. Van Riper's review of A. R. Luria and F. Yedovich, *Speech and the Development of Mental Processes in the Child* (London: Staples, 1959), in *Journal of Speech and Hearing Disorders,* 25 (1960): 211–212.

20. *Journal of Neurology and Psychopathology,* 8 (1927): 26: "The palilalia (as with stammering) disappears during pre-

formed speech automatisms, as, for instance, when the patient reads aloud, sings or recites."

1. Preambulations

1. For the present initial purpose, I define *stuttering,* in the spirit of the Stuttering Foundation of America, from "outside" the stuttering subject.

2. See, for example, Anne K. Cordes and Roger J. Ingham, "Stuttering Includes both Within-Word and Between-Word Disfluencies," *Journal of Speech and Hearing Research,* 38, no. 2 (April 1995): 382–386. The article reviews evidence supporting the contention that stuttering and normal disfluencies occur within, across, and between words. It also differentiates between a strong form of the within-word definition of stuttering and a weak form proposed by Edward G. Conture. See Conture's book *Stuttering* (Englewood Cliffs, N.J.: Prentice-Hall, 1982).

3. "Margaret O'Brien is drawn to a young James MacArthur, who comes to work for her father and poses as a deaf mute rather than reveal the speech impediment that afflicts him." *Tongues of Angels* (March 17, 1958), TV script, University of Iowa Library, Special Collections Department, Papers of Norman Felton, Box 50.

4. Ted Morgan, *Maugham* (New York: Simon and Schuster, 1980), p. 557.

5. "Disability": Marty Jezer, *Stuttering* (New York: Basic Books, 1997), p. xx: "I see stuttering not only as a disability that is challenging to live with and difficult to overcome, but as a metaphor for other impediments—physical and psychological, real and imagined—that inhibit so many peoples' lives."

"Cultural history": S. Brosch and W. Pirsig, "Stuttering in History and Culture," *International Journal of Pediatric Otorhinolaryngology,* 59, no. 2 (June 2001): 81–87.

6. James Malcolm Rymer, *The Unspeakable; or, The life and Adventures of a Stammerer* (London: Clarke and Beeton, 1855).

Benjamin Beasley, *Stammering, Its Treatment; and, Reminiscences of a Stammerer, Who Cured Himself after Suffering for More Than Thirty Years,* 17th ed. (Birmingham, England: Hudson, 1897).

Wendell Johnson, *Because I Stutter,* introduction by Lee Edward Travis (New York: Appleton, 1930).

James Sonnett Greene, comp. and ed., *I Was a Stutterer: Stories from Life; Autobiographic Sketches—Readjusted Personalities,* foreword by Albert Bigelow Paine (New York: Grafton Press, 1932). Greene was the founder and director of the National Hospital for Speech Disorders in New York.

Charles Pellman, *Overcoming Stammering,* foreword by Frederick Martin (New York: Beechhurst Press, 1947).

7. Ida E. Witten, *The Face of All the World Is Changed: An Autobiographical Study with the Focus on Stuttering* (Cincinnati: Privately printed, 1990).

8. Clarice Pont, *The Immediate Gift* (New York: David McKay, 1961); the main character graduates from college with a degree in speech pathology in the 1950s. In the movie *Waterboy* (1988), Bobby Boucher (Adam Sandler) is a socially inept thirty-one-year-old from the swamps of Louisiana, where he has been home schooled and sheltered by his overprotective mama. Presumably, this is one reason he stutters.

9. That is, a feeling of anxiety and panic when one is introduced to strangers.

10. *Zerkalo,* Tarkovsky's reminiscence of life as a child in Russia during World War II, focuses on a youngster whose search for a cure for his stuttering problem leads him to a hypnotist.

11. "Still much debated": See, for example, David B. Rosenfield and Howard S. Derman, "Physician Referral Patterns for Stutterers," Paper presented at the 43rd Annual Meetings of the Canadian Society of Otolaryngology–Head and Neck Surgery, Toronto, Canada, April 30–May 3, 1989.

"Regardless of intervention in childhood": This does not necessarily mean that children "simply outgrow" stuttering. The two groups of children—those who gain fluency and those who don't—may stutter *differently.* This is the argument presented in C. Stromstra, "A Spectrographic Study of Disfluencies Labeled as Stuttering by Parents," *De Therapia Vocis et Loquellae,* 1 (1965): 317.

12. See L. G. Stevenson, "The Surgery of Stammering: A Forgotten Enthusiasm of the Nineteenth Century," *Bulletin of the History of Medicine,* 42 (1968): 527–554; Edgar S. Werner, "Mutilation of Stutterers: Surgical Operations Which Have Been Performed for the Cure of Defects of Speech," *The Voice* (Albany, N.Y.), 3, no. 9 (September 1881): 127–128; ibid., no. 10 (October 1881): 146; and Gray Burdin, "The Surgical Treatment of Stammering, 1840–1841," *Journal of Speech Disorders,* 5 (1940): 43–64.

13. Alfred Charles Post, *Observations on the Cure of Strabismus, with an Appendix on the New Operation for the Cure of Stammering* (New York: Francis, 1841). Johann Friedrich Dieffenbach, *Die Heilung des Stotterns durch eine neue chirurgische Operation;* in English, *Memoir on the Radical Cure of Stuttering by a Surgical Operation,* trans. Joseph Travers (London: Highley, 1841).

14. In a number of studies, the ratio varies from about 2:1 to 4:1. David B. Rosenfield, "Stuttering," *Critical Reviews in Clinical Neurobiology,* 1, no. 2 (1984): 118.

15. Franklin H. Silverman, "The 'Monster' Study," *Journal of Fluency Disorders,* 13, no. 3 (June 1988): 225–231.

16. The Monster Study, so called because of the monstrous effect it had on its subjects, began with a simple premise: the researchers speculated that the genesis of stuttering is in the diagnosis. They theorized that parents, teachers, and therapists were inadvertently making young stutterers worse by calling attention to their problem. Further, they contended that a child's stuttering is worsened when one constantly corrects his or her speech. They speculated that if they could prove their theory through a valid scientific experiment, then they could publicize the results and end harmful diagnoses and treatment practices.

Their technique was simple: for six months a graduate student, Mary Tudor, regularly visited the orphanage and induced six children with normal speech patterns to believe that they were stutterers. The researchers initially were uncertain what the results would be, since the children ranged in age from five to fifteen—they were beyond the stage at which stuttering typically begins. Nevertheless, the youngsters acquired the classic symptoms of stutterers: they spoke less, and spoke more slowly; they became self-conscious; they believed something was wrong with them; and they responded physically with gestures such as covering their mouths when they spoke.

The researchers were so successful in proving the theory, that panicky orphanage employees contacted them after the study's end to say that the children's symptoms were getting worse. For eighteen months Mary Tudor visited the orphanage to deprogram the children. Jerry Halvorson, author of the novel *Abandoned: Now Stutter My Orphan* (Hager City, Wisc.: Halvorson Farms, 1999), which is based on the Monster Study and includes a foreword by Franklin Silverman, says it appears Tudor was unsuccessful with two of them. Halvorson believes the researchers were startled by the effects of the conditioning: "I don't think they realized how hard it would be to reverse." They suppressed the results.

Halvorson notes that in later years they tried to prove their theory through indirect research, but it took decades to persuade their colleagues of its validity. According to Halvorson, suppressing the Monster Study led to years of delay in the acceptance of a useful diagnostic tool for the treatment of stuttering. One obvious lesson, Halvorson says, is that "if you work with kids you shouldn't label them as stutterers" or try to make them speak in ways that are unnatural to them. "Most kids who are stuttering are better off being left alone, rather than being affected by people who don't know what they are doing." See "Fictionalized Work Unveils 'Monster Study,'" *This Week: A Newsletter for Faculty and Staff,* University of Wisconsin at River Falls, August 23, 1999 (www.uwrf.edu/thisweek/19990823.htm, accessed November 2004).

17. See the foreword to Halvorson's *Abandoned* by Franklin Silverman, who says that in the 1940s Wendell Johnson "apparently was concerned about how his professional colleagues and the general public would react to learning that he had turned orphans into stutterers, particularly at that time, when the Holocaust was going on in Germany and highly unethical medical experimentation was being done on inmates of concentration camps."

18. Hippocrates, *Epidemics,* trans. W. H. S. Jones (Cambridge, Mass.: Harvard University Press, 1957), Book 1, sect. 11.

19. Halvorson, as a child, was severely chastised by a teacher for his fear of reading aloud. His speech phobia would shape his life's work as teacher, therapist, and novelist.

20. See Silverman, "The 'Monster' Study."

21. Stutterers in my family include Leo, the firstborn son of my maternal grandfather Joseph; myself, likewise a firstborn son; and Kyam, the firstborn son of my sister Lieba. My paternal uncle Label stuttered partly because he was an epileptic—though family legend has it that his condition was also due to a trauma at birth.

22. See M. I. Buyanov, E. V. Bogdanova, R. A. Subbotina, and V. N. Trebuleva, "On Heredity in Stuttering" (written in Russian), *Defektologiya,* 3 (1987): 20–22. This article deals with the way in which the clinical picture of speech disorders relates to the presence or absence of such disorders in families. On the notion that stuttering runs in the family, see Oliver Bloodstein, *The Handbook of Stuttering* (San Diego: Singular Publishing, 1995), which reports on thirteen relevant studies. See also Jezer, *Stuttering,* p. 27.

23. Tourette's Syndrome is sometimes called "stuttering with one's hands and feet." See Larry Molt, "The Basal Ganglia's Possible Role in Stuttering: An Examination of Similarities between Stuttering, Tourette Syndrome, Dystonia, and Other Neurological-Based Disorders of Movement," Auburn University (Auburn, Alabama), September 1999, www.mnsu.edu/

comdis/isad2/papers/molt2.html, accessed June 2005. Investigations into the cause of stuttering have provided a wide variety of interesting etiological theories over the past century. Recent research utilizing Positron Emission Tomography (PET scans) has shown that people who stutter have greater than normal levels of blood flow in the corpus striatum region of the basal ganglia, evidence which indicates abnormal levels of activity in that region; see J. C. Wu, G. D. Riley, G. Maguire, A. Najafi, and C. Tang, "PET Scan Evidence of Parallel Cerebral Systems Related to Treatment Effects: FDG and FDOPA PET Scan Findings," in W. Hulstijn, H. F. M. Peters, and P. van Lieshout, eds., *Speech Production: Motor Control, Brain Research, and Fluency Disorders* (Amsterdam: Elsevier, 1997), pp. 329–339. The authors hypothesize that the corpus striatum may be involved in stuttering.

24. Warner Brothers' Porky Pig, created by Fritz Freleng, first came to the screen in 1935. See Will Friedwald and Jerry Beck, *The Warner Brothers' Cartoons* (Metuchen, N.J.: Scarecrow Press, 1981), p. xiv.

25. That is, the family believed his stuttering was caused by strokes and head injuries.

26. Andrew Boorde, *The Breviary of Health, for All Maner of Sickenesses and Diseases the Which May Be in Man or Woman, Doth Folowe: Expressyng the Obscure Termes of Greke, Araby, Latyn, and Barbary, in Englishe Concernyng Phisicke and Chierurgerie* (London, 1547), xli, 21: "If it [stuttering] do come with beying in the company of a stutter or stamerer, a man must refrayne the company of a stutter." Another such old such notion is that stuttering can be cured by silence. Mary Wortley Montagu wrote in a letter of 1741: "We must cure people of errors and lying, as they do of stuttering, by a long course of silence." The actor James Earl Jones followed this course of treatment, whether prescribed by himself or by others.

27. In Gary Wolf, *Who P-P-P-Plugged Roger Rabbit?* (New York: Villard Books, 1991), esp. p. 106.

28. John Mason Good, *The Study of Medicine,* 4 vols. (1822–

1829), vol. 1, p. 566. Also: "Children . . . ought never to be intrusted in the company of a stutterer, till their speech has become steady and confirmed" (ibid.).

29. All quotations from Anna Seward, *Memoirs of the Life of Dr. Darwin* (London: J. Johnson, 1804), pp. 2, 63, 62.

30. Robert Boyle, "Life" (1647), in Boyle, *Works,* 5 vols. (London: A. Millar, 1744), vol. 1, p. 6. Also in R. E. W. Maddison, *The Life of the Honorable Robert Boyle* (London: Taylor and Francis, 1969).

31. Edward Hoagland, "The Threshold and the Jolt of Pain," in *Heart's Desire: The Best of Edward Hoagland, Essays from Twenty Years* (New York: Summit Books, 1988), p. 130.

32. Egbert Joseph Spadino, *Writing and Laterality Characteristics of Stuttering Children: A Comparative Study of Seventy Grade School Stutterers and Seventy Matched Non-Stutterers* (New York: Teachers College, Columbia University, 1941).

33. Emma Luethy Hayhurst, *I Will!* (Hicksville, N.Y.: Exposition Press, 1978; 2nd ed. Canton, Ohio: Life Enrichment Publishers, 1982), p. 31.

34. Samuel Otway Lewis Potter, *Speech and Its Defects, Considered Physiologically, Pathologically, Historically, and Remedially* (Philadelphia: P. Blakiston, 1882). Potter devotes a chapter each to dyslalia, paralalia, and alalia; he defines paralalia on p. 33. His book, a foundational document in the field of speech disorders, won the Lea Prize of Jefferson Medical College, Philadelphia.

35. Dr. David B. Rosenfield (director of the Speech and Language Center, Department of Neurology, Baylor College of Medicine, Houston, Texas) is currently conducting research in this area. See David B. Rosenfield, W. Edwin Fann, and Nagalapura S. Viswanath, "Resolution of Stuttering Following Neurological Disease," in H. G. Bosshardt, J. S. Yaruss, and H. F. M. Peters, eds., *Fluency Disorders: Theory, Research, Treatment, and Self-Help,* Proceedings of the Third World Congress on Fluency Disorders, Nyborg, Denmark, August 7–11, 2000 (Nijmegen, Holland: Nijmegen University Press, 2001), pp. 99–101.

36. Jean Métellus, *La Parole prisonnière: Roman* (Paris: Gallimard, 1986), pp. 29–30, 41. Métellus is the president of the Groupe de Recherche sur l'Aphasie et les Altérations du Langage (GRAAL).

37. Abu Hamidi Muhammadi Al-Ghazzali lived from 1058 to 1111. There is a discussion of his tongue paralysis in William James, *The Varieties of Religious Experience* (New York: Random House, 1902), Lectures 16–17.

38. In *The Cowboys* (1972), cattle driver John Wayne hires a bunch of youngsters, including a boy of about ten who stutters. One of the kids gets thrown from his horse into the water. The stutterer runs to John Wayne for help but can't get out an intelligible word. By the time Wayne figures out what's wrong, the drowning boy has been saved by someone else. Wayne turns on the stutterer and begins yelling at him—not an uncommon event for young male stutterers. He tells the boy that he could talk fluently if he wanted to and that the boy has to stop "that stuttering" or leave the group. At that point, the "boy starts cursing at John Wayne—and while he's doing it, he doesn't stutter. He's cured!" See www.mnsu.edu/comdis/kuster/media/movie text.html cowboys.

39. Frederic Myers, *Catholic Thoughts on the Bible and Theology* (London, 1841–1848), 3.5.17.

40. Elizabeth Rice, "The Families of Children with Poliomyelitis," in *Poliomyelitis: Papers and Discussions Presented at the First International Poliomyelitis Conference* (Philadelphia: Lippincott, 1949), p. 312.

41. Reading aloud is usually a major topic of any memoir written by a stutterer. See, e.g., Jezer, *Stuttering,* pp. 90–91.

42. There are many disabilities that kept students out of school—obviously unfairly, in retrospect—and many were intellectually superior. In some cases it was difficult for students to speak (because of cerebral palsy), and in other cases they couldn't manage school stairs (because of muscular dystrophy, spina bifida, polio). It is the polio group that is of special interest because

there were so many children at once and they often came from wealthy or middle-class families.

43. See Joyce Hansen, *I Thought My Soul Would Rise and Fly: The Reconstruction Era Diary of Patsy, a Freed Girl* (New York: Scholastic, 1997). The book, intended for students aged nine to thirteen, is about a freed slave girl who stutters. She gets frustrated when people think she is stupid (which she is not).

44. Siobhan Hugh-Jones and Peter K. Smith, "Self-Reports of Short- and Long-Term Effects of Bullying on Children who Stammer," *British Journal of Educational Psychology,* 69, no. 2 (June 1999): 141–158.

45. According to Robert Lacey, cited in Margaret Drabble, "Public Speech and Public Silence," address to the British Stammering Association, October 18, 2001, Gulbenkian Lecture Hall, Oxford; reprinted in *Speaking Out,* publication of the British Stammering Association (Summer–Fall 2002).

46. For example Hansen, *I Thought My Soul Would Rise and Fly.* Although Patsy stutters, she has the courage to speak.

47. See Ethan S. Long, Raymond G. Miltenberger, and John T. Rapp, "A Survey of Habit Behaviors Exhibited by Individuals with Mental Retardation," *Behavioral Interventions,* 13, no. 2 (May 1998): 79–89. The authors measured the prevalence of major habit disorders (bruxism, trichotillomania, motor/vocal tics, and stuttering) and found that stuttering was the most prevalent, occurring in 32 percent of the subjects studied.

48. Norman J. Lass et al., "School Administrators' Perceptions of People Who stutter," *Language, Speech and Hearing Services in the Schools,* 25, no. 2 (April 1994): 90–93. The majority of reported adjectives were negative stereotypical personality traits. See also Franklin H. Silverman et al., "Teachers' Perceptions of Stutterers: A Replication," *Language, Speech and Hearing Services in the Schools,* 24, no. 2 (April 1993): 108.

49. Such concerns led to myriad studies early in the history of polio. See, for example, R. G. Gordon, John Alexander Fraser Roberts, and R. Griffiths, "Does Poliomyelitis Affect Intellectual

Capacity? An Investigation of 98 Cases," *British Medical Journal,* 2, no. 803 (October 21, 1939). This study showed that poliomyelitis, whether during or after an attack, does not impair intelligence as measured on the Stanford-Binet scale.

50. See Juvenal, *Satires,* 10.356.

51. On the extraordinary sort of tongue paralysis that one sometimes encounters in literature, philosophy, and religion, see (inter alia) James, *The Varieties of Religious Experience,* Lectures 16–17 (discussion of Al-Ghazzali).

Moebius' Syndrome (named for Paul Julius Moebius) is a rare disorder characterized by lifelong facial paralysis. See Jonathan Cole, *About Face* (Cambridge, Mass.: MIT Press, 1997).

52. A crux of many "self-help" discussions of stuttering and among stutterers in more recent years is: "Am I stutterer or a person who stutters?" (Jezer, *Stuttering,* p. 16). There are stutterers' handbooks that take this as a major theme. See, for example, Bryng Bryngelson, M. Chapman, and O. Hansen, *Know Thyself: An Objective Approach to Stuttering and Other Problems* (Minneapolis: Burgess, 1958); the book is discussed in Jezer, *Stuttering,* p. 138.

53. "Word-switching": See Peter Howell, James Au-Yeung, and Stevie Sackin, "Exchange of Stuttering from Function Words to Content Words with Age," *Journal of Speech Language and Hearing Research,* 42, no. 2 (April 1999): 345–354. Howell and his colleagues, according to their abstract, "tested whether function word dysfluencies in the speech of people who stutter occur when the plan for the subsequent word is not ready for execution and examined whether stuttering would arise when speakers abandon the use of a delaying strategy and attempt to produce the subsequent, partly prepared content word."

"Sound-based avoidance": See Colleen F. Martens and Dean C. Engel, "Measurement of the Sound-Based Word Avoidance of Persons Who Stutter," *Journal of Fluency Disorders,* 11, no. 3 (September 1986): 241–250. Abstract of article: "Analyzed the monolog samples of fifteen stuttering subjects (aged 14–34 years) to determine the percentage of words they chose that began with each phoneme. The distribution of initial sounds of words that stuttering subjects selected when formulating speech was compared with data gathered from forty nonstuttering adults. A profile was constructed of standard Z scores that permitted observation of an individual subject's deviation from the control group. Profiles of ten of the thirteen stuttering subjects who reported that they avoided words showed evidence of probable sound-based word avoidance. Sounds that subjects reported they were most likely to avoid were not highly related to the sounds they seemed to avoid."

54. See Albert Postma, *Stuttering and Self-Correction: On the Role of Linguistic Repair Processes in Disfluencies of Normal Speakers and Stutterers* (Nijmegen, Netherlands: Nijmegen Institute for Cognition and Information, 1991).

55. Likewise, in English-speaking Canada the word *silver*—which is the literal translation of *argent*—means pretty much the same as *small change.*

56. See the *Annales* of 1180 (Joannes Zonaras), in the seventeenth-century edition by Du Cange (Charles Du Fresne, sieur Du Cange): "God stirred up the spirit of a certain holy priest, a man of religion, who was called Lambert le Bègue (because he was a stammerer) of St. Christopher (in Liège), from whose surname women and girls who propose to live chastely, are called Beguines, because he was the first to arise and preach to them by his word and example the reward of chastity" (*Oxford English Dictionary,* s.v. "Beguine"). The *OED* (s.v. "beggar") associates begging with the Beguines etymologically: "A likely derivation is from the Old French *begart, begard,* and *begar,* medieval Latin *begardus* = *beghard,* or its synonym *beguin* and derivatives. Verb *beguigner,* 'to act the beguin.' It is known that the Beghards or Beguins were, or soon became, a lay mendicant order, and that in the thirteenth century mendicants calling themselves, or called, by these names, swarmed over Western Europe."

57. See Robert Calder, *Willie: The Life of W. Somerset*

Maugham (London: Heinemann, 1989), p. 283. "Maugham had rewritten the dialogue, removing all the difficult words," for a reading he was to do with Edward Weeks on the radio.

58. In a lecture entitled "Thankyou and Goodnight," Drabble says: "My broadcasting and lecturing style, if not my prose style, has been curiously affected by my choice of vocabulary. Like most stammerers, I know that there are some words with which I am almost certain to have difficulty. On innumerable occasions I have substituted the phrase *U.S.* for *America* or *TV* for *television*. This is clumsy and inelegant, but not disastrous. More problematic is the need to say *lady* instead of *woman*—this understandably causes offence and lands one in a pit of political incorrectness" (*Guardian,* October 20, 2001).

59. Marty Jezer, who is a different sort of stutterer from me, writes: "Many stutterers do what covert stutterers do and attempt to disguise their stuttering by anticipating words they think might give them trouble. They then substitute words they feel confident they can say without stuttering. That's why many stutterers develop large vocabularies" (Jezer, *Stuttering,* p. 10).

60. Arthur Chervin, *Des Phobies verbales* (Paris: Société d'Editions Scientifiques, 1895), pp. 2–3; quoted in René Bernard, *Le Bègue sur la scène française* (Paris: Droz, 1945), p. 30.

61. Jezer, *Stuttering,* p. 10.

62. Wolf, *Who P-P-P-Plugged Roger Rabbit?* pp. 239, 255.

63. Compare words which, on their own, sound like stutters, as when Porky Pig says, "Are you really the last of the dododos?"

64. *OED,* s.v. "hammer."

65. Additional lyrics:

> Now hey there, people, won't you lend an ear?
> 'Cause I've a story to tell and I'm telling it here
> I was born in a town in the great UK
> From a baby to a boy to a man today
> And I'm a musical man, and I'm a man of verse

But I've got a little problem and it's getting worse
Well my life was so well planned
Survivin' and a-jivin' in a f-f-funk band
'Cause rappin', it's my bread and butter
But it's hard to rap when you're born with a st-st-st, st, st-st, st, st-t, st-t, st-t, stutter!
Well no-one's ever seen what I mean
From the age of n-n-n-n-n-n-thirteen
We've all been caught in a m-m-mouth trap
So join with us and do the st-st-st-st-st-st-st-stutter rap.

Tony Hawks, "Stutter Rap (No Sleep till Bedtime)," sung by Morris Minor and the Majors (Virgin Music and Ten Records Ltd., 1988). Used by permission. Hawks, the lead singer, once played the role of a lisping food dispenser. See too the stutter rap of Thulani Ngcobo ("Pitch Black Afro") from Soweto.

66. Henry Creamer (lyrics) and Harry Warren (music), "Stop Stutterin', Sam" (Skidmore Music Company, 1924).

67. Seth Benardete, *Encounters and Reflections: Conversations with Seth Benardete,* ed. Ronna Burger (Chicago: University of Chicago Press, 2002), p. 48.

68. Abraham H. Kanter and Abe S. Kohn, *—And the Stutterer Talked* (Boston: Bruce Humphries, 1938), pp. 18–19.

69. For the word "unspeakable" in relation to stuttering, see James Malcolm Rymer, *The Unspeakable; or, The life and Adventures of a Stammerer* (London: Clarke and Beeton, 1855).

70. "That's why many stutterers . . . often speak with muddled syntax" (Jezer, *Stuttering,* p. 10).

71. One of Bryng Bryngelson's contributions to the field of stuttering therapy was his concept of "voluntary stuttering." Both Van Riper and Wendell Johnson were influenced by the work of Bryngelson at Iowa in the early 1930s (Bloodstein, *Handbook on Stuttering*). See, inter alia, Bryng Bryngelson, "A Phono-Photographic Analysis of the Vocal Disturbances in Stuttering" (Thesis, University of Iowa, 1931).

72. Jaan Pill (Peel District School Board and Canadian Association for People Who Stutter, Etobicoke, Ontario), "Einer

Boberg's Contribution to the Self-Help Movement," www.stutter.ca/jaanarticle.html (accessed June 2005).

73. Thomas Krall, keynote speech entitled "Thoughts" (in Bosshardt et al., *Fluency Disorders*), quoting a friend of his. Compare Friedrich Nietzsche's understanding of "stammering in a foreign tongue" in *The Birth of Tragedy,* in Nietzsche, *Werke in Drei Bänden,* ed. Karl Schlechta (Munich: Hanser, 1954–1956), vol. 1, p. 12, translated by Carol Jacobs in Jacobs, *The Dissimulating Harmony: The Image of Interpretation in Nietzsche, Rilke, Artaud, and Benjamin* (Baltimore: Johns Hopkins University Press, 1978), p. 3.

74. Pill, "Einer Boberg's Contribution to the Self-Help Movement."

75. William Perkins, *Tongue Wars: Recovery from Stuttering* (Reno, Nev.: Athens Press, 2000). This quotation from Perkins is, however, from the *National Stuttering Association Newsletter.* See Vikram Dayalu and Joseph Kalinowski, "Pseudofluency: An Illusion in Stuttering Therapy Is Challenged," *Journal of Speech, Language, and Hearing Research* (forthcoming). Kalinowski is the inventor of the "SpeechEasy" device, a delayed auditory feedback (DAF) machine.

76. For example, Jezer's relative lack of knowledge of French when living in Montréal had an important bearing on his unhappiness there with his stuttering. In his difficulty with communication, it seemed (I think) a sort of reiteration of one problem by the other (Jezer, *Stuttering,* p. 228).

77. R. Karniol, "Stuttering out of Bilingualism," *First Language,* 12, no. 36 (October 1992): 255–283. This paper, according to the abstract, "documents the development of a bilingual male child both before and after he started stuttering severely in both languages at twenty-five months, the point of transition to grammatical sentence construction. The subject's bilingual language awareness and the characteristics of Language 1 and Language 2 prior to and at the time of onset of stuttering are discussed."

78. Gary S. Neiman and Rebecca B. Rubin, "Changes in

Communication Apprehension, Satisfaction, and Competence in Foreign Dialect and Stuttering Clients," *Journal of Communication Disorders,* 24, nos. 5–6 (October–December 1991): 353–366. From the abstract: "Subjects were fifteen male foreign graduate students (mean age 30.6 yrs) and thirteen stuttering university students (mean age 24.4 yrs). Both foreign dialect and stuttering clients had significantly lower levels of communication apprehension and higher levels of communication competence after 3.5 months of their respective therapies."

79. See James Au-Yeung, Peter Howell, Steve Davis, Nicole Charles, and Stevie Sackin, "UCL Survey on Bilingualism and Stuttering," in Bosshardt et al., *Fluency Disorders.*

80. The relation between bilingualism and stuttering is a topic in many stuttering narratives; some people stutter in a second language and some don't. Jezer thinks this may have something to do with acting (Jezer, *Stuttering,* p. 105).

81. Lord Durham was addressing, in part, the constitutional and civil relationship between the English and French "races" (as the official courts then called them) in "Upper Canada" and "Lower Canada." See John George Lambton Durham, *Report on the Affairs of British North America,* ed. Charles Lucas, 3 vols. (Oxford, 1912). See Marc Shell, *Children of the Earth: Literature, Politics, and Nationhood* (New York: Oxford University Press, 1994), esp. ch. 3, "The Forked Tongue; or, The Road Not Taken in Québec."

82. John Earle, *The Philology of the English Tongue,* 5th ed. (Oxford: Clarendon, 1892; orig. pub. 1871). See also Oliver Farrer Emerson, "Prof. Earle's Doctrine of Bilingualism," *MLN,* 8, no. 7 (November 1983): 404–412.

83. Emerson, "Prof. Earle's Doctrine of Bilingualism," p. 406.

84. Ibid., p. 404.

85. Ibid., p. 405.

86. Porky's very name is already a "doublet": *porc* is the French word for *pig.*

87. Earle, *Philology of the English Tongue,* p. 407. My thanks to Scott Newstok for a Harvard term research project on this subject.

88. James Earl Jones, *Voices and Silences* (New York: Simon and Schuster, 1993), written with William Niven and Penelope Niven. See also Judy L. Hasday, *James Earl Jones: Overcoming Adversity* (Philadelphia: Chelsea House, 1998). Jones plays a stutterer in the movie *A Family Thing* (United Artists, 1996; written by Billy Bob Thornton and Tom Epperson; dir. Richard Pearce).

89. Jezer, *Stuttering,* p. 3.

90. Shakespeare, *Hamlet,* 1.2.

91. Jaan Pill writes: "I was consistently aware of Boberg's comment that avoidance, rather than overt stuttering, is the most salient feature of stuttering." Pill, "Einer Boberg's Contribution to the Self-Help Movement." Pill refers to such works as Einer Boberg and D. Kully, *Comprehensive Stuttering Program* (San Diego, Calif.: College-Hill Press, 1985).

92. According to one source, the anticipation of a beating by the cruel whip called "cat-o'-nine-tails" (a term often shortened to "cat") could *paralyze* a victim into silence. That is, presumably, why "Has the cat got your tongue?" came to mean "Are you unable to speak?"

93. On "compensation" as such, see Marc Shell, *Polio and Its Aftermath* (Cambridge, Mass.: Harvard University Press, 2005), pp. 218–226.

94. Viktor Shklovsky, "Art as Technique," in *Russian Formalist Criticism: Four Essays,* trans. and introd. Lee T. Lemon and Marion J. Reis (Lincoln: University of Nebraska Press, 1965).

95. On the theory that Shakespeare suffered from some sort of language dysfunction, see Marc Shell, *The End of Kinship* (Stanford, Calif.: Stanford University Press, 1988), esp. the Conclusion.

96. On the fact that William Butler Yeats was completely tone deaf, see Michael B. Yeats, *Cast a Cold Eye: Memories of a Poet's Son and Politician* (Dublin: Blackwater Press, 1998).

97. Although the story that Demosthenes put pebbles in his

mouth to improve his voice is probably only a legend, he seems to have been forced to overcome a weak voice and delivery. See Hans Holst, "Demosthenes' Speech Impediment," *Symbolae Osloenses,* 4 (1926): 11–25.

98. Potter, *Speech and Its Defects.* Culpepper tells us in his *Riverius* (1655) that "balbuties"—one of dozens of synonyms for stuttering that we will encounter in the following chapters—is "a kind of Stammering, which keepeth men from pronouncing of the Letter *R.*" Nicholas Culpepper, *The Practice of Physick: Being Chiefly a Translation of the Works of L. Riverius* [Lazare Rivière], *with a Physical Dictionary Explaining Hard Words* (London: Peter Cole, 1655). Compare the definition of the same word in Joseph E. Worcester, *A Dictionary of the English Language* (Boston, 1859): "Balbuties, stammering; vicious pronunciation, in which *b* and *l* are substituted for other consonants."

99. Certain scholars (e.g., David Elmer) suspect that this saying comes from a Roman writer, or, if not, from a Byzantine source. The spelling of the participle *rherhetoreumeno* might indicate Byzantium; it would have a *nu* on the end in good Attic Greek.

100. Guillaume Bouchet, *Les Sérées* (1615), Dialogue 35: "Mesme la langue prend encore quelque nature des eaux, que changent la voix et les langues, et faict que ceux que demeurent pres des rivieres, sont begues le plus souvent." Cited in Paul Cohen, "Mediating Linguistic Differences in the Early Modern French Atlantic World: Linguistic Diversity in Old and New France," International Seminar on the History of the Atlantic World, 1500–1825 (Harvard University), Working Paper 03–17 (2003): 9; see www.fas.harvard.edu/~atlantic/proghome.html.

101. Demosthenes said that Philip the Macedonian (father of Alexander the Great) was "not only no Greek, nor related to the Greeks, but not even a barbarian from any place that can be named with honors, but a pestilent knave from Macedonia, whence it was never yet possible to buy a decent slave" (Demosthenes, *Third Philippic*).

102. *The Alexiad of the Princess Anna Comnena: Being the History of the Reign of Her Father, Alexius I, Emperor of the Romans, 1081–1118 A.D.,* trans. Elizabeth A. S. Dawes (London: K. Paul, Trench, Trübner, 1928), 1:8.

103. Edward Hoagland, "The Threshold and the Jolt of Pain," in *Heart's Desire: The Best of Edward Hoagland—Essays from Twenty Years* (New York: Summit Books, 1988), p. 133.

104. See, for example, John Hutton, *A Glossary of Old and Original Words Now Used in the North of England.* Reprinted from *A Tour to the Caves, in the Environs of the Ingleborough and Settle in Yorkshire,* 2nd ed. (1781), p. 97. So far as the term *stammer* goes, both usages are included in *Promptorium parvulorum sive clericorum, lexicon Anglo-Latinum princeps* [1440] (London: Camden Society, 1843–1865), 472/1.

105. *Promptorium parvulorum sive clericorum, lexicon Anglo-Latinum princeps,* 471/2.

106. Richard Harvey, *Plaine Percevall, the Peace-Maker of England: Sweetly Indevoring, with His Blunt Persuasions to Botch up a Reconciliation between Mar-ton and Mar-tother* (1589), A.ij. The reference is to traulism.

107. Gervase Markham, *Cavelarice, or The English Horseman: Contayning All the Arte of Horse-manship, as Much as Is Necessary for Any Man to Vnderstand, Whether He Be . . . Horse-Ambler . . . or Sadler* (London: Printed for Edward White, 1607; 1617), p. 27.

108. John Stevens, trans. and ed., *The Comical Works of Don Francisco de Quevedo, Translated from the Spanish* (1707; 1709), p. 380. For other examples, see Robert Fergusson, *Hallowfair Poems* (1774; 1845), p. 16: "But if a birkie's oure weel sair'd [well served (with drink)] / It gars him often stammer / To ploys that bring to the Guard / And eke the Council Chammer." See also Robert Blakey, *An Essay Shewing the Intimate Connexion between our Notions of Moral Good and Evil, and Our Conceptions of the Freedom of the Divine and Human Wills* (Edinburgh: A. Black, 1831), p. 62: "The shot plied like hailstones round the old veteran. . . .

But he had the good fortune to escape unhurt, and when he was stammering back the Russians gave him three cheers."

109. Sylvester Judd, *Margaret: A Tale of the Real and the Ideal, Blight and Bloom* (Boston: Jordan and Wiley, 1845), ii.viii.

110. Terence, *The Eunuch,* trans. from the Latin by Richard Bernard (Cambridge, 1598), ii.iii.133.

111. Bob Dylan and Robert Hunter, "The Ugliest Girl in the World," in *Down in the Groove* (Columbia Records, 1987/1988).

112. John Struthers, "The Poor Man's Sabbath: A Poem," in Struthers, *Poetical Works,* 2 vols. (London: A. Fullarton, 1850), vol. 1, p. 43.

113. This is taken from Bianca Plouffe's stutter poem, "Ma Lutte." The entire poem is posted on Plouffe's website, www.geocities.com/HotSprings/1085/malutte.html (accessed June 2005).

114. In Shakespeare's *King Henry IV, Part II* (2.3), Lady Percy says about Hotspur's manner of walking and talking: "He had no legs that practised not his gait; / And speaking thick, which nature made his blemish, / Became the accents of the valiant; / For those that could speak low and tardily."

115. Philip eventually has an operation which all but removes his impediment.

116. Reported in Morgan, *Maugham,* p. 16.

117. *OED,* s.v. "walkie-talkie": "I thought it was a proper big doll you'd lost. . . . Like one of them walkie-talkies." Quoted from Jenifer Wayne, *The Day the Ceiling Fell Down* (London: Heinemann, 1961), p. 72.

118. Alberta Armer, *Screwball* (New York, 1963), pp. 32, 74.

119. Jan Mark, *The Ennead* (New York: Crowell, 1976).

120. On Emmett Till, see Stephen J. Whitfield, *A Death in the Delta: The Story of Emmett Till* (New York: Free Press, 1988).

121. On March 13, 1991, Australian senator John Tierney gave an address that described how he had initially been attracted to his country's Liberal Party: "Turning on the radio one evening

in 1958, I heard Robert Menzies deliver a speech at the opening of a poultry farmers' conference. The occasion was very ordinary, but the speech was extraordinary. This eloquent man outlined with such grace his vision for Australia, *and there was I, a boy with a bad stutter recovering from the effects of polio,* totally intrigued, listening and drawn to the Liberal vision of an Australia built on a deep respect for the dignity and the freedom of the individual, of an Australia where one could be rewarded for effort and where enterprise would be encouraged, and of an Australia where there is real equality of opportunity and choice." (Source: www.senatortierney.com/speeches/show.asp?id=18. Accessed December 2004; italics added.)

122. The Peruvian Rotarians Gustavo Gross and Julio Ruíz, who brought the teenaged boy from his village to Lima, said that he arrived sick, with a stutter. At the time, he took classes with a speech therapist to overcome language problems, and he did exercises to strengthen his leg muscles.

123. Walter Scott wrote: "I have a hideous paralytic custom of stuttering with my pen" (Scott, *Journal,* April 5, 1831).

124. "Psellism," in *Household Words,* 348 (November 22, 1856): 464–469; quoted from *Household Words: A Weekly Journal Conducted by Charles Dickens,* 14, nos. 330–353 and the number-and-a-half for Christmas, July 19, 1856, to December 27, 1856 (London: Office 16, Wellington Street North, 1856).

125. Ibid., p. 465.

126. See Tore Wolff, "En teori om hur stamning uppkommer" [in Swedish] (A Theory about the Cause of Stuttering), *Psykisk Haelsa,* 30, no. 1 (1989): 45–49. Wolff interprets stuttering as a consequence of a strong, unconscious reluctance to talk that is caused by a lack of confidence in the ability to communicate, which is itself caused by traumatic childhood experiences.

127. Mark S. George and R. Bruce Lydiard, "Social Phobia Secondary to Physical Disability: A Review of Benign Essential Tremor (BET) and Stuttering," *Psychosomatics,* 35, no. 6 (November–December 1994): 520–523.

128. Norman Fenton, *Shell Shock and Its Aftermath* (St. Louis: C. V. Mosby, 1926), p. 156, tells of a train of "war neurotics" on which one man had a stutter: "when they detrained the next day almost all of them stuttered." See Margaret R. Higonnet, "Authenticity and Art in Trauma Narratives of World War I," *Modernism/Modernity,* 9, no. 1 (2002): 103.

129. From *The Definitive Paul Hardcastle,* CD (Connoisseur Records, 1993). Words and music by Mike Oldfield, Paul Hardcastle, William Couturie, and Jonas McCord. Copyright © 1985 EMI Virgin Music Ltd. and Oval Music. All rights for EMI Virgin Music Ltd. in the United States and Canada controlled and administered by EMI Virgin Music, Inc. All rights reserved. International copyright secured. Used by permission.

130. See William Russel MacAusland, *Poliomyelitis, with Especial Reference to the Treatment* (Philadelphia: Lea and Febiger, 1927), p. 84. MacAusland refers to Smith Sly Jelliffe and William A. White, *Diseases of the Nervous System* (Philadelphia: Lea and Febiger, 1923); and John Ruräh and Erwin E. Mayer, *Poliomyelitis in All Its Aspects* (Philadelphia: Lea and Febiger, 1917).

131. Arthur C. Clarke, "Painful Memory of a Silent Stalker," *Times Higher Education Supplement,* History of Science (June 29, 2001): 34.

132. Enid Foster, *It Can't Happen to Me* (Cape Town, South Africa: Howard Timmins, 1959), p. 104.

133. See MacAusland, *Poliomyelitis,* p. 94.

134. Susan Sontag, *Styles of Radical Will* (New York: Farrar, Straus and Giroux, 1969), p. 9. Idem, *Illness as Metaphor* (New York: Farrar, Straus and Giroux, 1978). Idem, *AIDS and Its Metaphors* (New York: Farrar, Straus and Giroux, 1989).

135. See Shell, *Polio and Its Aftermath,* esp. the Preface.

136. Gilles Deleuze, in *L'Abécédaire de Gilles Deleuze,* an eight-hour series of interviews with Claire Parnet, filmed by Pierre-André Boutang in 1988–1989 (broadcast 1994–1995), transcript by Charles J. Stivale. See www.langlab.wayne.edu/CStivale/D-G/ABC1.html, accessed June 2005.

137. See, for example, Marcel Proust, "Dialogues," 149, from *By Way of Sainte-Beuve.*

138. "That which stutters": Gilles Deleuze and Félix Guattari, *Qu'est-ce que la philosophie?* (Paris: Minuit, 1991). In English, *What Is Philosophy,* trans. Hugh Tomlinson and Graham Burchell (New York: Columbia University Press, 1994).

Gilles Deleuze, "He Stuttered," in Constantin V. Boundas and Dorothea Olkowski, eds., *Gilles Deleuze and the Theatre of Philosophy* (New York: Routledge, 1994), pp. 239, 24–25, 28. See too Olkowski, "Beside Us, in Memory," *Man and World,* 29 (1996): 283–292.

139. Gilles Deleuze and Claire Parnet, *Dialogues,* trans. Hugh Tomlinson and Barbara Habberjam (New York: Columbia University Press, 1987), pp. 1–19.

140. See Carol Jacobs, "Nietzsche—The Stammering Text: The Fragmentary Studies Preliminary to *The Birth of Tragedy,*" in Jacobs, *The Dissimulating Harmony: The Image of Interpretation in Nietzsche, Rilke, Artaud, and Benjamin* (Baltimore: Johns Hopkins University Press, 1978), ch. 1.

141. Hoagland, "The Threshold and the Jolt of Pain," p. 133.

142. Jean-Jacques Courtine and Claudine Haroche, "Silences du langage," prefatory essay to Joseph Antoine Toussaint Dinouart, *L'Art de se taire* [1771] (Montbonnot-Saint-Martin, France: J. Millon, 1987), p. 30.

143. On the term *Possum,* see Shell, *Polio and Its Aftermath,* p. 224. On Ben'ari: ibid., 122.

144. Hoagland, "The Threshold and the Jolt of Pain," p. 130.

145. "Stutterers are not aphasics": David B. Rosenfield, "Stuttering," *Critical Reviews in Clinical Neurobiology,* 1, no. 2 (1984): 118.

146. See Rosemary D. Hammond, "Distinguishing Stutterers from Nonstutterers on the Basis of Their Handwriting" (1984).

147. There is one sequence in the movie where the jester (Danny Kaye), dressed as an old grandfather, is trying to fool the

king's troops into releasing him and his granddaughter Maid Jean (Glynis Johns). The granddaughter is supposedly deaf and can communicate only by feeling her grandfather's lips and by talking in sign language. At one point a soldier asks a question, which Danny Kaye repeats to his granddaughter as she reads his lips. She signs a long answer, which Danny Kaye interprets simply as "No." When the soldier asks why she took so long to say this and used so many hand signals, Danny Kaye says simply, "She stutters." (Elin Edwards, personal communication, February 2, 2000).

148. See J. G. Lockhardt, *Narrative of the Life of Sir Walter Scott* (New York: Dent, 1906), p. 5, editor's note.

149. Dickinson's mother was paralyzed in 1875. See Kamilla Denman, "Emily Dickinson's Volcanic Punctuation," *Emily Dickinson Journal* (1993), especially on Alan Helms's reading of Dickinson's poem "After great pain, a formal feeling comes—." Compare also the explicit theme of paralysis in Dickinson's "I've dropped my Brain—My Soul is numb—."

150. *OED,* s.v. "dash," citing Ronald Sutherland Gower, *My Reminiscences* (London: K. Paul, Trench, 1883), II.28.259: "Who the Dash is this person . . . and what the Dash does he here?"

151. Anna Nicholas, *An Idyl of the Wabash and Other Indiana Stories* (Indianapolis: Bowen-Merrill, 1899), p. 64.

152. *The Institutes of Gaius and Rules of Ulpian,* trans. James Muirhead (Edinburgh: T. and T. Clark, 1880), p. 13.

153. Anne Clark, *Lewis Carroll: A Biography* (London: Dent, 1979), p. 105. Drabble, "Thankyou and Goodnight." John Updike, "Getting the Words Out," in Updike, *Self-Consciousness: Memoirs* (New York: Knopf, 1989), p. 87. For more on Lewis Carroll, whom I discuss in terms of name-changing and punning, see Shell, *Polio and Its Aftermath,* p. 53.

154. Quotations concerning James are from Simon Nowell-Smith, comp., *The Legend of the Master* (London: Constable, 1947), pp. 13, 134, 10.

155. Ibid., p. 35 (testimony of James's contemporary Ger-

trude Atherton). Definitions here are from the *OED,* s.v. "er" and "uh."

156. Nowell-Smith, *The Legend of the Master,* p. 40.

157. Joseph Conrad, *Lord Jim: A Tale* (Edinburgh: William Blackwood, 1900), ch. 6.

158. Nowell-Smith, *The Legend of the Master,* p. 41.

159. Updike, "Getting the Words Out," p. 81n. Espousing the view of Joseph Sheehan, Updike believes that his stuttering is precipitated when "I feel myself in a false position," such as guilty of being "in the wrong." See Benson Bobrick, *Knotted Tongues: Stuttering in History and the Quest for a Cure* (New York: Simon and Schuster, 1995).

160. Quoted in Calder, *Willie.*

161. Morgan, *Maugham,* p. 15.

162. Updike, "Getting the Words Out," p. 87.

163. "Euphemism": substitution of an agreeable or at least nonoffensive expression for one whose plainer meaning might be harsh or unpleasant. "Anadiplosis" ("doubling back"): the rhetorical repetition of one or several words; specifically, repetition of a word that ends one clause at the beginning of the next. Throughout, for definitions, I have used the *OED* and sometimes also *A Glossary of Rhetorical Terms with Examples,* by Ross Scaife (www.uky.edu/ArtsSciences/Classics/rhetoric.html). The Francis Bacon quotation is from Bacon, *The Essays, or Counsels,* XI: "Of Great Place."

164. "Anaphora": the repetition of a word or phrase at the beginning of successive phrases, clauses, or lines (Scaife, *A Glossary of Rhetorical Terms*). The quotation is from Winston Churchill, Speech before the House of Commons, June 4, 1940.

165. "Anacoluthon": lack of grammatical sequence; a change in the grammatical construction within the same sentence. "Had ye been there—for what could that have done?" Milton, "Lycidas," in John Milton, *The Major Works* (New York: Oxford University Press, 2003), p. 41.

166. "Aposiopesis": a form of ellipsis by which a speaker

comes to an abrupt halt, seemingly overcome by passion (fear, excitement, etc.) or modesty. Scaife, *A Glossary of Rhetorical Terms.*

167. "Such rebels I—" (Virgil, *Aeneid,* 1.135; Neptune is speaking). "O judgment! thou art fled to brutish beasts, / And men have lost their reason. Bear with me, / My heart is in the coffin there with Caesar, / And I must pause till it come back to me" (Shakespeare, *Julius Caesar,* 3.2.104–107).

168. "Brachylogy": a general term for abbreviated or condensed expression; specific types of brachylogy include asyndeton and zeugma. "Ellipsis" is often used as a synonym. The suppressed word or phrase can usually be deduced from the surrounding context. "Aeolus haec contra" ("Aeolus thus [spoke] in reply"; Virgil, *Aeneid,* 1:76). "Non Cinnae, non Sullae longa dominatio" ("The despotisms of Cinna and Sulla were brief"; Tacitus, *Annals,* 1.1, trans. Alfred John Church and William Jackson Brodribb).

169. "Synecdoche": understanding one thing by means of another; the use of a part for the whole, or the whole for the part; a type of metonymy.

170. "Paronomasia": use of similar-sounding words; often, etymological wordplay. Quotation is from Matthew 16:18.

171. "Praeteritio" (or "paraleipsis"): pretended omission for rhetorical effect. The quotation is from Thucydides, "Funeral Oration of Pericles," *The History of the Peloponnesian War,* trans. Richard Crawley (New York: Dutton, 1950), pp. 122–123.

172. "Paraprosdokian": a surprising or unexpected ending of a phrase or series.

173. "Irony": an expression of something which is contrary to the intended meaning; the words say one thing but mean another. Quotation is from Shakespeare, *Julius Caesar,* 3.2.95–96.

174. When a text intended to be ironic is not seen as such, the effect can be disastrous. Defoe's contemporaries took his "Shortest Way with the Dissenters" literally and jailed him for it (the pamphlet satirized intolerance by calling for the suppression

of dissent at all costs, no matter how cruel the means). The case of Billy Budd (in Herman Melville's novella) is partly analogous.

175. Neurologists see palilalia as a symptom of Parkinsonism (especially the type that develops in the wake of encephalitis), in which a word or syllable is repeated and the flow of speech is interrupted.

On palilalia and schizophrenia, see Abe Bert Baker, *Clinical Neurology,* 4 vols. (New York: Hoeber-Harper, 1955), vol. 1, p. 376, quoting J. M. Nielsen: "Palilalia is a repetitive disturbance encountered in Parkinsonism and in encephalitis (as representatives of organic causes), and in schizophrenia."

On the connection with brain injuries, see Walter Russell Brain, *Speech Disorders: Aphasia, Apraxia, and Agnosia* (London: Butterworth, 1961), p. 107: "I have once met with palilalia as a temporary phenomenon in a patient who suffered from compression of the medulla."

176. *OED,* s.v. "emphasis." John Smith, *The Mysterie of Rhetorique Unvail'd* (London: G. Evershaw, 1657). Thomas Urquhart, "Ekskubalauron; or, The Discovery of a Most Exquisite Jewel" (1652), in Urquhart, *Works* (Edinburgh, 1834), p. 292.

177. *Journal of Neurology and Psychopathology,* 8 (1927): "The palilalia (as with stammering) disappears during pre-formed speech automatisms, as, for instance, when the patient reads aloud, sings or recites."

178. Unsigned editorial, "Palilalia and Gertrude Stein," *Journal of the American Medical Association,* 103, no. 22 (December 1, 1934): 1711–12. The writer here is considering the case of the author Gertrude Stein. See also *OED,* s.v. "palilalia"; and E. H. Bensely, "Gertrude Stein as a Medical Student," *Pharos,* 47 (Spring 1984): 36–37.

2. Testing the Word

1. Robert Phillipson and Tove Skutnabb-Kangas, "Linguicide," *The Encyclopedia of Language and Linguistics,* 10 vols.

(New York: Pergamon, 1994), pp. 2211–12. See also Tove Skutnabb-Kangas and Sertac Bucak, "Killing a Mother Tongue: How the Kurds are Deprived of Linguistic Human Rights," in Tove Skutnabb-Kangas and Robert Phillipson, eds., with Mart Rannut, *Linguistic Human Rights: Overcoming Linguistic Discrimination* (New York: Mouton de Gruyter, 1994), pp. 347–370. See too Jaroslav Rudnyc'kyj, *Linguicide,* 3rd rev. ed. (Winnipeg: Ukrainian Technological University, 1976); and Liudmyla Kovalenko, *Linguicide in Bad Ems, 1876,* Texts in Ukrainian and English, English translations by Ol'ha Woycenko (Winnipeg: n.p., 1976).

2. "Fostbraedrasaga, or Fóstbrœðra Saga," in Guðbrandur Vigfússon and F. York Powell, eds. and trans., *Origines Islandicae: A Collection of the More Important Sagas and Other Native Writings Relating to the Settlement and Early History of Iceland,* 2 vols. (Oxford: Clarendon Press, 1905), 2.5.

3. Earle Stanley Gardner, *The Case of the Stuttering Bishop* (New York: Pocket Books, 1936).

4. William S. Gilbert and Arthur S. Sullivan, *The Mikado* (1885), Act 1, "I Am So Proud." Sung simultaneously by Ko-Ko, Pooh-Bah, and Pish-Tush.

5. Concerning this pun-laden line, Panagiota Batsaki writes: "It is very hard for a Greek to enunciate this phrase well" (personal communication, November 2003).

6. Tachyphemia is speech that is unintelligible due to rapid speaking rate and erratic rhythm.

7. Among the relevant works by Alexander Melville Bell would be *Observations on Defects of Speech, the Cure of Stammering, and the Principles of Elocution,* new ed. (1883); *The Faults of Speech: A Self-Corrector and Teachers' Manual* (Salem, Mass.: J. P. Burbank, 1880); *The Principles of Speech and Vocal Physiology, and Dictionary of Sounds, Embracing a Full Theoretical Development for the Guidance of Parents, Teachers, Public Speakers, &c., with Minute Practical Directions and Exercise for the Cure of Stammering,* and *All Impediments and Faults of Articulation,* new ed. (London: Hamilton, Adams, 1863).

Among works by Alexander Graham Bell, see *Establishment for the Study of Vocal Physiology, for the Correction of Stammering and Other Defects of Utterance, and for Practical Instruction in "Visible Speech"* (Boston: Rand, Avery, 1872).

8. In John Milton's *Samson Agonistes,* the Chorus tells the tale this way: "Thy words to my remembrance bring / How Succoth and the fort of Penuel / Their great deliverer contemned, / The matchless Gideon, in pursuit / Of Madian, and her vanquished kings; / And how ingrateful Ephraim / Had dealt with Jephtha, who by argument / Not worse than by his shield and spear, / Defended Israel from the Ammonite, / Had not his prowess quelled their pride / In that sore battle when so many died / Without reprieve, adjudged to death / For want of well pronouncing *Shibboleth.*"

9. Francis Marion Crawford, *The Rulers of the South: Sicily, Calabria, Malta* (New York: Macmillan, 1900–1901), p. 321.

10. John Cleveland, *The Rustick Rampant; or, Rurall Anarchy Affronting Monarchy in the Insurrection of Wat Tiler* (London: Printed for F.C., 1658), p. 36.

11. James Heath, *Flagellum; or, The Life and Death, Birth and Burial of Oliver Cromwel, Faithfully Described in an Exact Account of His Policies and Successes, Not Heretofore Published or Discovered, by S.T.* (London: Printed for L.R., 1663), p. 123.

12. Henry Cassels Kay, *Yemen: Its Early Medieval History* (London, 1892), p. 36.

S. Lane Poole, *History of Egypt in the Middle Ages* (Karachi: S. M. Mir), p. 300.

The emphatic voiced alveolo-palatal spirant *r* may be unique to Thaqovelith, one of the twenty varieties of Berber. As such, it often serves as a shibboleth, in that speakers of Arabic and French pronounce it as an "ell." See Gregory Paul Schaltz, *A Descriptive Phonology of Thaqovelith* (Diss., Illinois Institute of Technology, 1980).

13. Edwidge Danticat, *The Farming of Bones: A Novel* (New York: Soho Press, 1998). Rita Dove, *Selected Poems* (New York:

Vintage, 1993). For a historical account, see R. Michael Malek, "The Dominican Republic's General Rafael L. Trujillo and the Haitian Massacre of 1937: A Case of Subversion in Inter-Caribbean Relations," *Annals of the Southeastern Council on Latin American Studies,* 11 (March 1980): 137–155; and Michelle Wucker, *Why the Cocks Fight: Dominicans, Haitians, and the Struggle for Hispaniola* (New York: Hill and Wang, 1999).

14. The first book illustrated by Dr. Seuss was Alexander Abington, ed., *Boners: Being a Collection of Schoolboy Wisdom, or Knowledge as It Is Sometimes Written, Compiled from Classrooms and Examination Papers* (New York: Viking, 1931).

15. See Curtis F. Jones, *The Army Specialized Training Program: Gateway to the Foreign Service,* www.unc.edu/depts/diplomat/AD_Issues/amdipl_6/jones_astp.html. In the years 1936–1938, cartoonist Rube Goldberg had a cartoon strip called *Lala Palooza.*

16. Patricia Beatty, *Charley Skedaddle* (New York: Morrow, 1987). Charley Quinn, former member of a New York City street gang, is determined to avenge the death of his older brother who was killed at the Battle of Gettysburg. Too young to enlist as a soldier in the Union Army, he sneaks onto a troop ship and becomes a drummer boy. His eagerness to kill fades when he sees men dying all around him and even shoots one Confederate soldier himself. Charley "skedaddles" into the wilderness and is reluctantly taken in by a tough old mountain woman. She does not trust him at first, and he must hide his identity from the mountain folk, who would shoot him at the first sound of his northern accent.

Skedaddle, in its current sense ("scram," "vamoose," "exit unceremoniously"), was first recorded in the 1860s, during the Civil War. It could be a frequentative form of *skip,* in which case its ultimate source would be the Old French *esquiper,* "to leave by ship," and it would be cognate with *ship* and *skiff.* Yet *skedaddle* was also a dialect word in the north of England long before the 1860s; it meant "to spill." See William B. Stark, "The Great Skedaddle," *Atlantic Monthly,* 162 (July 1938): 86.

17. Abraham Tucker, *The Light of Nature Pursued* (1834; orig. pub. 1768–1774), 2.622. Raphael Holinshed, *The Firste (Laste) Volume of the Chronicles of England, Scotlande, and Irelande* (1577–1587), 2.13/1.

18. In *A Collection of Psalms and Hymns from Various Authors: For the Use of Serious and Devout Christians of All Denominations* (London: J. and W. Oliver, 1774).

19. William Beveridge, *Sermons* (London: Arthur Bettesworth and William Innys, 1729; orig. pub. 1680) 1.111. Robert Sanderson, *Sermons* (London, 1620), 1.157.

20. See *Cornhill Magazine* (October 1866): 464. "The affected, lisping, and haw-haw fool."

21. Jehan Palsgrave, *Lesclarcissement de la langue françoyse* (1852; orig. pub. 1530), 612.2.

22. Richard Steele, *Tatler,* no. 27 (1709): 5. "She has naturally a very agreeable Voice and Utterance, which she has chang'd for the prettiest Lisp imaginable." Compare Lady Mary Wortley Montagu, Letter to Countess Mar, November 21, 1716: "They all affect a little soft lisp" (*Letters, 1709–1762* [London: J. M. Dent, 1906]). See also Charles Dickens, *Dombey and Son* (London, 1848), p. 36: "A young lady of sixty-five . . . who spoke with an engaging lisp."

23. Thomas Gataker, *A Mistake or Misconstruction, Removed* (London, 1646), p. 31.

24. From the CD *My Name Is Joe* (Jive, 2000).

25. Doris Lessing, *The Golden Notebook,* cited in Margaret Drabble, "Public Speech and Public Silence," address to the British Stammering Association, October 18, 2001, Gulbenkian Lecture Hall, Oxford; reprinted in *Speaking Out,* publication of the British Stammering Association (Summer–Fall 2002).

26. Johann Georg Hamann to Immanuel Kant, late December 1759, in *The Cambridge Edition of The Works of Immanuel Kant,* trans. and ed. Arnulf Zweig (Cambridge: Cambridge University Press, 1999).

27. John Updike, *Getting the Words Out* (Northridge, Calif.:

Lord John Press, 1988). Reprinted in John Updike, *Self-Consciousness: Memoirs* (New York: Knopf, 1989), ch. 3. Quoted in Drabble, "Public Speech and Public Silence."

28. Thomas Middleton, *Father Hubburds Tales; or, The Ant and Nightingale,* in Middleton, *Works,* ed. Arthur Henry Bullen (New York: AMS Press, 1964; orig. pub. 1604), 8.80: "She had a humour to lisp often, like a flattering wanton."

29. Joanna Baillie, *Count Basil,* 2.4, in Baillie, *Works* (London: Longman, Brown, Green, 1851), p. 27: "The lisp'd flattery of a cunning child."

30. Fanny Burney, *Diary,* August 13, 1786: "Lady Charlotte is very handsome, . . . she unfortunately lisps very much."

31. Drabble, "Public Speech and Public Silence."

32. For other "explanations" of the Castilian lisp, see André Martinet, "The Unvoicing of Old Spanish Sibilants," *Romance Philology* (1951). According to one version of the story, King Ferdinand had some sort of physical defect that affected the way he spoke.

33. Shakespeare, *King Henry IV, Part II* (2.3):

> There were two honours lost, yours and your son's.
> For yours, the God of heaven brighten it!
> For his, it stuck upon him as the sun
> In the grey vault of heaven, and by his light
> Did all the chivalry of England move
> To do brave acts: he was indeed the glass
> Wherein the noble youth did dress themselves:
> He had no legs that practised not his gait;
> And speaking thick, which nature made his blemish,
> Became the accents of the valiant;
> For those that could speak low and tardily
> Would turn their own perfection to abuse,
> To seem like him: so that in speech, in gait,
> In diet, in affections of delight,
> In military rules, humours of blood,
> He was the mark and glass, copy and book,
> That fashion'd others.

34. Thomas Fuller, *The History of the Worthies of England* (1662; orig. pub. 1661), "Leicester," 2.126. "Lisping accent": Samuel J. Pratt, *The Pupil of Pleasure* (1777; orig. pub. 1776), 1.27.

35. Battista Guarini, *Il Pastor Fido: The Faithfull Shepheard, with an Addition of Divers Other Poems,* trans. Richard Fanshawe (London, 1646), p. 142.

36. Edward Hoagland, "The Threshold and the Jolt of Pain," in *Heart's Desire: The Best of Edward Hoagland—Essays from Twenty Years* (New York: Summit, 1988), p. 131.

37. René Bernard, *Le Bègue sur la scène française* (Paris: Droz, 1945). Maurice Sand, *Masques et Bouffons* (Paris: A. Levy Fils, 1862), 2.325–332. More generally on Tartaglia, see Giacomo Oreglia, *The Commedia dell'Arte,* trans. Lovett F. Edwards, introd. Evert Sprinchom (London: Methuen, 1968), passim.

38. Ruby Rohrlich, *The Puerto Ricans: Culture Change and Language Deviance* (Tucson: University of Arizona Press, 1974). Joseph Letie Stewart, *The Problem of Stuttering in Certain North American Indian Societies* (Washington, D.C.: American Speech and Hearing Association, 1960).

39. Anna Seward, *Memoirs of the Life of Dr. Darwin* (London: J. Johnson, 1804), pp. 63, 64. Charles Robert Darwin himself also stuttered. His son Francis wrote: "When puzzled in talking, [Charles Robert Darwin] had a peculiar stammer on the first word of a sentence" (Francis Darwin, ed., *The Life and Letters of Charles [Robert] Darwin, Including an Autobiographical Chapter,* 3 vols. [London: John Murray, 1887], vol. 1, p. 59). Charles Robert Darwin records a relevant anecdote in his autobiography: "One evening a poor young man got up, and after stammering for a prodigious length of time, blushing crimson, he at last slowly got out the words, 'Mr. President, I have forgotten what I was going to say'" (*Life and Letters,* vol. 1, p. 18).

40. Simon Nowell-Smith, comp., *The Legend of the Master, Henry James* (New York: Oxford University Press, 1985), pp. 32, 43.

41. Johann Dolaeus, *Encyclopaedia Chirurgica Rationalis* (Venice, 1711).

42. Ted Morgan, *Maugham* (New York: Simon and Schuster, 1980), p. 15. "Maugham had not stuttered while he lived in France."

43. Robert Calder, *Willie: The Life of W. Somerset Maugham* (London: Heinemann, 1989), p. 11.

44. Benjamin Humphrey Smart, *A Practical Grammar of English Pronunciation: On Plain and Recognized Principles, Calculated to Assist in Removing Every Objectionable Peculiarity of Utterance Arising from Either Foreign, Provincial, or Vulgar Habits, or from a Defective Use of the Organs of Speech . . . ; Together with Directions to Persons Who Stammer in Their Speech; Comprehending Some New Ideas Relative to English Prosody* (London: John Richardson and J. Johnson, 1810).

45. Grace A. McCullough and Agnes V. Birmingham, *Correcting Speech Defects and Foreign Accent* (New York: Scribner's, 1925).

46. When I read Shakespeare's *Merchant of Venice* for the first time, it seemed to me that the play was a drama in which people who were not Venetian simply couldn't speak well, or rather properly, with Venetians—and so they were abused. I understood Portia to be calling her suitors animals because they did not speak proper Italian. And above all, there was the speech of the alien Shylock—his terrifying and threatening language, his punning, quasi-barbaric, and virtually stuttering use of standard "Italian" to reveal and revel in the hidden truth about Italy—patterns that were of the greatest interest to me and that caused the Italians around him to call him a half-animal, indeed a werewolf. Such aliens cannot hear the music of Italian—do not have the music in them. And this turns out to be a great problem for Shylock's daughter, Jessica.

47. Glen J. Doman, *What To Do About your Brain-injured Child, or Your Brain-Damaged, Mentally Retarded, Mentally Deficient, Cerebral-Palsied, Emotionally Disturbed, Spastic, Flaccid, Rigid,*

Epileptic, Autistic, Athetoid, Hyperactive Child, illus. David Melton (Garden City, N.Y.: Doubleday, 1974).

48. Elizabeth Stucley, *The Contrary Orphans* (New York: Franklin Watts, 1961).

49. Arthur C. Clarke, "Painful Memory of a Silent Stalker," *Times Higher Education Supplement,* History of Science (June 29, 2001): 34.

50. *OED,* s.v. "rattle." "Persons are said to have the 'death-rattle' or 'ruttle' in their dying moments": C. Clough Robinson, *The Dialect of Leeds and Its Neighbourhood* (1862), p. 396.

51. The tension between activity and passivity was already embedded in the stuttering literature of the time, including that for children. An example is Ruth Arthur, *Miss Ghost* (New York: Athenaeum, 1979), a novel about a little girl named Elphie. "Stuttering is referred to as stammering in this story, and although Elphie does not stutter often, it is clearly a cause of dismay when her 'wretched stammer' occurs. Elphie stutters during painful or difficult conversations. . . . She refers to stuttering as 'something that happens to her, not as something that she does.'" Tahirih Bushey and Richard Martin, "Stuttering in Children's Literature," *Language, Speech and Hearing Services in the Schools,* 19, no. 3 (July 1988): 235–250.

52. *Johnny Rocco* (1958), directed by Paul Landres, is based on the story "I Led Three Lives," by the actor Richard Eyer, who plays the young boy Johnny Rocco in the movie.

53. A. M. Drummond, ed., *Studies in Rhetoric and Public Speaking, in Honor of James Albert Winans, by Pupils and Colleagues* (New York: Russell and Russell, 1962). In addition to essays on Plato and Aristotle, on medieval preaching, by Francis Bacon on political oratory, by De Quincey on public speaking, and on the "literary criticism of oratory" by Herbert August Wichelns (who first published this important piece in the Cornell tradition of rhetoric in 1925), this volume also contains Smiley Blanton's "Stuttering" and Margaret Gray Blanton's "Speech Defects Other Than Stuttering."

Andrew Comstock, *Remarks on Stammering, from a Lecture on Elocution Delivered Before the American Lyceum, May 6, 1837* (Philadelphia, 1837).

54. This question is also raised in the 1937 Warner Brothers movie *The Case of the Stuttering Bishop*, based on a 1936 book in the Perry Mason series by Earle Stanley Gardner. This murder mystery concerns a large inheritance, and the key figure is a bishop from Australia who asks for Perry Mason's help. But as he tells his story, it is obvious that he is a stutterer. Immediately, Mason begins to doubt his veracity. The following scene (which inspired the 1959 episode in the TV series *Perry Mason*) occurs between Mason and his secretary.

Secretary: Well, Chief, how do you figure?
Mason: Della, bishops don't stutter.
Secretary: That's what I thought when he barged in here. But you wouldn't listen.
Mason: Bishops have to talk in public. If a man stutters, he won't even become a minister let alone a bishop.

At the end of the movie, the bishop provides an explanation:

Mason: I hope you'll pardon a personal question. Isn't it a bit unusual for a bishop to stutter?
Bishop: It's a defect which I overcame in my childhood, Mr. Mason. It never comes back to me except when I'm under some emotional shock.

Before he boards a ship back to Australia, the bishop is kissed farewell by some very attractive women. Flustered by this, he exclaims, "G-G-Goodness gracious!" And the movie ends on a light note.

55. Abraham Herbert Kanter and Abe Samuel Kohn, *—And the Stutterer Talked* (Boston: Bruce Humphries, 1938), p. 91.

56. See Robert B. Ray, *How a Film Theory Got Lost, and Other Mysteries in Cultural Studies* (Bloomington: Indiana University Press, 2001), ch. 1.

57. André Bazin, "L'Evolution du langage cinématogra-

phique," from three of his articles—the first for the book *Vingt ans de cinéma à Venise* (1952), the second, "Le Découpage et son évolution," from *L'Age nouveau,* 93 (July 1955), and the third from *Cahiers du cinéma,* 1 (1950), in *Qu'est-ce que le cinéma?* vol. 1: *Ontologie et langage* (Paris: Cerf, 1958), pp. 131–148, and in *Qu'est-ce que le cinéma?* single-volume edition (Paris: Cerf, 1975), pp. 63–80. Translated as "The Evolution of the Language of Cinema," in Hugh Gray, *What Is Cinema?* vol. 1 (Berkeley: University of California Press, 1967), pp. 23–40.

58. James Hynes, *Publish and Perish: Three Tales of Tenure and Terror* (New York: Picador, 1997).

59. Randle Cotgrave, *A Dictionarie of the French and English Tongues* (London: Adam Islip, 1611), s.v. "narquois": "the gibbridge, or barbarous language used among them [Gypsies]." See too Homer's *Iliad* in William Cowper's translation (1791), ii.1063: "The Carians, people of a barbarous speech."

60. From the preface to the King James Version of the Bible (1611): "The Scythian counted the Athenian, whom he did not understand, barbarous."

When anglophones say, "That person was abbobed" (i.e., astonished), they employ a particular adaptation of *balbus.* See W. B. D. D. Turnbull, ed., *Arthour and Merlin: A Metrical Romance, Now First Edited from the Auchinleck Ms.* [1330] (Edinburgh: Abbotsford Club, 1838), line 1969: "The messangers were abobbed tho, Thai nisten what thai mighten do." On cognates, the *OED,* s.v. "barbarous," says: "The Greek word had probably a primary reference to speech, and is compared with Latin *balbus* (stammering). The sense-development in ancient times was (with the Greeks) 'foreign, non-Hellenic,' later 'outlandish, rude, brutal'; (with the Romans) 'not Latin nor Greek,' then 'pertaining to those outside the Roman empire'; hence 'uncivilized, uncultured,' and later 'non-Christian,' whence 'Saracen, heathen'; and generally 'savage, rude, savagely cruel, inhuman.' One has to account here for the *l–r* change. . . . It will be noted that some of these contortions involve also an interchange between *l* and *r,* which is not so general a sound-change, but which is exemplified in some differences between Greek and Latin (e.g., Greek *leirion,* 'lily,' Latin *lilium;* Greek *barbaros,* 'a non-Greek-speaker,' Latin *balbus,* stammerer." Cf. etymology of *Hottentot.*

61. William Bonde, *A Devoute Treatyse in Englysshe, Called the Pylgrimage of Perfeccyon* (London: W. de Worde, 1531; orig. pub. 1526), p. 2: "My wytte is grosse . . . and my tonge very barbarouse." Andrew Boorde, *The Introduction of Knowledge* (London: W. Copland, 1547), p. 221: "Barbarouse Latin doth alter from trew Latins." Thomas Starkey, *England in the Reign of Henry the Eighth: A Dialogue between Cardinal Pole and Thomas Lupset Lecturer in Rhetoric at Oxford* (London, 1538), p. 193: "To see al our law . . . wryten in thys barbarouse langage" (i.e., Old French).

62. John Ruskin, *Political Economy of Art* (London: Smith, Elder, 1857), p. 19.

63. John Hill Burton, *The Scot Abroad* (Edinburgh: Blackwood, 1864), 2.178.

64. John Marston, *Scourge of Villanie* (London, 1598), iii.ix.G.8.b.

65. Procopius of Caesarea, *History of the Wars,* 7 vols., trans. from the Greek by H. B. Dewing (Cambridge, Mass.: Harvard University Press, 1914; rpt. 1953–1954), 2.11–23.

66. Jerome, *Letters and Select Works* (Letter 127, to Principia), vol. 6 of *Nicene and Post-Nicene Fathers: Second Series,* ed. Philip Schaff and Henry Wace (Peabody, Mass.: Hendrickson, 1994).

3. Animals That Talk

1. These days, I have my doubts.

2. *Caxton's Aesop* (1484), ed. Robert Thomas Lenaghan (Cambridge, Mass.: Harvard University Press, 1967).

3. John Vanbrugh, *Aesop* (London: Thomas Bennet, 1697), 2.1.

4. Some writers deny the existence of such a person as Aesop, and it is true that we have but scanty details on his life and

work. Even his appearance is in dispute. According to a monk of Constantinople named Maximus Planudes, writing in the fourteenth century, Aesop was an ugly, deformed dwarf; the famous marble statue at the Villa Albani in Rome shows him in this guise. But Plutarch, writing some 1,300 years earlier, says nothing about his appearance. Indeed, the Athenians are said to have put up a noble statue in honor of Aesop.

5. From A. André Ntonfo, cited in Françoise Naudillon, *Jean Métellus* (Paris: Harmattan, 1994), p. 144: "Après avoir donc écrit *La Parole prisonnière* sur le plan de l'état et des conditions de vie politique haïtienne, j'ai décrit les conditions de vie qui interdisent la parole."

6. Isaiah 28:11. The same verse was quoted in Chapter 2, in another translation.

7. Dwight N. Hopkins and George C. L. Cummings, *Cut Loose Your Stammering Tongue: Black Theology in the Slave Narratives* (Maryknoll, N.Y.: Orbis Books, 1991).

8. See Jack C. Horn and Jeff Meer, "The Pleasure of Their Company: *PT* Survey Report on Pets," *Psychology Today* (1984): 52–59. This fraction does not include those who use animal-training commands with "working animals." In "How to Say 'Fetch!'" (*Raritan,* 3 [Fall 1983]: 12), Vicki Hearne writes—concerning her relationship to her dog Salty—that "love, of course, is getting into things," but does not define the precise quality of her love or speech as trainer. See, too, Vicki Hearne, "Moral Transformation of the Dog, and Other Thoughts on the Animals among Us" (*Harper's,* 268 [January 1984]: 57–67), also written from the trainer's viewpoint.

9. James Russell Lowell, *Letters* (1894), 2.465: "My dog . . . looks up at me as who should say, 'You are become unspeakable [cf. *infantile*] as one of us, poor old fellow!'"

10. On hippotherapy and stuttering, see Marc Shell, *Polio and Its Aftermath* (Cambridge, Mass.: Harvard University Press, 2005), pp. 92–98. Hippotherapy, from the Greek *hippos* (horse)—sometimes also called "equine assisted therapy"—relies on prosthetic

as well as natural affiliations between human and animal movement.

11. Stephen Cosgrove, *Creole* (Los Angeles: Price Stern Sloan, 1983), a book for children aged 5–9. The central character is an alligator who stutters. See also Kristín Steinsdóttir, *Ármann og Blíða* (Armann and Gentle; 1994). The book is about Armann, who is six years old and stutters, and his cat, Gentle. Originally written in Icelandic, it has been translated into English and is available from the Stuttering Foundation of America.

12. I was first introduced to Stevenson's work in 1957, by way of a dramatization of *Treasure Island.* This children's drama was written by Jules Eckert Goodman, an author already well known from *The Silent Voice.* It appears in Montrose Jonas Moses, ed., *Another Treasury of Plays for Children* (Boston: Little, Brown, 1926), pp. 3–95.

13. Friedrich Max Müller, *Natural Religion* (London: Longmans, Green, 1889), p. 361.

14. Robert Arthur, *The Mystery of the Stuttering Parrot,* illustrated by Harry Kane (New York: Random House, 1964). Leo Edwards (Edward Edson Lee), *Poppy Ott and the Stuttering Parrot,* illustrated by Bert Salg (New York: Grosset and Dunlap, 1926).

15. Low German *tateln:* "to gabble," "to cackle," like a goose.

16. Irene Pepperberg, *The Alex Studies: The Cognitive and Communicative Abilities of Grey Parrots* (Cambridge, Mass.: Harvard University Press, 1999).

17. Gary K. Wolf, discussing the making of the movie *Who Framed Roger Rabbit?* Wolf, who wrote the book on which this movie was based, says that the actor who supplied Roger's voice "tried a lisp, a slobber, etc and finally came up with the stuttered *p.* That wasn't in my book, but it works perfectly."

18. Dr. Seuss, *Gerald McBoing Boing: Told by the Great Gildersleeve,* 45-rpm record (Hollywood: Capitol Records, 1950). The animated cartoon was originally released by United Productions of America in 1951, and won an Academy Award. The book, il-

lustrated by Mel Crawford, was first published in 1952 and was reissued by Random House in 2000.

19. Lewis Carroll, *Sylvie and Bruno* [1889], in *The Complete Works of Lewis Carroll* (New York: Barnes and Noble, 1994), ch. 14, p. 264.

20. The film *Once in a Lifetime* was an adaptation of the play by Moss Hart and George S. Kaufman.

21. See *OED,* s.v. "dub," v5.

22. A bit of trivia: Some complicated dubbing went on behind the scenes. Kathy was supposed to dub Lina's singing voice, but that was done by someone other than Debbie Reynolds. And Kathy's dubbing of Lina's speaking voice was actually dubbed by—surprise!—Jean Hagen. Jean Hagen had more stage experience than Debbie Reynolds and was considered a better choice.

This merry mixup of real-life dubbing was addressed in Ray Hagen's article on Jean Hagen in *Film Fan Monthly* (December 1968): "In the film, Debbie Reynolds has been hired to re-dub Hagen's dialogue and songs in the latter's first talking picture. We see the process being done in a shot of Reynolds . . . matching her dialogue to Hagen's and synchronizing it while watching a scene from the film. But the voice that is used to replace Hagen's shrill, piercing one is not Reynolds' but Hagen's own quite lovely natural voice, meaning that Jean Hagen dubs Debbie Reynolds dubbing Jean Hagen! To further confuse matters, the voice we hear as Hagen mimes 'Would You?,' supposedly supplied by Reynolds, is that of yet a third girl, [Betty Royce]." See Laura Wagner, "'I Dub Thee': A Guide to the Great Voice Doubles," *Classic Images,* 281 (November 1998), www.classicimages.com/1998/november98/idibthee.html.

23. My own favorite examples of such dubbing concern two polios. In *Interrupted Melody* (1955), opera singer Eileen Farrell did the singing for Eleanor Parker, who portrays the opera singer Marjorie Lawrence, felled by polio. Peg La Centra did the sing-

ing for the real-life polio Ida Lupino in two films: *The Man I Love* (1946), in which Lupino plays the singer Petey Brown, and *Escape Me Never* (1947), in which Lupino plays Gemma Smith.

24. The song also alludes to the fact that Moses paints Aaron's toes red with the blood of a ram. Here, some might see that there are two "Moseses" in opposition: the one who supposes and the one who knowses. Others, in discussing this "nursery rhyme" per se, point to Leviticus 22–24, where the "dummy" Moses, using the blood of a ram, paints the toes of his "ventriloquist" brother Aaron red.

25. On Muybridge's studies of horses and other animals in motion, see Shell, *Polio and Its Aftermath,* pp. 96, 131, 134–135.

26. Walt Disney was probably inspired by *Dinner Time* when he made his own first sound cartoon, but he and his company failed to give the film the credit it deserved.

27. Gerald F. Johnson, "A Clinical Study of Porky Pig Cartoons," *Journal of Fluency Disorders,* 12 (1987): 235–238. Porky Pig's stuttering topography includes stuttering when he talks to animals.

28. I. Biran and I. Steiner, "The Speech Disorder of Doc in Walt Disney's *Snow White and the Seven Dwarfs,*" *Neurology,* 57 (2001): 363.

29. Mel Blanc, *That's Not All, Folks* (New York: Warner Books, 1988), pp. 65, 66.

30. Ibid., p. 64. Eventually, someone else also played the role of the bull (p. 68).

31. On Barney Rubble's laugh, see Blanc, *That's Not All, Folks,* p. 222.

The word for "stutter" in Jèrriais (a Norman dialect spoken on the Isle of Jersey) is *aheuqu'ter,* which sounds like the French word *hoqueter,* meaning "hiccup." Perhaps, for the residents of the Isle of Jersey, it connotes not only hiccupping but also stuttering. Historically, certain cultures seem to have regarded stuttering and hiccupping as similar breathing disorders.

32. Blanc, *That's Not All, Folks,* pp. 7, 5.

33. Ibid., pp. 102, 106, 223.

34. Ibid., p. 66; cf. 115–117. Speedy Gonzales first appeared in 1953.

35. Ibid., p. 114.

36. R. Tincoff and M. D. Hauser, "Cognitive Basis for Language Evolution in Nonhuman Primates," in K. Brown, ed., *Encyclopedia of Language and Linguistics,* 2nd ed. (Oxford: Elsevier, forthcoming), cited in Carmen Gloria Iguina, "Primate Vocal Communication: Evidence for Adjustment in Response to Auditory Feedback" (Senior Honors Thesis, Harvard College, 2005).

37. Warner Brothers–Looney Tunes, *Porky's Poppa,* black-and-white animated feature directed by Robert Clampett, produced by Leon Schlesinger, animated by Chuck Jones, written by Ben Harrison, music by Carl W. Stalling (originally released January 15, 1938).

38. Anonymous, "Stutterers Object to Porky Pig Ad," *Lansing State Journal* (December 8, 1991): 51. This Associated Press article, which deals with a Warner Brothers catalog, quotes Ira Zimmerman of the National Stuttering Project.

39. A few once-influential theorists of stuttering have claimed that certain cultures have no stuttering; see, for example, W. Johnson, "The Indians Have No Word for It: Stuttering in Children," *Quarterly Journal of Speech,* 30 (1944): 330–337. But this position has been disproved many times—e.g., by Joseph L. Stewart, *The Problem of Stuttering in Certain North American Indian Societies,* Speech and Hearing Disorders monograph suppl. 6 (Washington, D.C.: American Speech and Hearing Association, 1960).

40. Initials or nicknames referring to the acquaintance of Elgar's whose personality is ostensibly suggested accompany each variation in the *Enigma Variations.* The variations offer glimpses into Elgar's relationships with several people. "Dorabella" (Variation 10, composed in 1899) is probably named after a character from Mozart's opera *Così fan tutte,* but it was also Elgar's nick-

name for his young acquaintance Dora Penny. She had a stutter, which Elgar may be alluding to with his lilting interruptions in the woodwinds. Mozart likewise alludes to stuttering in *Così,* when he has Don Alfonso deliver bad news to the sisters Dorabella and Fiordiligi:

> How to break the awful news!
> Stammer, stutter . . . it is no use.
> Woe is me, my tongue is tied
> And the words are stuck inside.
> What solution? What to do?
> Such a dreadful thunderbolt!
> Though I'd speak, my lips revolt.
> How my heart goes out to you,
> Hopes and dreams all gone askew.

(Trans. Donald Pippin; www.pocketopera.org/libs/cosi.htm.)

41. Emanuel Schikaneder, *Der Königssohn aus Ithaka* (The King's Son from Ithaka; Vienna, 1795), with music by Franz Anton Hoffmeister: "Ich schickte mich herrlich darein / Ein Paperl, ein Paperl zu seyn" ("I'd be suited so wonderfully well / A Polly, a Polly to be"). Quoted in Kurt Honolka, *Papageno: Emanuel Schikaneder, Man of the Theater in Mozart's Time,* trans. Jane Mary Wilde (Portland, Ore.: Amadeus Press, 1984), p. 166.

42. See Thomas-Simon Gueullette, ed., *Théâtre des boulevards, ou Recueil de parades,* 3 vols. (Paris: A. Mahon, 1756), esp. *Caracataca et Caracataqué,* in vol. 1.

43. So demonstrated the work of Fernando Nottebohm. See Michael Specter, "Rethinking the Brain: How the Songs of Canaries Upset the Fundamental Principle of Science," *New Yorker* (July 23, 2001): 42.

44. See David B. Rosenfield, "Stuttering," *Critical Reviews in Clinical Neurobiology,* 1, no. 2 (1984): 130. Actually, this is an old theory put forward in L. E. Travis, *Speech Pathology* (New York: Appleton-Century, 1931).

45. A. J. Doupe and P. K. Kuhl, "Birdsong and Human

Speech: Common Themes and Mechanisms," *Annual Review of Neuroscience,* 22 (1999): 567–631.

46. Specter, "Rethinking the Brain," p. 52, quoting Fernando Nottebohm.

47. In the research literature, the ratio of male stutterers to female stutters varies from about 2:1 to 4:1 (Rosenfield, "Stuttering," p. 133). On songmaking in male and female canaries, see Specter, "Rethinking the Brain," p. 44.

48. For an argument that they do, see A. L. Foundas, A. M. Bollich, D. M. Corey, M. Hurley, and K. M. Heilman, "Anomalous Anatomy of Speech-Language Areas in Adults with Persistent Developmental Stuttering," *Neurology,* 57 (2001): 207–215.

49. Jean Aitchison, *The Seeds of Speech: Language Origin and Evolution* (Cambridge: Cambridge University Press, 1996).

50. See Pepperberg, *The Alex Studies.*

51. See William Yate, *An Account of New Zealand* (London, 1835), ii.52, commenting on the Tui: "This remarkable bird, from the versatility of its talents for imitation, has by some been called 'the Mocking Bird.'" On avian mimicry in general, see Maxwell Knight, *Talking Birds,* illustrated by David Cornell (London: G. Bell, 1961).

52. Donald Mackenzie Wallace, *Russia* (London: Cassell, Petter and Galpin, 1877), p. 413: "the 'monkeyism' and 'parrotism' of those who indiscriminately adopted foreign manners and customs." See likewise Maria Edgeworth, *Ennui* (London: J. Johnson, 1809), where she laments that some people are "the mere puppets and parrots of fashion."

53. Max Müller, *Lectures on the Science of Language* (London: Longman, Green, 1861), p. 352.

54. The *mixophyes balbus,* also called the Southern Barred Frog, is indigenous to Australia.

55. Iguina, "Primate Vocal Communication," pp. 68, 75.

56. Ibid., pp. 11, 33, 45. See also A. Leonardo and M. Konishi, "Decrystallization of Adult Birdsong by Perturbation of Audi-

tory Feedback," *Nature,* 399 (1999): 466–470; and J. Cynx and U. Von Rad, "Immediate and Transitory Effects of Delayed Auditory Feedback on Bird and Song Production," *Animal Behavior,* 62 (2001): 305–312.

57. Robert R. Provine, "Laughter," *American Scientist,* 84 (1998): 38–45, esp. 40. See also idem, *Laughter: A Scientific Investigation* (London: Faber, 2000). On the evolution of the human vocal tract as a factor in language development, see Philip Lieberman, *The Biology and Evolution of Language* (Cambridge, Mass.: Harvard University Press, 1984).

58. *OED,* s.v. "spink," n1, 3; and s.v. "pink," n6, 1: "An imitation of the note of the chaffinch (often reduplicated: pink-pink); hence, by transference, a local name of the bird itself."

59. Leonardo and Konishi, "Decrystallization of Adult Birdsong by Perturbation of Auditory Feedback."

60. The figure of 7 percent has been confirmed in studies carried out by David B. Rosenfield, director of the Speech and Language Center, Baylor College of Medicine. None of the finches he studied had stuttering parents.

61. See Matthew M. Vriends, *Zebravinken en andere kleine Exoten* (Bussum: Van Dishoeck, 1967); and idem, *The Zebra Finch: An Owner's Guide to a Happy Healthy Pet* (Hoboken, N.J.: Wiley, 1997).

62. Charles Darwin, *Descent of Man* (London: Murray, 1971), p. 33.

63. Rousseau, Diderot, Rameau, and Condillac all made this link. For an early twentieth-century argument, see Otto Jespersen, *Language: Its Language, Nature, and Development* (London: Allen, 1922).

64. Rosenfield, "Stuttering," p. 124.

65. Daniel Rock, *The Church of Our Fathers, as Seen in St. Osmund's Rite for the Cathedral of Salisbury* (London, 1853), III.ii.21: "This drawing out of the notation for the Alleluia, they called the 'sequence.'"

66. See Aldous Huxley, *Island: A Novel* (London: Chatto and

Windus, 1962), p. 242: "long-drawn, almost bird-like melismata on a single vowel sound."

67. Notker Balbulus of St. Gall, *Notkeri poetae liber ymnorum* [*Liber hymnorum*] (Bern: Francke Verlag, 1960), pp. 6–9. Ekkehard says that Notker was "delicate of body but not of mind, stuttering of tongue but not of intellect."

68. For information about Notker's work, see John Stevens, *Words and Music in the Middle Ages* (New York: Cambridge University Press, 1986); and Jeremy Yudkin, *Music in Medieval Europe* (Englewood Cliffs, N.J.: Prentice Hall, 1989).

69. See the preface to Notker's *Liber hymnorum:* "When I was yet young and could not always succeed in retaining in my memory the long-drawn melodies on the last syllable of the Hallelujah, I cast about in my mind for some method of making them easier to remember. Now it happened that a certain priest from Gimedia [Jumièges] came to us who had an Antiphonarium, wherein were written some strophes to these melodies, but indeed by no means free from faults. This put it into my mind to compose others for myself after the same manner. I showed them to my teacher, Yso, whom they pleased on the whole, only he remarked, that as many notes as there were in the music, so many words must there be in the text. At this suggestion I went through my work again, and now Yso accepted it with full approbation, and gave the text to the boys to sing." This translation appears in Catherine Winkworth, *Christian Singers of Germany* (London: R. Clay Sons and Taylor, n.d.), pp. 12–13.

70. The oldest known chess game was a match between as-Suli (author of the first book about *shatranj,* an early form of chess) and al-Lajlaj. See H. J. R. Murray, *A History of Chess* (Oxford: Clarendon, 1913).

71. Henri Bergson, *Laughter: An Essay on the Meaning of the Comic,* trans. Cloudesley Brereton and Fred Rothwell (Los Angeles: Green Integer, 1999; orig. pub. London, 1911). Bergson also writes: "Is not something of the same kind found in the following sally of Figaro's (though here an attempt is perhaps made

to suggest the image of an animal rather than that of a thing): 'Quel homme est-ce?—C'est un beau, gros, court, jeune vieillard, gris pommelé, rusé, rasé, blasé, qui guette et furette, et gronde et geint tout à la fois.' ('What sort of man is here?—He is a handsome, stout, short, youthful old gentleman, iron-grey, an artful knave, clean shaved, clean "used up," who spies and pries and growls and groans all in the same breath.')"

72. Ibid., ch. 1, part 5. As I understand it, after the first performance of the opera *Le Nozze di Figaro* (1786), Mozart seemed to think that the magistrate Curzio should have been presented as a stutterer in the great sextet of Act 3. Likewise, some people have interpreted the woodwinds in the overture in terms of stuttering. "Mozart employs comic touches, such as the chattering woodwinds supposedly suggesting the magistrate Don Curzio's loose dentures and resultant stutter." Henry Wyatt, Program notes for concert at the Mason Gross School of the Arts, June 14, 2003 (Rutgers University, New Brunswick, N.J.).

73. "So science has determined that if you're going to tell a talking-animal joke, make it a duck." Richard Wiseman, quoted in Tad Friend, "What's So Funny? A Scientific Attempt to Discover Why We Laugh," *New Yorker* (November 11, 2002): 79. Wiseman is a professor at the University of Hertfordshire.

74. Blanc, *That's Not All, Folks,* p. 95; for examples, see p. 98.

75. Rosenfield, "Stuttering."

76. On the way in which the pulmonic air-stream mechanism (inhaled air modified to produce speech sounds) is used in Tsou, see Michael Fuller, "Pulmonic Ingressive Fricatives in Tsou," *Journal of the International Phonetic Association,* 20, no. 2 (1990): 9–14. Such sounds on inhalation are to be distinguished from stridor—a harsh vibrating noise produced by a bronchial, tracheal, or laryngeal obstruction. Therapists often note that stutterers try to talk on inhalation and treat that as a symptom of stuttering instead of (also) an attempt to cure it.

77. Bruce Baghemil, "The Morphology and Phonology of Katajjait (Inuit Throat Games)," *Canadian Journal of Linguistics /*

Revue Canadienne de Linguistique, 33, no. 1 (1988): 1–58; see esp. the section called "Pulmonic Egressive." Empty morphology is characteristic of certain other alternative speech forms found in the world, especially "ludlings" (game languages). It is clear that the Katajjait constitute just such a game language. See also Margarita Mazo, "Lament Made Visible: A Study of Paramusical Elements in Russian Lament," in Bell Yung and Lam Joseph, eds., *Themes and Variations: Writings on Music in Honor of Rulan Chao Pian* (Paris: Orphée, 1994), pp. 164–211. Mazo compares vocal production in lament with that in speech and singing, taking special note of voiced inhalations and (voiced) gasping exhalations at the ends of phrases. She remarks that many vocal effects in lament, such as vocal fry ("the use of a creaky, raspy-sounding voice") and glottal coup ("a spectral turbulence"), "have been observed in pathological rather than regular speech" (p. 196).

78. On stuttering and whoops, see Thomas Clifford Allbutt, ed., *A System of Medicine, by Many Writers* (New York, 1896–1899), 7.452.

79. Charles Darwin, *The Expression of the Emotions in Man and Animals* (London: John Murray, 1872), p. 129: "The purr of satisfaction, which is made during both inspiration and expiration." We now know that cats produce the purr through intermittent signaling of the laryngeal and diaphragmatic muscles. They purr during both inhalation and exhalation with a consistent pattern and a frequency of 25–150 hertz.

Hester Lynch Piozzi, *Observations and Reflections Made in the Course of a Journey through France, Italy, and Germany* (London: A. Strahan and T. Cadell, 1789), II.231: "An English lady once made me observe, that a cat never purrs when she is alone."

80. The *glottalic* air-stream mechanism uses the glottal stop. Many polio survivors—who have a good deal of experience with enforced caesuras (for example, in the iron lung) and with glosso-pharyngeal breathing (called "frog-breathing" or "air-stacking")—are quite good at speaking this way. There is also the

gastric air-stream mechanism, which uses air burped up from the stomach.

4. Moses' Tongue

1. *OED,* s.v. "sheva," "schwa," and "murmur."

2. The Ten Commandments are variously listed at Exodus 20:2–17, Exodus 34:12–26, and Deuteronomy 5:6–21. Compare the Latin: "Non adsumes nomen Domini Dei tui in vanum nec enim habebit insontem Dominus eum qui adsumpserit nomen Domini Dei sui frustra."

3. Ezekiel 13:6–9: "They have seen vanity and lying divination, saying, The Lord saith: and the Lord hath not sent them: and they have made others to hope that they would confirm the word. Have ye not seen a vain vision, and have ye not spoken a lying divination, whereas ye say, The Lord saith it; albeit I have not spoken? Therefore thus saith the Lord God; Because ye have spoken vanity, and seen lies, therefore, behold, I am against you, saith the Lord God. And mine hand shall be upon the prophets that see vanity, and that divine lies: they shall not be in the assembly of my people, neither shall they be written in the writing of the house of Israel, neither shall they enter into the land of Israel; and ye shall know that I am the Lord God."

4. See Marty Jezer's memoir, *Stuttering: A Life Bound Up in Words* (New York: Basic Books, 1997), p. 91.

5. For example, Dr. Einer Boberg, professor of speech pathology and cofounder of the Institute for Stuttering Treatment and Research, was a severe stutterer, and was so afraid of being teased that he quit school at age fifteen. Eventually he managed to conquer his fears and continue his education.

6. See the case of "Bill," a stutterer who turned down an opportunity to study at Oxford. "The oral dissertation required of him he could not fulfill. He was too broken to make the attempt." Abraham Herbert Kanter and Abe Samuel Kohn, *—And the Stutterer Talked* (Boston: Bruce Humphries, 1938), p. 157.

7. For Abraham's responses, see Genesis 22:1 and 22:7; see also Isaiah 6:8.

8. Neil Schmitz, "To the Speech Clinic," *International Quarterly* 3, no. 2 (1998): 36–39.

9. Geneva Bible (1560), Isaiah 32:4. In the 1611 edition of the King James Version, the term used in this passage is *stammerer.* Compare Richard Whitlock, *Zootomia* (1654), p. 150: "What mighty lines hath Isaiah? Read, and confesse Demosthenes and Cicero but Stammerers at Eloquence."

10. Exodus 3:13, trans. Robert Young, in *Young's Literal Translation of the Holy Bible* (rev. ed., 1898; rpt. Grand Rapids, Mich.: Barker Book House, 1953), brackets inserted by Young.

11. See James Malcolm Rymer, *The Unspeakable; or, The Life and Adventures of a Stammerer* (London: Clarke and Beeton, 1855).

12. W. Alan Froggatt, "I Am I Am According to Dr. Seuss" (poem), *Theology Today,* 48, no. 4 (January 1992): 465. Froggatt was a minister of the Congregational Church in Bridgewater, Connecticut.

13. George M. Lamsa, *The Holy Bible from Ancient Eastern Manuscripts: George M. Lamsa's Translations from the Aramaic of the Peshitta* (Philadelphia: Holman, 1957; orig. pub. in segments 1933, 1939, 1940, 1955).

14. "You know that I talk slowly and don't use the best words" (English Version for Deaf, 1978).

"I speak slowly, and I become tongue-tied easily" (God's Word, 1995).

"I am weak in speech, and slow-tongued" (English Septuagint, 1870).

"I have no command of words" (Moffatt New Translation, 1926).

"I am slow of speech and of an awkward tongue" (New Berkeley Version, 1969).

"I speak slowly and can't find the best words" (New Century Version, 1986).

"I'm clumsy with words" (New Living Translation, 1996).

"I am slow in talking and it is difficult for me to speak" (New Life Version, 1969).

"I am slow and hesitant" (Revised English Bible, 1989).

"I am slow of speech and slow in expressing my ideas" (The Shorter Bible, 1925).

"For heavy of mouth and heavy of tongue I am" (Restoration of Original Sacred Name, 1976).

"I am a poor speaker, slow and hesitant" (Today's English Version, 1971).

"I am a slow speaker and not able to speak well" (Jerusalem Bible, Catholic, 1966).

"When I get up before a crowd my tongue sticks to the roof of my mouth" (The Word Made Fresh, 1988).

15. These would include "unskilled in speech" (New American Standard Bible, 1963), "of deficient and impeded speech" (Amplified Bible, 1958), and "no orator" (New Living Translation, 1996). French translators offer "moi qui n'ai pas la parole facile" (Louis Segond, 1910) and "je n'ai pas la parole facile" (Bible de Semeur, 1992). German translations include "Ich bin einfach ein zu schlechter Redner" (Hoffnung für Alle).

16. This is the rendering given in the English Standard Version (1952), New International Version (1979), King James Version (1611), Twenty-First Century King James Version (1994), American Standard Version (1901), Young's Literal Translation (1862), and Darby Translation (1890).

17. "Uncircumcised lips'" *(aral sefatayim)* occurs at Exodus 6:12 and Exodus 6:30. Rashi, commenting on Exodus 6:12, says *aral sefatayim* or *atum sefatayim* (one whose lips are blocked). "Likewise, I [Rashi] say that all instances of the term *orla* mean 'blocked.'" Rashi gives six examples (Yirmiyahu, Habakuk). Rambam uses *aral sefatayim,* as opposed to *ragil.* An *aral sefatayim* is not learned and is unable to say Tefilla *(la'arokh Tefilla)* and praises. In some way his lips are "blocked," uncircumcised. Jeer 6:10 says: "To whom shall I speak, and give warning, that they

may hear? Behold, their ear is uncircumcised, and they cannot hearken: behold, the word of Yahweh is unto them a reproach; they have no delight in it."

Circumcision appears as a symbol of purity (Isaiah 52:1). We read of uncircumcised lips (Exodus 6:12, 30), ears (Jeremiah 6:10), and hearts (Leviticus 26:41). The fruit of a tree that is unclean is spoken of as uncircumcised (Leviticus 19:23).

Circumcision also signifies purification of the heart, inward circumcision effected by the Spirit (Deuteronomy 10:16, 30:6; Ezekiel 44:7; Acts 7:51; Romans 2:28; Colossians 2:11).

18. As Moses is making his way to Egypt, there occurs one of the most mysterious episodes in the Bible. Yahweh, for some reason, tries to kill Moses, and it is Tzipporah who comes to the rescue: with a sharp stone she circumcises "her son"—which one is not specified—and holds the severed foreskin to Moses' genitals (euphemistically called "feet") while saying, "Surely a bloody husband art thou to me." As a result, Yahweh spares Moses, with Tzipporah reiterating, "A bloody husband thou art, because of the circumcision." Is Yahweh angry enough to kill him because Moses—raised as an Egyptian—is uncircumcised? And does Tzipporah therefore circumcise Moses vicariously?

19. How difficult it must have been for Moses to hold up his hands during the battle of the Israelites and the Amalekites! He needs help—from Aaron and Hur. As long as the arm was up, the battle went well for the Israelites. "[9]: And Moses said unto Joshua, Choose us out men, and go out, fight with Amalek: to morrow I will stand on the top of the hill with the rod of God in mine hand. [10]: So Joshua did as Moses had said to him, and fought with Amalek: and Moses, Aaron, and Hur went up to the top of the hill. [11]: And it came to pass, when Moses held up his hand, that Israel prevailed: and when he let down his hand, Amalek prevailed. [12]: But Moses' hands were heavy; and they took a stone, and put it under him, and he sat thereon; and Aaron and Hur stayed up his hands, the one on the one side, and the other on the other side; and his hands were steady until the going

down of the sun. [13]: And Joshua discomfited Amalek and his people with the edge of the sword. [14]: And the Lord said unto Moses, Write this for a memorial in a book, and rehearse it in the ears of Joshua: for I will utterly put out the remembrance of Amalek from under heaven. [15]: And Moses built an altar, and called the name of it Jehovah-nissi: [16]: For he said, Because the Lord hath sworn that the Lord will have war with Amalek from generation to generation [Exodus 17]."

20. The Amalekites lived in the desert, south of Canaan around Kadesh (Genesis 14:7), otherwise known as the northern part of the Negev (Numbers 13:29; 14:25, 14:43). Amalek was the son of Eliphaz (Esau's eldest boy) by a concubine named Timna (Genesis 36:12) and became a "clan leader" or "chief" in the tribe of Esau (Genesis 36:15). Thus, the Amalekites were distant cousins of the Israelites. It is quite possible they knew that the land of Canaan had been promised to Esau's twin brother, Jacob; so they should not have felt any threat to their interests in the Negev, had this promise been remembered and taken seriously. After all, the promise was to be a means of blessing Amalek, along with all the other nations (Genesis 12:3), if only they, like Abraham, had believed. Instead, they "came" *(wayyabo')* and attacked Israel at Rephidim, some distance south of the north-central region in the Sinai where they lived (Exodus 17).

21. On Esau as Jacob's wrestling partner, see Marc Shell, *Polio and Its Aftermath* (Cambridge, Mass.: Harvard University Press, 2005), pp. 80–81. Compare Shakespeare, *Merchant of Venice,* 1.3: "If I can catch him once upon the hip . . ." On other analogies between Shylock and Jacob, see Marc Shell, "The Wether the Ewe," in Shell, *Money, Language, and Thought* (Berkeley: University of California Press, 1982).

22. Richard Wiseman, *Treatise on Wounds* (1672), I.ix.120. John Fisher (1469–1535), *English Works,* ed. John E. B. Mayor (London: N. Trübner for the Early English Text Society, 1876), I.356.

23. Philip Glass suggests that, according to the archeological

records, the Egyptian ruler Aknaten (or Akhenaten) was "distorted physically, that is, had a physical distortion." See, *inter alia,* John Richardson, "Refractions of Masculinity: Ambivalence and Androgyny in Philip Glass's Opera *Aknaten* and Selected Recent Works," *Jyväskylä Studies in the Arts* (1995): 49.

24. Sigmund Freud, *Moses and Monotheism* (1939), vol. 23 of *The Standard Edition of the Complete Psychological Works,* ed. James Strachey (London: Hogarth, 1960). See also Jan Assman, *Moses the Egyptian: The Memory of Egypt in Western Monotheism* (Cambridge, Mass.: Harvard University Press, 1997); and James Breasted, "De hymnis in solem sub rege Amenophide IV" (Diss., Berlin, 1894), which, like Freud's work, devotes much attention to Akhenaten's monotheism.

25. Freud, *Moses and Monotheism,* p. 25.

26. Asclepias studied the art of healing from the centaur Cheron. Cheron is often represented with a serpent *(askalabos)* coiled around his staff. The name "Asclepias" may be derived from the Greek word *askalabos.* Since that time, Asclepias' knotted staff, whose origin can be traced to the magician's wand used by the Egyptians and by Moses, has a single serpent entwined around it. For centuries this staff, known also as the caduceus, the winged staff of Hermes-Mercury, the messenger of the gods, is depicted with two entwining serpents and has been the symbol of the medical profession.

27. On Jacob wrestling, see Shell, *Polio and Its Aftermath,* pp. 80–81.

28. Some writers claim that when the time came for Israel (*né* Jacob) to confer the blessing, he did it "leaning upon his staff." This posture was a symbol of that night of wrestling with God and the resulting change in his life (see Hebrews 11:21). On his crossing the Red Sea, see Genesis 32:10. Cf. Exodus 14:16 and Midrash Yelamdenu (Yalkot) on Ps. ex. sect. 869.

29. *Pirke D'Rebbe Eliezer,* 40 (a Midrashic work composed by the school of Rebbe Eliezer ben Hyrcanus around 100 C.E.), gives the history of this amazing staff: "Created at twilight, before

the Sabbath, it was given to Adam in the Garden of Eden. Adam gave it to Chanoch (Enoch), who gave it to Metushelach (Methuselah); he in turn passed it on to Noach (Noah). Noach bequeathed it to his son Shem, who transmitted it to Avraham (Abraham). From Avraham to Yitzchak (Isaac), and then to Ya'akov (Jacob), who took it with him to Egypt. Ya'akov gave it to Yosef (Joseph); upon Yosef's death, all his possessions were removed to Pharaoh's place. Yitro (Jethro), one of Pharaoh's advisors, desired it, whereupon he took it and stuck it in the ground in his garden in Midian. From then on, no one could pull out the staff until Moshe (Moses) came. He read the Hebrew letters on the staff, and pulled it out readily. Knowing then that Moshe was the redeemer of Israel, Yitro gave him his daughter Tzipporah (Zepporah) in marriage." Later, Hashem (a shepherd to Yitro), while investigating the phenomenon of the burning bush, says to Moses, "What is that in your hand?" *Pirkê de Rabbi Eliezer (The Chapters of Rabbi Eliezer, the Great): According to the Text of the Manuscript Belonging to Abraham Epstein of Vienna,* trans. Gerald Friedlander, 4th ed. (New York: Sepher-Hermon Press, 1981).

30. The etymology of "Pesach" is uncertain. Some derive it from a Hebrew root meaning "to leap, limp, hobble" (as in the tale of Jonathan's lame son in 2 Samuel 4:4; or the ambivalent Israelites' fence-sitting on Mount Carmel in 1 Kings 18:21). But the explanation given in Exodus 12:13, 23, 27 is that Yahweh "passed over," "left out," or "protected" the dwellings of the Israelites. Yahweh struck Egypt, but He spared those Israelites who were under the protection of the blood of a substitute lamb. See J. B. Segal, *The Hebrew Passover, from the Earliest Times to A.D. 70* (London: Oxford University Press, 1970); and Roland de Vaux, *Ancient Israel: Social Institutions,* vol. 1 (New York: McGraw-Hill, 1965).

The meaning of *pesach* is debated along predictable lines. Some have tried to connect the word to the Hebrew verb of the same radical that means "to halt, leap, limp, stumble." See 1 Kings 18:21, where *pesach* describes the priests of Baal cavorting around the altar; also 2 Samuel 4:4, where it describes a crippled child. Others connect it to the Akkadian *passahu,* which means "to appease, make soft, placate." Still others link it to an Egyptian word that commemorates the harvest (Segal, *The Hebrew Passover,* pp. 95–100). The verb occurs in Isaiah 31:5 with the connotation "to protect." Brevard S. Childs, *Exodus: A Commentary* (London: S.C.M. Press, 1974), p. 183, note 11, suggests that this was already influenced by the Exodus tradition.

31. On Mephibosheth, see Shell, *Polio and Its Aftermath,* p. 60; and 2 Samuel 4, 9, 16, and 21.

32. The relationship between the Israelites and a group of lepers who had been expelled is taken up in Eduard Meyer, *Aegyptische Chronologie: Abhandlungen der Preussischen Akademie der Wissenschaften* (Leipzig: Hinrichs, 1904), esp. pp. 92–95. Cf. Assmann, *Moses the Egyptian,* esp. p. 29.

33. Assman, *Moses the Egyptian,* p. 21.

34. Tacitus, *Historia,* 53.

35. In many Greek and Roman stories, it is a plague (some say leprosy—a most serious problem of pollution among the Jews as well—others say a disease that leads to bodily deformities) that separates the Egyptians from the aliens, and then it is the plague that gives rise in some ways to the latter's Jewishness. Leprosy, one should add, often leads to paralysis. The same doctors often work on both; an example is the nineteenth-century Harvard professor William Lloyd Aycock.

36. "Plurimi auctores consentiunt orta per Aegyptum tabe quae corpora foedaret, regem Bocchorim adito Hammonis oraculo remedium petentem purgare regnum et id genus hominum ut invisum deis alias in terras avehere iussum" (Tacitus, *Historia,* 5.3).

37. Exodus Rabbah 1:26. Compare *Encyclopedia Judaica,* 12:396. Islamic tradition has a similar story, as reported in *Encyclopedia Judaica,* 12:403. In the famous incident during Moshe's childhood in which Pharaoh tests the young lad who has taken off the ruler's crown (see *Parshat Shemos*), Pharaoh is unable to

discover that Moshe is the redeemer of the Jews. Moshe injures his own mouth, affecting his power of speech. Muslim commentators say that Moses, when a child, burned his tongue with a live coal. The same story is found in *Midrash Jalkut* on Exodus 166; and in Gedaliah Ibn Yahya, *Shalsheleth Hakabalah* (Amsterdam, 1697; orig. pub. 1587), p. 5.

38. On this term, see Marty Jezer, *Stuttering,* p. 222. Jezer is described this way by his daughter.

39. Commentary on the Mishnah entitled *Tiferet Yisrael,* commentary to *Kiddushin* (Talmudic tractate), end, note 77 (*Encyclopedia Judaica,* 12:400).

40. *Encyclopedia Judaica,* 12:400.

41. Acts 7:22 (King James Version) is part of a quote from Stephen: "And Moses was learned in all the wisdom of the Egyptians, and was mighty in words and deeds." The New Century Version reads: "The Egyptians taught Moses everything they knew, and he was a powerful man in what he said and did."

42. Freud, *Moses and Monotheism.* See also John Toland, *Adeisidaemon, sive Titus Livius a superstitione vindicatus. . . . Annexae sunt ejusdem Origines Judaicae* (The Hague: Thomas Johnson, 1709).

43. Johann Wolfgang von Goethe, "Israel in Wüste" (Israel in the Desert; 1819), in Goethe, *Noten und Abhandlungen zu besserem Verständnis des West-östlichen Divans,* in *Goethe: Divan, Noten und Abhandlungen,* in *Goethes Werke,* ed. Erich Trunz, 14 vols. (Munich: Beck, 1981), 2:207–225. See also Konrad Burdach, "Faust und Moses," *Sitzungsberichte der Königlichen Preussischen Akademie der Wissenschaft* (1912), 1:358–403.

44. See Nachum Sarna, *Exploring Exodus: The Heritage of Biblical Israel* (New York: Schocken, 1986).

45. For the relevant psychoanalytic authors, see Michel de Certeau, *The Writing of History,* trans. Tom Conley (New York: Columbia University Press, 1988), pp. 340–341.

46. Francis Bacon, "Experiment Solitary Touching Stutting," *Sylva Sylvarum,* in *The Works of Francis Bacon,* ed. James Spedding,

Robert Leslie Ellis, and Douglas Denon Heath (London, 1857–1874), vol. 2, no. 386, p. 470. Bacon is apparently referring to Aristotle, *Problems,* 11.54, throughout his "Experiment."

47. According to the *Encyclopedia Judaica,* 12:404, this work is preserved in the writings of Eusebius of Caesarea, ed. J. Bloch (1929). See, too, Benjamin Stillingfleet, *Moses and Zipporah* (1765); and William Sinclair (often attributed to Samuel B. H. Judah), *The Maid of Midian* (1833), which is more interesting but was never staged, because of the way it treats the slaying of the Midianite captives (Numbers 31:2–18).

48. According to some commentators, even the Torah suggests that Jethro is the "father-in-law" of the Jewish religion, since he sketched out its political organization and the like. He was also apparently the first to praise God after the liberation.

49. Zora Neale Hurston, *Moses, Man of the Mountain* (Urbana: University of Illinois Press, 1984; orig. pub. 1939); on the language issue, see esp. ch. 31.

50. Moses therefore told God that since he had left Egypt at an early age and was now eighty, he lacked fluency in the Egyptian language and would have to stutter to find the proper words (Rashbam 4:10).

51. Halakhah 4; see David Cohen, *Sefer Avraham Yagel Yitzchak Yeranen* (Brooklyn, N.Y.: Artscroll Mesorah, 2000), 126; citing *Even HaEzer* and *Talmud Yerushalmi* (Shabbat).

52. This is the translation of Moses' words to God in *The Word Made Fresh.*

53. B. de Boysson-Bardies, L. Sagart, and C. Durand, "Discernible Differences in the Babbling of Infants According to Target Language," *Journal of Child Language,* 11 (1984): 1–15.

54. Rambam's own emigration history is worth recalling here. His family fled Almohad Spain for Fez, Morocco, and eventually settled in Forstatt, Egypt. Regarding the explanation I report in the text, Rambam may be alluding to his understanding of Moses' protest in Shemot 6: rather than the conventional un-

derstanding (that Moses felt he would stutter), Rambam may think Moses was claiming he wasn't fluent in *diplomatic* speech.

55. When God told Moses to deliver a message to Pharaoh, Moses assumed he was to speak in the Egyptian language. Hashem told him, "I have appointed you a master over Pharaoh. Thus, he is your inferior, and you are the head of a major empire. Consequently, in accordance with proper protocol, you will address him in *lashon hakodesh* ["the holy tongue," i.e., Hebrew]. Do not be concerned about his inability to understand Hebrew, because Aaron will be your interpreter." Moshe Bogomilsky, *Vedibarta Bam—And You Shall Speak of Them: A Compilation of Selected Torah Insights* (Brooklyn, N.Y.: M. Bogomilsky, 1995–), Exodus 6:30–7:1.

56. Exodus Rabbah 3:16. Compare *Encyclopedia Judaica,* 12:396.

57. Isaac Disraeli, *Commentaries on the Life and Reign of Charles the First, King of England,* new rev. ed., 2 vols. (London: Henry Colburn, 1851), 1.11.

58. Leonard Kriegel, *Falling into Life* (San Francisco: North Point Press, 1991), p. 161. In his essay "From the Burning Bush," the polio survivor Kriegel calls Aaron "a kind of verbal aide-de-camp," which, Kriegel suggests, makes Aaron the world's "first editor."

59. See Assmann, *Moses the Egyptian,* p. 18.

60. Certeau, *The Writing of History,* p. 269. See also Freud, *Moses and Monotheism.*

61. See esp. http://home.nycap.rr.com/porush/DaveWeb/HTML%20FIles/Moses%20Alphabet-Bringer.html (accessed June 2005). On *aleph-tov,* see Robert K. Logan, *The Alphabetic Effect: The Impact of the Phonetic Alphabet on the Development of Western Civilization* (New York: Morrow, 1986). There is debate about the Proto-Sinaitic script found at Serabit el Khadim; see note 72 below. The Israelites have already seized all of the animals and goods of the Midianites and burned their towns.

62. The fragment by Eupolemus is included in Felix Jacoby,

ed., *Fragmente der griechischen Historiker* (Leiden: E. J. Brill, 1958). See, too, Ben Zion Wacholder, *Eupolemus: A Study of Judaeo-Greek Literature* (Cincinnati: Hebrew Union College and Jewish Institute of Religion, 1975). For Grimme's views, see Hubert Grimme, *Die altsinaitischen Buchstabeninschriften* (Berlin, 1929), pp. 21–22, 100–109.

63. *Encyclopedia Judaica,* 12:403.

64. The engraving is a copy of Rembrandt's painting *Moses Smashing the Tables of the Laws* (1659), now in the Gemäldegalerie, Berlin.

65. William Horman, *Vulgaria,* sentences in English and Latin (London: Richard Pynson, 1519), p. 75. See also *OED,* s.v. "happer.127"128

66. Alternate transcriptions are Hathoor, Het-heru, and Het-Hert.

67. An acrophonic writing system is one that uses the initial sound (acrophone), rather than the entire syllable. Thus, the letter for the sound "bee" could stand for /bee/, /bah/, /boe/, /beh/, and so on. A picture of a bee and simplified representations of it might be acrophonic pictograms.

68. In *Moses und Aron* (1926–1932), Schoenberg uses the twelve-tone system and *Sprechstimme* (a blend of speaking and singing) to explore the events of the Book of Exodus and the meaning of God. Moses (John Tomlinson, in the Met's 1999 production) is a bass-baritone, barking out the Word of God in *Sprechstimme,* unable to convey to the people his vision of an all-powerful, invisible deity. Aaron (the name was shortened by the superstitious Schoenberg to prevent the title of the opera from having thirteen letters) is a lyric tenor who "sells" Moses' visions to the Israelites with conjuring tricks and visible miracles—water that turns to blood, a staff that becomes a serpent, a pillar of fire, and most famously the Golden Calf.

69. Trans. Allen Forte.

70. Gielen is the conductor on a fine recording of this opera (Phillips, 1974), which is the soundtrack for the movie *Moses und*

Aron, directed by Jean-Marie Straub and Danièle Huillet (Germany: Janus Films, 1974). He is also a composer in his own right and was a student of Josef Polnauer (who studied with Schoenberg).

71. Exodus 37:28–36: "Then there passed by Midianites merchantmen; and they [Joseph's brothers] drew and lifted up Joseph out of the pit, and sold Joseph to the Ishmeelites for twenty pieces of silver: and they brought Joseph into Egypt. . . . And the Midianites sold him into Egypt unto Potiphar, an officer of Pharaoh's, and captain of the guard."

72. A crucial tablet/idol was discovered there in 1905 by Sir Flinders Petrie. See William Albright, *The Proto-Sinaitic Inscriptions and Their Decipherment* (Cambridge, Mass.: Harvard University Press, 1966), p. 12. Albright says that in "discussing the proposed Semitic adaptations of Egyptian appellations of divinity, [the scholar Herbert] Donner might have recalled the 'fact' that all the Proto-Sinaitic carved panels and sculptures bear inscriptions. In 1988 a doctoral dissertation was completed at Tel Aviv University by Benjamin Sass titled, "The Genesis of the Alphabet and Its Development in the Second Millennium B.C." (Ägypten und Altes Testament, Band 13). It appeared in Kommission bei Otto Harrassowitz (Wiesbaden), *The Origin of the Phoenician Letters [and even moreso the Old Negev letters] in the Proto-Canaanite and Proto-Sinaitic Scripts;* and the borrowing of most, if not all, letter forms in the latter script from Egyptian hieroglyphics on the basis of acrophony are now seen as indubitable facts (cf. Snyczer 1974, p. 9)."

73. Martin Luther, *A Commentary on St. Paul's Epistle to the Galatians,* trans. Theodore Graebner (Grand Rapids, Mich.: Zondervan, 1939), regarding verse 3: "The conscience ought to know only Christ. To say this is easy, but in times of trial, when the conscience writhes in the presence of God, it is not so easy to do. As such times we are to believe in Christ as if there were no Law or sin anywhere, but only Christ. We ought to say to the

Law: 'Mister Law, I do not get you. You stutter so much. I don't think that you have anything to say to me.'"

74. See Konrad Burdach, "Faust und Moses," *Sitzungsberichte der Königlichen Preussischen Akademie der Wissenschaft,* 1.358–403.

75. Herodotus, *Inquiries,* 4.150–156; compare Pindar, *Pythian Odes,* 4.10.

76. Alternate spellings include Dekanahwidah and Dekanawidah. He convinced each of the fifty leaders of the Iroquois nation to sit as a "brother among brothers" at a grand council to work out problems peacefully. In this way, some people say, he created the world's first representative government. Benjamin Franklin, who studied the Iroquois, proposed that the fledgling United States adopt a similar system.

77. See Alice Beck Kehoe, *North American Indians: A Comprehensive Account,* 2nd ed. (Englewood Cliffs, N.J.: Prentice Hall, 1992).

78. Consider, too, Bohemund III, Prince of Antioch (1163–1201), who was called "the Stutterer."

79. In Hilary Mantel's novel *A Place of Greater Safety* (London: Viking, 1992), Danton seems to argue that Camille Desmoulins' stutter was a key to understanding him: "In the old days, [Camille] claimed that his stutter was a complete obstacle to successful pleading [in court]. Of course, when one is used to it, it might discomfit, irritate or embarrass. But Hérault has pointed out that Camille has wrung some extraordinary verdicts from distraught judges. Certainly I have observed that Camille's stutter comes and goes. It goes when he is angry or wishes forcibly to make a point; it comes when he feels put upon, and when he wishes to show people that he is in fact a nice person who is really not quite able to cope" (p. 402).

See also Susanne Alleyn's play *A Far Better Rest* (New York: Soho Press, 2000).

80. See Jacques Janssens, *Camille Desmoulins: Le Premier Républicain de France* (Paris: Perrin, 1973).

81. The supposed "Déclaration de Camille Desmoulins aux Parisiens" (July 12, 1789) is in Gilles Baillat et al., eds., *Histoire, géographie, education civique: Cycle 3, Niveau 3,* Collection Gulliver (Paris: Nathan, 1996).

82. René Farge, *Un Episode de la journée du 12 juillet 1789: Camille Desmoulins au jardin du Palais-Royal* (Paris: E. Leroux, 1914).

83. The numeric values of the Hebrew letters in the word *tzit-tzit* add up to 600. If you then add five knots and eight strings, the total sum is 613, which is the number of *mitzvos* (laws).

84. In the holy books, this is made clear: "My Beloved is like a gazelle or a young deer. [I thought He had abandoned me forever, but] behold, He was near the entire time, standing behind our wall, supervising from the windows, peering [*me-tzitz*] through the lattices." The related verb is *tztaz* ("to peer or gaze"). Impure reduplicatives might include such words as *boogie-woogie, double trouble, fancy-schmancy, flower power, hanky-panky, harum-scarum, heebie-jeebies, helter-skelter, herky-jerky, higgledy piggledy, hoity-toity, hurdy-gurdy, itsy-bitsy, mumbo-jumbo, namby-pamby, powwow, super-duper, teeny-weeny, tutti-frutti, walkie-talkie, willy-nilly.* There are also such titles as *Chitty Chitty Bang Bang* (movie), *Cox and Box* (operetta by Sir Arthur Sullivan), *Humpty Dumpty, Rikki-Tikki-Tavi,* and *Rin-Tin-Tin.*

85. Leonard Cohen, "The Window" (1979), on the album *Recent Songs* (Stranger Music, 1979; Sony, 1990).

86. See also Numbers 20:12. On the legends about the striking of the rock, see Louis Ginzberg, *The Legends of the Jews,* 7 vols. (Philadelphia: Jewish Publication Society of America, 1909–1938), vol. 3 (trans. Paul Radin), esp. pp. 609–619.

87. Robert Anderson Hall, *Introductory Linguistics* (Philadelphia: Chilton, 1964), p. 42.

88. On the glottal stop in the Chumash language, see www.chumashlanguage.com. On this language and its stops, see also

the two relevant essays in *Proceedings of the Meeting of the Society for the Study of the Indigenous Languages of the Americas, July 2–4, 1993* (Columbus, Ohio, 1993); and Margaret Langdon, ed., *Hokan-Penutian Workshop, July 3, 1993* (Berkeley, Calif.: Survey of California and Other Indian Languages, 1994).

89. Hall, *Introductory Linguistics,* p. 42.

90. Henry Sweet, *A History of English Sounds from the Earliest Period* (Oxford: Clarendon, 1888), p. 1: "The glottal stop is produced by a sudden shutting or opening of the glottis, as in a cough." See also Henry Sweet, *A Handbook of Phonetics* (Oxford: Clarendon Press, 1877), 2.6: "The most familiar example of this 'glottal catch' is an ordinary cough."

91. John F. A. Sawyer, *A Modern Introduction to Biblical Hebrew* (Boston: Oriel, 1976), p. 8: "Aleph is not pronounced, except between vowels, where it stands for a glottal stop. See *OED,* s.v. "aleph": "Hebrew and Phoenician *āleph,* literally 'ox'; the character may have developed from the hieroglyph of an ox's head."

92. This poem appears in Paul Celan, *Fadensonnen* ("Thread-Suns") (Frankfurt: Suhrkamp, 1968). In English, *Glottal Stop: 101 Poems by Paul Celan,* trans. Nikolai Popov and Heather McHugh (Middletown, Conn.: Wesleyan University Press, 2000).

93. Popov and McHugh, preface to Celan, *Glottal Stop: 101 Poems.*

94. "World to be stuttered after" is John Felstiner's translation of the title of Celan's poem "Die nachzustotternde Welt." John Hamilton did the translation of these lines from "Tübingen, Jänner." The fifteenth-century gargoyle known as the *Lällekönig* is in Basel's Historical Museum. The lullaby is from Shakespeare, *A Midsummer Night's Dream,* 2.2. *Lall:* "When stammering attains such a grade that the speech is thereby rendered very indistinct or entirely unintelligible, it is called lalling *(lallatio)*" (Hugo von Ziemssen, ed., *Handbuch der speciellen pathologie und therapie;* in English, *Cyclopaedia of the Practice of Medicine,* trans.

Albert H. Buck and others [New York: W. Wood, 1874–1881], 14:844).

5. Marilyn's Duh

1. Milton Berle, alias the Thief of Bad Gags, dubbed himself "Uncle Miltie" during a television episode of *The Texaco Star Theater* (1949). The nickname stuck.

2. Cecil Hunter (1909–1986), a talented mimic of animal sounds, became popular on the radio in the 1930s. One of his regular routines in subsequent years was to stammer and stumble onstage, and he acquired the nickname "Stuttering Sam." Hunter worked with Cal Farley on Farley's daily radio program in 1936. See Beth Feagles Day, *A Shirttail to Hang To: The Story of Cal Farley and His Boys Ranch* (New York: Holt, 1959); and Nipsey Russell, *The Funny Side of Nipsey,* LP (Humorsonic, early 1960s). This recording contains six comedy classics, including Hunter's "Stuttering Sam."

3. Unable to teach Clément to talk and walk like a dodo, Berle tries to teach him another comic routine. This one involves the deliberate mispronunciation of the English word *kill.*

4. Perhaps he was thinking of the long tradition in dance—harking back to the 1890s and extending into the 1950s—where people imitate animals: the "panoply" of popular "animal dance movements" that arose during the period of earlier polio epidemics and that included the Turkey Trot, Camel Walk, Lame Duck, Bunny Hop, Bunny Hug, Grizzly Bear, and, around 1912, the early forms of Foxtrot known as the Horsetrot and Fishwalk, as well as the famous Chicken Reel.

5. On the Cajun dance *fais-dodo,* see Lauren C. Post, *Cajun Sketches from the Prairies of Southwest Louisiana* (Baton Rouge: Louisiana State University Press, 1962). One relevant French-language song goes: "Fais dodo, Colas, mon p'tit frère / Fais dodo, t'auras du lolo." Another goes: "Do, do, l'enfant do / L'enfant dormira bien vite."

On doo-wop (or du-wop), see *Johnny Keyes and Du-Wop* (Chicago: Vesti, 1987).

T. S. Eliot, *The Waste Land,* section 5, "What the Thunder Said," lines 399–400. A translation of "Datta, dayadhvam, damyata" would be "Give, sympathize, restrain yourselves."

Edgar Bergen (ventriloquist): "Do you have a flair for writing?" Mortimer Snerd (dummy): "Duh, no, Mr. Bergen. Just a pencil and paper."

6. Dictionaries suggest that there are several alternatives for *d'oh,* among them *doy.*

7. *OED,* s.v. "daw." "To play the daw" means "to play the fool." There is an allusive connection to Aesop's fable of the jackdaw.

8. John Earle, *Philology of the English Tongue,* 2nd ed. (Oxford, 1873), sect. 138, p. 139.

9. Margaret Drabble, "Public Speech and Public Silence," address to the British Stammering Association, October 18, 2001, Gulbenkian Lecture Hall, Oxford; reprinted in *Speaking Out,* publication of the British Stammering Association (Summer–Fall 2002).

10. *Let's Make Love,* directed by George Cukor (20th Century Fox, 1960; DVD, 2002).

11. According to the *OED,* the use of "dough" to mean "money" is at least as old as 1851.

12. Samuel Butler, *Erewhon; or, Over the Range* (London: Trübner, 1872), ch. 15: "The Musical Banks."

Does *doh* as "the first note of the musical scale" help lead up to the need for Bing Crosby the singing specialist? The term is *do,* or *doh,* and both mean *ut*—the first note in the system of hexachords devised by Guido d'Arezzo in the eleventh century and the first note of the octave in modern solmization, the note C in the natural scale of C major. In Guthrie's song, the pun involves *dough* (meaning "money").

13. Marty Jezer, *Stuttering* (New York: Basic Books, 1997), p. 68.

14. Ibid., p. 138, discussing Bryng Bryngelson, Myfanwy Chapman, and Orvetta Hansen, *Know Yourself: A Workbook for Those Who Stutter,* 3rd ed. (Minneapolis: Burgess, 1958).

15. *Cancellation* means pausing after a stutter and repeating the stuttered word. *Pullouts* involve slowing down speech or prolonging it. In "fluent stuttering," instead of switching over to another word, one sticks with the same word but does it by the method of cancellation or pullout. Another method, taken from Wendell Johnson (Jezer, *Stuttering,* p. 74), was the *bounce*—a simpler method of "voluntary stuttering."

16. Bobby L. Childers II, *Stuttering: What It Is and Isn't,* PowerPoint presentation for Emergency Services Personnel (2000), www.nettak.com/bobby/Presentation_Notes.htm. In one fictional interview with Marilyn Monroe, stuttering is a major feature. See www.stonecircle.com/cdouglas/marilyn.html, text by Carole Nelson Douglas (August 15, 1999):

"The Actress addresses the unseen interviewer, her voice an aging contralto. Occasionally a breathless, girlish quality emerges.

"*The Actress:* Thank God I didn't die! I was this close. No kidding. Of course, I might as well have died, for all anyone ever saw of me for almost thirty years. Hollywood.

"[*She slaps rouge under and over her cheekbones, then stops to stare at her feverish reflection.*] You know, that's one thing I found out in Korea when I entertained the troops on our honeymoon. Wow, that sounds . . . Joe's and my honeymoon. Joe hated my jaunt to the frontlines, but it showed me I could do more than I thought, though I didn't really know it until much, much later. Those boys were so sweet. They were with me all the way, and I was something special to them. Something more than a pinup or a sex symbol. Oh, I was that all right, and I played it to the hilt. Gosh, it was cold! Took real acting talent to wear that slinky spaghetti-strapped dress and not turn into one big goose bump. And those kind of bumps they weren't interested in! But the craziest thing is, I wasn't scared! All those men, that sea of faces I couldn't even focus on I was shivering so much, but I didn't freeze or forget. Or stutter. Women seldom stutter, you know. It's a male chromosome thing usually. Unless some youthful trauma kicks in, and my youth was all trauma. That's why I went in for Drama. [*Laughs self-mockingly.*]

"I don't stutter now. When I finally got off the shrinks—and I had to in the outback where I lived all those years—and got into self-help, that's when I finally understood it, me, after all those years. Attention, of course. I was seeking male attention in an industry where the father figures were studio heads who kept harems of starlets in 'stables' like race horses. Ran us until we dropped, or turned thirty."

17. See the website www.dystonia-support.org/LA-Voice-Speech-Breathing%20Exercises.htm (accessed January 2005).

18. The song "Heat Wave" was originally from Irving Berlin's Broadway revue *As Thousands Cheer* (1933).

19. In 1937, Cole Porter's legs were severely injured when he was pinned under a horse. Eventually he had to have his right leg amputated. It was during this period that he wrote the song "Can-Can" and the musical of the same name (1953).

20. In *The Man Who Shot Liberty Valance*—a Western made in 1962 starring James Stewart, John Wayne, and Lee Marvin—there is a minor character who stutters severely and thereby provides "comic relief" throughout the film.

21. Helen Glover, Joseph Kalinowski, and Michael Rastatter, "Effect of Instruction to Sing on Stuttering Frequency at Normal and Fast Rates," *Perceptual and Motor Skills,* 83, no. 2 (October 1996): 511–522.

22. "Psellism," in *Household Words,* 348 (November 22, 1856): 464–469; quoted from *Household Words: A Weekly Journal Conducted by Charles Dickens,* 14, nos. 330–353 and the number-and-a-half for Christmas, July 19, 1856, to December 27, 1856 (London: Office 16, Wellington Street North, 1856).

23. Simon Nowell-Smith, comp., *The Legend of the Master* (London: Constable, 1947), p. 48.

24. Carly Simon quoted in Thomas David Kehoe, *Stuttering: Science, Therapy, and Practice—The Most Complete Book about Stuttering* (Boulder, Colo.: Casa Futura Technologies, 1997), citing Marie Brenner, "I Never Sang for My Mother," *Vanity Fair,* 58 (August 1995): 128. See also the site www.stutteringf.org/famous people%20who%20stutters.htm (accessed June 2005).

25. On Tillis, see M. Tillis and W. Wager, *Stutterin' Boy* (New York: Rawson Associates, 1984). On Mather, see Benson Bobrick, *Knotted Tongues* (New York: Simon and Schuster, 1995), pp. 72–75; and Cotton Mather, "*Ephphatha:* Some Advice to Stammerers," in Mather, *The Angel of Bethesda* (Barre, Mass.: American Antiquarian Society and Barre Publishers, 1972).

26. "Why, let the stricken deer go weep, / The hart ungalled play; / For some must watch, while some must sleep: / So runs the world away" (*Hamlet,* 3.2). "Words, words, words" (*Hamlet,* 3.2). On perseveration and stuttering, see Robert West, "A Perseverative Theory of Stuttering," in Jon Eisenson, ed., *Stuttering: A Symposium* (New York: Harper, 1958).

27. Yet another example: Bedrich Smetana's opera *The Bartered Bride* (1866) famously includes a pathetic stutterer named Vasek.

28. Ritchie York, "John and Yoko and Year One," *Rolling Stone,* 51 (February 7, 1970).

29. Alvin Lucier, *I Am Sitting in a Room* (Lovely Music, Ltd.; CD 1013). Composed 1970; recorded 1980.

30. "Oh, Helen" (1918) was written by Charles MacCarron and Carey Morgan. "Tell Her I Stutter" (1922) was written by Billy Rose and Cliff Friend. "K-K-K-Katy" (1918) was written by Geoffrey O'Hara.

31. Henry Harington, "Goody Groaner: The Celebrated Stammering Glee," score arranged for the pianoforte (London: Duncombe, 1825).

32. More specifically, Porky Pig's stuttering consists of the insertion of the *schwa*-vowel, part-word and whole-word repeti-

tions, word substitutions and circumlocutions, insertions of unrelated syllables and sounds, struggle, and retrials.

33. See Marc Shell, "Portia's Portrait: Representation as Exchange," *Common Knowledge,* 7, no. 1 (Spring 1998): 94–144. Aman-da uses the word *potatoes* in her half-spoken prologue to the song "Specialization" in *Let's Make Love.* See also H. T. Lowe-Porter's translation of Thomas Mann's *Magic Mountain* (1927), II.vii.787: "If some first-class excitement doesn't come along every day, you pull a face as though you were saying: 'H'm, small potatoes *and* few in the hill!'" Art Buchwald, *How Much Is That in Dollars?* (Greenwich, Conn.: Fawcett Crest, 1962), p. 122: "Mary Soo, by tradition but not contract, has the garbage concession of all United States Navy ships entering Hong Kong, which out here is no small potatoes."

34. It is worth adding here that Mime, in Wagner's opera *Siegfried* (scene 3), is concerned with stuttering: "Was du doch falsch mich verstehst! / Stamml' ich, fasl' ich wohl gar?" ("But how is it that you misunderstand me! / Am I stammering, am I really just driveling?"—Trans. John Hamilton.)

35. See especially Karl Marx, "The Power of Money in Bourgeois Society," in Marx, *Economic and Philosophic Manuscripts of 1844* (New York: International Publishers, 1980).

36. Dionysius of Miletus made this remark to Avidius Heliodorus, who had charge of the emperor Hadrian's correspondence. Noted in Cassius Dio Cocceianus, *Roman History,* book 69.

37. The song was written by Cole Porter for his two-act musical comedy *Leave It To Me* (1938–1939), book by Bella Spewack and Samuel Spewack, based on their play *Clear All Wires* (1932). The plot of *Leave It To Me* is worth summarizing. Bathtub manufacturer Alonzo P. Goodhue, socially and politically the best horseshoe pitcher in Topeka, Kansas, is appointed U.S. ambassador to Russia, largely through the maneuverings of his ambitious wife. An envious J. H. Brody, publisher of the *Paris*

and Chicago World-Tribune, orders his best correspondent, Buckley Thomas, to see that Goodhue is disgraced and recalled. As it turns out, the unassuming Goodhue is himself eager to be shipped home, and so he and Thomas join forces. Goodhue delivers an antagonistic speech, kicks the German ambassador in the belly, and attempts to assassinate a prince—and in each case he is proclaimed a hero. Finally, Thomas, realizing that only *good* deeds go unrewarded, has Goodhue deliver an optimistic speech expressing hope for a unified world. Goodhue is promptly recalled. Other characters include Colette, Thomas' old flame, and Dolly, an incorrigible flirt (originally played by Mary Martin, in her first role on Broadway; she sang "My Heart Belongs to Daddy" about two-thirds of the way through the second act.)

38. Eddy Duchin and His Orchestra, vocal by Mary Martin, "My Heart Belongs to Daddy" / "Most Gentlemen Don't Like Love," 78-rpm (Brunswick, 1938).

39. Jack Hylton and His Orchestra, vocal by Pat Kirkwood, "Most Gentlemen Don't Like Love" / "My Heart Belongs to Daddy," 78-rpm (HMV, 1938). Count Basie, vocal by Helen Hulmes, "My Heart Belongs to Daddy," 78-rpm (Decca, 1939). Chick Webb and His Orchestra, vocal by Ella Fitzgerald, "My Heart Belongs to Daddy," 78-rpm (Decca, 1939). Valaida Snow, "My Heart Belongs to Daddy," 78-rpm (Sonora, 1939). Larry Clinton and His Orchestra, vocal by Bea Wain, "My Heart Belongs to Daddy" / "Most Gentlemen Don't Like Love," 78-rpm (Victor, 1938).

40. Eddie DeLange and His Orchestra, "My Heart Belongs to Daddy," 78-rpm (Bluebird, 1938).

41. One reviewer wrote of O'Day: "My favorite album from this challenging singer is the Giuffre set. 'My Heart Belongs to Daddy' absolutely throbs with sex. What a wonderful lyric." See www.mosaicrecords.com / prodinfo.asp?number=188-MD-CD (accessed January 2005).

42. See Della Reese (*née* Deloreese Patricia Early), *Della*

Della Cha Cha Cha (LP, RCA Victor, 1960; reissued on CD), which includes "My Heart Belongs to Daddy."

43. See Glenn Meredith Loney, *Unsung Genius: The Passion of Dancer-Choreographer Jack Cole* (New York: F. Watts, 1984). See also *Catalogue of the Jack Cole Collection of Books and Pictures on the Dance . . . Which Will Be Sold by Auction by Sotheby Parke Bernet and Co. . . . Days of sale, Monday, 16th July, 1979, Tuesday, 17th July, 1979* (London: Sotheby Parke Bernet, 1979).

44. Some versions had no introduction; others had apparently "private" introductions such as the following:

> I used to fall in love with all
> Those boys who maul refined ladies,
> But now I tell each young gazelle
> To go to hell, I mean *Hades.*
> For since I've come to care
> for such a sweet millionaire.

45. John Russell Bartlett, *Dictionary of Americanisms: A Glossary of Words and Phrases Usually Regarded as Peculiar to the United States,* 2nd ed. (Boston: Little Brown, 1859), s.v. "good": "English travellers have repeatedly noticed the adverbial use of this word. 'He cannot read good.' 'It does not shoot good.'"

46. *OED,* s.v. "well," adverb 5.

47. Ibid., s.v. "well," adverb 6c.

48. Ibid., s.v. "well," adverb 6d.

49. Ibid., s.v. "well," adverb 12.

50. Both definitions ibid., s.v. "swell."

51. Ibid., s.v. "guff": "2. slang (orig. U.S.). Empty talk, nonsense, 'stuff,' 'blather.' *Scribner's Magazine* (August 1888): 219.1: 'I tell you all this talk is guff, and it just comes down to the money.' G. B. Shaw, *Apple Cart* (1930), II.78: 'You cant run them [power stations] on patriotic songs . . . and guff and bugaboo.' John Dos Passos, *Best of Times* (1966; rpt. 1968), iv.144: 'Whether it was politics or literary work or painting he [Ernest Hemingway]

would take the guff out of a situation with a wellplaced fourletter word.'"

52. Richard Huloet, *Abcedarium anglico latinum, pro tyrunculis* (London: G. Riddel, 1522).

53. In *Some Like It Hot* (1959), Joe/Josephine (Tony Curtis) and Jerry/Daphne (Jack Lemmon) disguise themselves as "ladies" until they are revealed to be "laddies." In one of Mary Martin's several recorded versions of "My Heart Belongs to Daddy," Martin refers to the laddies as "under-graddies"—as opposed to real daddies.

54. Philip Larkin, "Next Please" (1955), in Larkin, *Collected Poems,* ed. A. Thwaite (New York: Farrar Straus Giroux, 1988), p. 52.

55. In many works about stuttering, the example for stuttering as part-word or syllable repetition is *DadaDadady.* See Peter R. Ramig's comments on the *schwa*-vowel, in his open letter "To the Parent of the Nonfluent Child" (University of Colorado, Boulder, Department of Communication Disorders and Speech Science, 1993), www.mnsu.edu/comdis/kuster/Parents/ramig parents.html.

56. "Control your desire to curse / While I crucify the verse / The tin-pan-ti-thesis of melody / Me re do so mi do la si." That is how Sarah Vaughn sings the song.

57. *OED,* s.v. "uh": "U.S. Expressing hesitation: = *er.* J. D. MacDonald, *Only Girl in Game* (1962), vi.85: '"Are you cashing cheques?" . . . The man hesitated. "Uh . . . Yes, we are."' National Observer (U.S.) (February 3, 1973): 'He wanted most awfully to see the one in the advertisement about being, uh, well, you know.' *New York Review of Books* (August 4, 1977), 32.4: '"Perhaps we should, uh, wait," I said.'"

58. *OED,* s.v. "uh": "Repr. the indefinite article in the speech of U.S. blacks. H. A. Shands, *Some Peculiarities of Speech in Mississippi* (1893), 65. *Uh,* the common negro form for the indefinite article *a.* Dialect writers generally write this *er,* but no sound of *r* is ever apparent in the negro pronunciation. *Publ.*

Texas Folklore Society, 11 (1933), 105: 'Dey's jes' ez good uh fish in de creek ez evah been caught.' *Black World* (October 1973), 74: 'Locking up folks lives for stealing less than uh hundred dollars.'"

59. *OED,* s.v. "uh": "*Uh-uh* is often a spoken affirmative or noncommittal response to a question or remark; 'yes,' 'oh yes?' See *Dialect Notes,* 5 (1924), 278: '*Uh-húh,* yes.') A feeling of reticence can be indicated at the same time. See too Nicholas Blake, *Minute for Murder* (London: Published for the Crime Club by Collins, 1947), v.111: 'You ought to go on the movies, Blount.' 'Uh-huh?'"

60. David Dalby writes: "African usage can also explain the frequent use by Americans of the interjections *uh-huh* for 'yes' and *uh-uh* for 'no.' Similar forms, especially for 'yes,' occur in scattered parts of the world, but nowhere as frequently and as regularly as in Africa." In Alan Dundes, comp., *Mother Wit from the Laughing Barrel: Readings in the Interpretation of Afro-American Folklore* (Englewood Cliffs, N.J.: Prentice-Hall, 1973), p. 1391.

61. John Christopher Wells, *Accents of English* (New York: Cambridge University Press, 1982), III.vi.556: "There are also the grunts sometimes spelt *uh-huh* and *uh-uh,* respectively. The first, 'yes,' is . . . nasal or nasalized; it usually has a rising tone pattern. . . . The second, 'no,' is not necessarily nasal, and has an accented final syllable, with an obligatorily falling tone pattern."

62. *OED,* s.v. "infant." The etymologies usually claim the term derives from *in* ("not") and *fari* ("to speak").

63. There were earlier movies in which Monroe had or may have had bit, uncredited, or cut-out parts: *Scudda Hoo! Scudda Hay!* (1948; a.k.a. *Summer Lightning*) and *The Shocking Miss Pilgrim* (1947). Here are the words for "Ev'ry Baby Needs a Da-Da-Daddy":

> It was cold outside of Tiffany's
> I was shivering in the storm
> I walked in and asked a gentleman
> Could I please keep warm
> He asked me how come baby doll

Has no coffee place to go
So I told that kindly gentleman
My tale of woe
Every baby needs a Da-Da-Daddy
To keep her worry free
Every baby needs a Da-Da-Daddy
But where's the one for me
Rich or poor I don't care who
if he hasn't got a million then a half'll do
Every baby needs a Da-Da-Daddy
Could my Da-Da-Daddy be you.

64. A "reconstruction" of the incomplete 1962 movie, which runs 37 minutes and stars Dean Martin as well as Marilyn Monroe, is featured in a two-hour AMC documentary, *Marilyn Monroe: The Final Days* (2001; directed by George Cukor). *Something's Got to Give* was a remake of the classic *My Favorite Wife* (1940); it was "completed"—actually taken over—by Doris Day and James Garner, and appeared in moviehouses after Marilyn Monroe's death as *Move Over, Darling* (1963).

65. Jan Jones, *Billy Rose Presents—Casa Mañana* (Fort Worth, Tex.: TCU Press, 1999).

66. Lyrics by Henry Creamer, music by Harry Warren (Skidmore Music Co., 1924). Harry Warren often worked with Rose.

67. Lyrics by Sidney D. Mitchell, music by Maceo Pinkard (New York: Broadway Music Corp., 1922). "Little Freddie Ray / is a very bashful chap / still I'm here to say / that Freddie isn't any sap. / *Chorus:* He whispers 'I love, lu lu lu lu lu love you dear, indeed I do.'"

68. The two were depicted on the cover of *Life Magazine* and other publications. Legend has it that there was much sexual tension between the stars. At about the same time, Arthur Miller—to whom Marilyn Monroe may allude in the Yiddish *meshugennah* in *Let's Make Love* and who wrote the screenplay for *Let's Make Love* with Norman Krasna and Hal Kanter (though he's uncredited)—was writing the script for Marilyn Monroe's last

completed movie, *The Misfits* (1961), which costarred Clark Gable. Gable was likewise a stutterer who was relatively fluent on stage.

69. See Norman Mailer, *Marilyn* (New York: Grosset and Dunlap, 1973). Marilyn Monroe was working with Michael Chekhov at the time.

70. Shakespeare, *King Lear,* 1.1: "Unhappy that I am, I cannot heave / My heart into my mouth: I love your majesty / According to my bond; no more nor less."

71. Harold Wentworth and Stuart Berg Flexner, *Dictionary of American Slang* (New York: Crowell, 1967), s.v. "daddy."

72. The term *daddy* largely replaced *sugar daddy* during the 1930s. See ibid.

73. One story has it that Wilder described making this movie as follows: "I knew we were in midflight, and there was a nut on the plane."

74. See *OED* for examples of the various senses. "Money": Rolf Boldrewood, *A Colonial Reformer* (1890; ed. 1891), 308: "He's always got the sugar, consequence he always gets the worth of his money." "Drugs," including medicaments intended to make one fall in love, or fall out of love, as well as heroin: A. J. Pollock, *Underworld Speaks* (1935), 116.2: "*Sugar and salt,* poisonous habit-forming drugs; any of the white narcotics." "Brothel district": *Sugar* implies *Sugar Hill,* meaning "a district with African-American brothels." "Sugar hill": Wentworth and Flexner, *Dictionary of American Slang.* "Sugar baby": Margaret Mitchell, *Gone with the Wind* (1936), xxvi.455: "Scarlett said gratefully: 'Thank you, Sugarbaby.'"

75. J. Manchon, *Le Slang: Lexique de l'anglais familier et vulgaire* (Paris: Payot, 1923), p. 300. Throughout the twentieth century, *to sugar* meant "to flatter." See Raymond Chandler, *The Big Sleep* (1939), ii.25: "It won't get you anything. Sugaring them never does." See also William Faulkner, *The Reivers* (1962), x.219: "When I sugars up a woman, it aint just empty talk."

76. *OED:* "*Dada,* interjection: A childish and familiar ex-

pression for 'Good-bye!'; the earlier form of *ta-ta*. A: Interjection: A nursery expression for 'Good-bye'; now also in general colloquial use. Cf. *tatty-bye*."

77. T. S. Eliot, *The Waste Land* (1933), 2.26: "Goonight Bill. Goonight Lou. Goonight May. Goodnight. Ta ta. Goonight." George Bernard Shaw, *Buoyant Billions* (1949), IV.52: "I must go now to see about Father's lunch. Tata." See, too, Lynne Reid Banks, *The L-Shaped Room* (1960), xxiii.297: "Charlie'll come up in a few minutes and see how you're getting on. Tata for now." All examples from the *OED*.

78. *Times* [London] (July 13, 1973), *Motor Racing Supplement*, iii.2: "The oil and petrol companies, for a long time the sugar-daddies of top-class motor racing." Ibid. (September 20, 1973), 3.7: "Norma Levy, a prostitute, had a 'sugar daddy' called Bunny who paid her rent and gave her a Mercedes car." All examples from the *OED*.

79. *The Cop and the Anthem* (1952) was based on the novel by O. Henry, directed by Howard Hawks, and narrated by John Steinbeck. It is one of the five short films in the feature *O. Henry's Full House* (1952).

80. M. M. Kaye, *House of Shade* (1959), xii.163: "A nice kind sugar-daddy of the adoring door-mat type."

81. "I'm Gonna File My Claim": "I've looked around the country and I've seen it all, / And what I want, I'm ready to name! / It's big and strong and handsome and it's six feet tall, / I'm gonna file my claim!"

82. Likewise, when Marilyn Monroe—or her "impersonator" Cynthia Basinet—sings the song "Santa Baby," she addresses herself to a sugar daddy bearing gifts to the babe that is herself. Cynthia Basinet (often mistaken for Marilyn Monroe) sings "Santa Baby," written by J. Javits and P. Springer and originally sung by Eartha Kitt.

83. *Athenaeum* (August 13, 1920): 222–223, cited in the *OED*. For an even more extreme formulation, see D. Gascoyne,

Short Survey of Surrealism (1935), p. 25: "The Dada spirit was something shared by a number of extreme individualists of various nationalities, all of whom were in revolt against the whole of the epoch in which they lived."

84. Sung Hwan Kim, *A-da-da,* film presented at the Rencontres Internationales (Paris and Berlin, 2003). The film attempts to represent visually the verbal repetitions of a stutterer.

85. *Etre sur son Dada* was the name of the Dadaist movement's journal; the title means something like "to ride one's hobbyhorse." The review, which first appeared in Zurich in 1916, was founded by Tristan Tzara (a Romanian poet), Hans Arp (a German artist from Alsace), and Richard Huelsenbeck (a German poet).

86. Gilbert Murray, *The Classical Tradition in Poetry* (London: Oxford University Press, 1927), ix.254.

87. *Journal of Abnormal and Social Psychology,* 32 (1927): 15. In *Nigger Heaven* (1926), p. 25, Carl Van Vechten uses the word *daddy* to mean "husband or lover." And Jack Kerouac, in *On the Road* (1957), I.vii.44, refers to "a waitress . . . slightly hung-up on a few sexual difficulties which I think you can manage, you fine gone daddy you."

88. See Cole Porter, "Is It the Girl (or Is It the Gown)?" (1944):

> You see a perfect Juliet enter.
> She so drives you mad
> That you wish you had
> Just a cottage cool
> By a swimming pool
> With her waiting there for *Daddy.*
> Well, before you grow fonder,
> Stop and ponder, *laddie.*

89. Vladimir Nabokov, *Lolita* (Paris: Olympia Press, 1955).

90. Likewise, Mary Martin dropped the line. So did Della Reese, Peggy Lee, and Julie London.

91. The journal *American Speech,* 37 (1962): 35, reports: "*Daddy* has a history beginning much earlier than 1935 as a term meaning simply 'lover' in Negro songs and blues."

92. Likewise, many singers add or drop these lines: "Though other dames at football games / May long for a strong under-graddy, / I never dream of making the team / 'Cause my heart be-longs to Dad-dy."

93. See Marc Shell, "The Want of Incest in Christian Doctrine," unpublished paper.

94. See esp. Wentworth and Flexner, *Dictionary of American Slang,* s.v. "dad": "Mark Twain, *Huckleberry Finn* (1884), xxxiv.354: 'It's de dad-blame' witches.' *Dialect Notes* (Boston, U.S.), *Kentucky Words* (1890), II.64: '*Dad, dod,* for *God,* in certain curses.' *Word Study,* 7.2 (February 1978): 'Darn it,' 'dad gum it,' 'heck.'"

95. English words by John Turner and Geoffrey Parsons (1953); music and original lyrics by Paul Burkhyard (1948), "O Mein Papa."

96. Aman-da saves Clément's skin when she tells the "ghost behind the ghost" that she saw "Alexander" buying a joke for ten dollars. So it is that the meeting of Clément and Aman-da, whose name means "loving Da," is the defining moment of *Let's Make Love.*

97. Is this papal Pa-Pa Aman-da's real *propriétaire?* That would make him a property owner more powerful than the new owner of the theater building. Clément, who gets 51 percent control of the satirical revue, is now somehow both of these—director and owner—but, unlike the great landlord in the sky, only on the earthly level.

98. 1 Timothy 6:10–11. "For the love of money is the root of all evils; it is through this craving that some have wandered away from the faith and pierced their hearts with many pangs. But as for you, man of God, shun all this; aim at righteousness, godliness, faith, love, steadfastness, gentleness."

99. *OED,* s.v. "jack," 18b: "In *Dialect Notes,* 3 (1908), 323:

'*Jack*, . . . a piece of metal with five tines or protuberances, used in the game of jacks. *Jacks*, an indoor catching game played with small five-tined metal pieces.' Alice Corbin Sies, *Spontaneous and Supervised Play in Childhood* (New York: Macmillan, 1922), 293: '*Jacks* is a game in which throwing and catching are not the main centers of interest; rather are the attention and interest focussed on what is done between catches.'"

100. *OED*, s.v. "jack," 19b. "Slang (orig. U.S.). See Malcolm Townsend, *U.S., An Index to the United States of America: Historical, Geographical and Political: A Handbook of Reference Combining the 'Curious' in U.S. History* (Boston: D. Lothrop, 1890), 427: 'The . . . verbal wealth of the United States language is illustrated in an inquiry for a loan of money; by using any of the following words in conjunction with the inquiry, Have you any . . . Jacks, [etc.].'"

101. Compare the end of the song "A Little Girl from Little Rock" (from the movie *Ladies of the Chorus*):

> For a kid from a wrong street
> I did very well on Wall Street
> Though I never owned a share of stock!
> And now that I'm known in the biggest banks
> I'm going back home and give my thanks
> To the one who broke my heart
> The one who broke my heart
> The one who broke my heart, in Little Rock!
> Little Rock.

102. To those not "in the know," Clément appears to have perfect Arabic, Chinese, German, French, and English. And, of course, Yves Montand was Italian.

103. *OED*, s.v. "dud": "A counterfeit thing . . . applied spec. to an explosive shell that failed to explode; hence . . . applied contemptuously to any useless or inefficient person or thing."

104. *OED*, s.v. "patter," esp. n.1 and v.

105. Dinah Maria Mulock Craik, *John Halifax, Gentleman* (London: Hurst and Blackett, 1856), p. xxvi.

106. On a 1906 sheet-music song published by Chappell and

Co. (copyright copy, Library of Congress), it was termed an "Old Irish Air," arranged by Herbert Hughes, when it appeared as the tune for "The Stuttering Lovers." The latter, although counted an Irish folksong, is a completely expurgated version of a song published from a manuscript copy of 1633 in John Wardroper, ed., *Love and Drollery* (London: Routledge and Kegan Paul, 1969), no 320.

107. *The Writings of Clement of Alexandria,* trans. William Wilson (Edinburgh: T. and T. Clark, 1867–1869): "Tis ho sozomenos plousios."

6. Hamlet's Pause

1. The spelling of "Hamlet" varies a good deal: "Amlothi" (in Saxo Grammaticus' *Gesta Danorum*), "Amleth" (in François de Belleforest's *Histoires tragiques*), and "Ambletus" (in Albert Krantz's *Chronica regnorum aquilonarium,* which mentions the Danish Ambletus and the Roman emperor Claudius on the same page). The general meaning seems to be, as E. Cobham Brewer suggests in his *Dictionary of Phrase and Fable* (London, 1894), "a daft person; from Icelandic, *amlod.*" On Lucius Junius Brutus, see Marc Shell, *Children of the Earth: Literature, Politics, and Nationhood* (New York: Oxford University Press, 1993), esp. pp. 107, 122.

2. Hamlet would *not* be Nero, who committed incest with his mother and killed her: "Soft, now to my mother. / O heart, lose not thy nature; let not ever / The soul of Nero enter this firm bosom. / Let me be cruel, not unnatural" (Shakespeare, *Hamlet,* 3.3.377–380). See Shell, *Children of the Earth,* pp. 110–112.

3. Shakespeare, *Hamlet,* 4.3: "And, England, . . . / Since yet thy cicatrice looks raw and red / After the Danish sword, and thy free awe / Pays homage to us."

4. Heinrich [Henry] Bullinger, *Sermonum decades quinque*

(1557), in English, *The Decades of Henry Bullinger,* trans. H.I., ed. Thomas Harding (London, 1592), p. 296.

5. Hamlet (3.3):

> Up, sword; and know thou a more horrid hent:
> When he is drunk asleep, or in his rage,
> Or in the incestuous pleasure of his bed;
> At gaming, swearing, or about some act
> That has no relish of salvation in't;
> Then *trip* him, that his heels may kick at heaven,
> And that his soul may be as damn'd and black
> As hell, whereto it goes.

6. Shakespeare, *Hamlet,* Second Quarto (1604), 3.1.150: "You gig and amble, and you list, you nickname Gods creatures, and make your wantonnes ignorance."

7. John M. Jephson and L. Reeve, *Brittany* (1859), p. 111: "The usual pace of these animals [mules] is an amble, which consists in lifting both legs on the same side at once."

8. Cyril Tourneur, *The Revengers Tragedy* (1607), 4.5.84: "Put a Reueller Out of his Antick amble."

9. Dr. Carlos Espinel of Georgetown University has studied the cripple depicted in this painting. He believes that the lesion causing the man's impairment has not harmed vertebrae C1–C3 (the upper vertebrae are identified as C1—the one closest to the brain—down to C8), because this is the location of the phrenic nerve, which controls breathing. Because the man in the painting is shown flexing his forearms, C5–C6 are probably intact. But he seems unable to extend his wrists or use his hands, gestures that depend on neuronal activity at C6–C7. Dr. Espinel therefore surmises that the man's polio lesion is located between C6 and C7. See Carlos Espinel, "Masaccio's Cripple: A Neurological syndrome: Its Art and Medicine," *Lancet,* 346 (1995): 1684–86.

10. In Masaccio's painting, the men at left seem to be recovering from their illnesses and are rising to their feet as Saint Peter walks by. (Saint Peter's own grandmother was supposedly cured

by Christ himself.) See also the biblical story about Ananias and his wife, Sapphira, and their dealings with Peter (Acts 5:1–16).

11. This is not quite the same thing as to say that Shakespeare's supposedly "hunchback" Richard III, a *locus classicus* for some schools of disability studies (in some ways an all too obvious one and in many ways too nondialectically reflective of common historical "prejudices"), suffers from "Sprengels deformity."

12. *Hamlet,* New Globe Theatre, directed by Giles Block (London, 2000). The cast featured Mark Rylance, artistic director of the New Globe Theatre, in the title role.

13. Michael Lawrence and David M. Barclay, "Stuttering: A Brief Review," *American Family Physician* (May 1, 1998).

14. See Robert West, "A Perseverative Theory of Stuttering," in Jon Eisenson, ed., *Stuttering; A Symposium,* introd. Wendell Johnson (New York: Harper, 1958).

15. Francis Bacon, "Experiment Solitary Touching Stutting," *Sylva Sylvarum,* in *The Works of Francis Bacon,* ed. James Spedding, Robert Leslie Ellis, and Douglas Denon Heath (London, 1857–1874), vol. 2, no. 386, p. 470. Bacon is apparently referring to Aristotle, *Problems,* 11.54, throughout his "Experiment."

16. Johann Georg Hamann, *Briefwechsel,* ed. Walther Ziesemer and Arthur Henkel, 8 vols. (Frankfurt: Insel Verlag, 1955–1975), vol. 5, 177.16–21.

17. If, as I am suggesting, Hamlet does/should stutter, where would it be? How about here: "I am but mad north-north-west: when the wind is / southerly I know a hawk from a handsaw." Hamlet double-puns on *hawk* and *handsaw:* both words have double meanings involving birds and carpenters. At one and the same time, therefore, Hamlet's statement means that he knows one bird from another, one carpenter's tool from another, a bird from a carpenter's tool, and a carpenter's tool from a bird. Is it "sane"—i.e., not mad—to know these things? When Hamlet speaks, is he sane or not? He says only that he is mad when the wind is from the northwest. Might that mean Norway? Is south-

erly, then, from Wittenberg? But Hamlet stutters (perseverates, repeats) on "north-west," doubling the word *north.*

18. Compare the lines "Imperious Caesar, dead and turned to clay . . ." (5.1), with their different rhyme scheme (*a-a-b-b*).

19. Marshall McLuhan speaking with John Lennon, quoted in Ritchie York, "John and Yoko and Year One," *Rolling Stone,* 51 (February 7, 1970).

20. *OED,* s.v. "pause": "A character denoting an interval of silence; a rest."

21. *Hamlet,* 4.4: "Be thou assured, if words be made of breath, / And breath of life, I have no life to breathe / What thou hast said to me."

Just before the duel between Hamlet and Laertes, the doubly duplicitous Claudius tosses poison into the cup and claims publicly, "The king shall drink to Hamlet's better breath" (5.2). Gertrude soon afterward remarks that Hamlet is "scant of breath" (5.2).

22. On the Clares' vow of silence, see Marc Shell, *The End of Kinship* (Stanford, Calif.: Stanford University Press, 1988), p. 182.

23. See John Palsgrave, *Lesclarcissement de la langue francoyse* (London: Richard Pynson and Johan Haukyns, 1530).

24. Jacques Du Bosc, *L'Honneste femme,* part 1 (Paris: P. Billaine, 1632), translated by Walter Montague as *The Accomplish'd Woman* (London: Gabriel Bedell and Thomas Collins, 1656), p. 17.

25. Locked-In Syndrome is a neurological disorder that afflicts the body's voluntary muscles, leaving the individual mute and paralyzed except for eye movements.

26. See Shakespeare, *Othello* (1604), 4.1, stage direction: "[Othello] Falls in a Traunce."

27. Henry Rogers, *The Eclipse of Faith* (Boston: Crosly, Nichols, 1863; orig. pub. 1852), p. 296: "Paulus thinks that Christ was only in a trance when he seemed to be dead."

28. Huon de Bordeaux, *Histoire de Huon de Bordeaux* (13th

century), in English as *The Boke of Duke Huon of Burdeux,* trans. John Bourchier, Lord Berners (London: Wynkyn de Worde, 1533), p. 215.

29. See Aubrey de Sélincourt, *Six Great Thinkers: Socrates, Saint Augustine, Lord Bacon, Rousseau, Coleridge, John Stuart Mill* (London: Hamish Hamilton, 1958).

30. John Lydgate, *The Assembly of Gods* (1420), ed. Jane Chance (Kalamazoo, Mich.: Medieval Institute Publications, 1999), p. 15.

31. To put the matter otherwise: Hamlet would not do what he knows he wants to do. You might even say he is aware of two sides of himself—the conscious and the unconscious, as Freud called them. But what Freud says Hamlet does not know is what Freud does not know about Hamlet. This is what Hamlet says—and in some ways the statement should remind us of the situation of a paralyzed person or a stutterer. "I will speak daggers to her, but use none. / My tongue and soul in this be hypocrite" (3.2.381–382).

32. See, for example, the famous vase painted by Kleophrades: an Attic red-figure hydria (ca. 480 B.C.E.), in the Museo Nazionale, Naples.

33. *Hamlet,* 2.2.470. On Pyrrhus' and Hamlet's state of neutrality, see also Harry Levin, "An Explication of the Player's Speech," in Shakespeare, *Hamlet: An Authoritative Text,* ed. Cyrus Hoy (New York: Norton, 1963), esp. p. 230.

34. My references to this speech in *Hamlet* and to surrounding ones are taken from all three versions of the play: Q1, Q2, and F.

35. The name "Pyrrhus" should be understood here not only in the usual way—as the son (of Pyrrhus the father), i.e., the Greek Achilles, also called Pyrrhus, who killed Priam as Hecuba watched. The name should also be interpreted as Pyrrhus the son, i.e., Neoptolemus, also called Pyrrhus, who was the son of Achilles and who killed his mother or stepmother Polyxena at the bidding of Achilles' ghost. Neoptolemus is called Pyrrhus in

Thomas Cooper's *Achilleus* (1565). Compare Christopher Marlowe and Thomas Nash, *The Tragedie of Dido, Queene of Carthage: Played by the Children of his Majesties Chappell* (1594), possibly one source of the "Aeneas speech" in *Hamlet.* Finally, see Horace Howard Furness' remark on this matter in his variorum edition of Shakespeare's *Troilus and Cressida* (Philadelphia: Lippincott, 1953), pp. 451–452. Epirus is on the northwestern coast of Greece; the kings there were supposedly descended from that Pyrrhus (or Neoptolemus) who was the son of Achilles.

36. John Lydgate, *Troy Book, A.D. 1412–1420,* ed. Henry Bergen (London: Early English Text Society and K. Paul, Trench, Trübner, 1906–1935), 2.4648.

37. *OED,* s.v. "truce": "A suspension of hostilities for a specified period between armies at war (formerly also between combatants in a private feud or quarrel); a temporary peace or cessation from arms; an armistice; also, an agreement or treaty."

38. Robert Burton, *Anatomy of Melancholy* (Oxford: Henry Cripps, 1621), 1.2.1.4.77. What is missing at the ellipsis is: "and are balde."

39. On Virgil as a stutterer, see Benson Bobrick, *Stuttering in History and the Quest for a Cure* (New York: Simon and Schuster, 1995), p. 63.

40. Barbara Levick, *Claudius* (London: Batsford, 1990), pp. 13ff.

41. Suetonius (*Claudius,* 2.1) emphasizes various physical and mental problems in childhood and youth.

42. See Lucia Graves, "The Poetry of Robert Graves, from the War to *The White Goddess,*" *Miscelánea: A Journal of English and American Studies* (Universidad de Zaragoza, Spain), 12 (1991). For an account by Robert Graves interwoven with one by his daughter, Lucia, see also Lucia Graves, *A Woman Unknown: Voices from a Spanish Life* (London: Virago, 1999).

43. Bernard Bergonzi, "Soldiers, Poets, Survivors," address at the conference *Mars in Ascendant: The Great War and the Twentieth Century,* University College, London, July 31–August 4, 2001.

Bergonzi argues that Graves was afflicted by something like shell-shock at least as severely as Siegfried Sassoon, and that Graves did not "exorcize" his war experience in his war poetry but rather used his later prose to achieve this exorcism.

44. See Patrick Quinn, *The Great War and the Missing Muse: The Early Writings of Robert Graves and Siegfried Sassoon* (Selinsgrove, Penn.: Susquehanna University Press, 1994).

45. Robert Graves, *Claudius the God and His Wife Messalina: The Troublesome Reign of Tiberius Claudius Caesar, Emperor of the Romans (Born B.C. 10, Died A.D. 54), as Described by Himself; Also His Murder at the Hands of the Notorious Agrippina (Mother of the Emperor Nero) and His Subsequent Deification, as Described by Others* (London: A. Barker, 1934). Robert Graves, *I, Claudius: From the Autobiography of Tiberius Claudius . . . Emperor of the Romans, Born B.C. 10, Murdered and Deified A.D. 54* (New York: H. Smith and R. Haas, 1934).

46. Sternberg's unfinished film was remade as a thirteen-part TV series for Masterpiece Theater in 1977, which is when I first saw it. *The Epic That Never Was* (1965) was the title of the Thames TV reconstruction narrated by Dirk Bogarde, with surviving footage from the film, which also starred Emlyn Williams, Merle Oberon, and Dame Flora Robson.

47. C. Tranquillus Suetonius, *The Lives of the Twelve Caesars,* trans. Alexander Thomson (New York: R. Worthington, 1883), "Claudius," section 38: "He did not scruple to speak of his own absurdities, and declared in some short speeches which he published, that he had only feigned imbecility in the reign of Gaius, because otherwise it would have been impossible for him to have escaped and arrived at the station he had then attained. He could not, however, gain credit for this assertion."

"Indifference" and "unconcern" translate *oblivio* and *inconsiderantia,* respectively (Suetonius, "Claudius," 39). The Latin term *inconsiderantia* is rare; it is in Salvian, *De gubernatione Dei,* 1.11, and possibly in Cicero, *Ad Quintum fratrem,* 3.9.2.

48. *I, Claudius,* TV series (BBC, 1976–1977), episode 4,

n TV, running almost continuously, with various on different networks, from 1937 to 1956. On the ncho los Amigos, see Virginia Lee Counterman *Tragedy of 1941* (n.p., 1999), p. 19.

ar Allan Poe, "The Premature Burial" (1844), in *The e Late Edgar Allan Poe,* ed. N. P. Willis, J. R. Lowell, and swold (New York: Redfield, 1850), 1:325–338.

ne Boyle Needham, *Looking Up,* as told to Rosemary New York: Putnam, 1959), p. 54.

Gummo eventually dropped out of the act with the Marx brothers, Groucho, Harpo, Chico, and Zeppo. He ed with his uncle Heine Schoenberg (Harry Shean) in riloquism act. One version of the story goes as follows: mo would sit on his uncle's knee while wearing a papier- é head and answering his uncle's jokes. "His uncle would both of Gummo's legs into one leg of the dummy's pants. would then stab the other one with a long hat-pin." Gummo ilton) Marx also says that he and his uncle Harry Shean "con- cted an act which consisted of a ventriloquist's dummy, in hich I was inside. The head was over my head and I operated he mechanical part as well as speaking. Uncle Harry just stood there." Quoted from an interview in Richard Anobile, with Groucho Marx, *The Marx Brothers' Scrapbook* (New York: Darien House, 1973); and Simon Louvish, *Monkey Business: The Lives and Legends of the Marx Brothers* (London: Faber and Faber, 1999), p. 45. See also Groucho Marx, "Why Harpo Doesn't Talk," *Los Angeles Times* (December 12, 1948).

66. J. G. Hamann to Immanuel Kant, Late December 1759, in Kant, *The Cambridge Edition of the Works of Immanuel Kant,* trans. and ed. Arnulf Zweig (Cambridge: Cambridge University Press, 1999), p. 62: "I don't like wine for its own sake but because it loosens my tongue enough to tell you the truth as I sit drunkenly on my donkey." See also ibid., p. 65.

67. "I'm fifty-eight years old, and if I stutter while giving Candice Bergen a direction, who cares? If [the stuttering] is re-

"What Shall We Do about Claudius?" Derek Jacobi, who played Claudius in the TV series, also played the stuttering codebreaker Allan Turing in the stageplay *Breaking the Code* (1986; film version, 1996). Alan Turing was the British mathematician who broke the Enigma Code during World War II.

49. In the seventh and sixth centuries B.C.E, the Etruscans controlled the major part of the Italian peninsula, living in walled city-states set on hilltops. Their art shows influences of earlier Italic cultures, the eastern Mediterranean, and Greece, but their style is unique.

50. That is how Immanuel Kant puts a similar matter in "What Is Enlightenment?" in Kant, *On History,* ed. Lewis White Beck, trans. Lewis White Beck, Robert E. Anchor, and Emil L. Fackenheim (Indianapolis: Bobbs-Merrill, 1963), p. 8.

51. Concerning Claudius' Shavian-like alphabet reforms, Suetonius ("Claudius," 41.3) references their appearance and indicates their adoption, though the precise nature of the biographer's distinctions remains somewhat elusive. Claudius, he says, "invented three new letters, and added them to the alphabet, maintaining that they were greatly needed; he published a book on their theory when he was still in private life, and when he became emperor had no difficulty in bringing about their general use. These characters may still be seen in numerous books, in the daily gazette, and in inscriptions on public buildings." *The Lives of the Twelve Caesars,* trans. J. C. Rolfe (London: Heinemann, 1914).

52. See W. J. T. Mitchell, "Ekphrasis and the Other," in Mitchell, *Picture Theory: Essays on Verbal and Visual Representation* (Chicago: University of Chicago Press, 1994).

53. As Mitchell points out, the tongue was not the only organ that the mutes in Turkish seraglios were missing. Gotthold Lessing's fear of literary emulation of the visual arts is not only fear of muteness or loss of eloquence, but also fear of castration, a threat which is re-echoed in the transformation from "superior being" to "doll," a mere feminine plaything. See Murray Krieger, "The Ekphrastic Principle and the Still Moment of Poetry; or,

Laokoön Revisited," in idem, *The Play and Place of Criticism* (Baltimore, Md.: Johns Hopkins University Press, 1967). This essay is incorporated in Krieger, *Ekphrasis: The Illusion of the Natural Sign* (Baltimore, Md.: Johns Hopkins University Press, 1992).

54. See http://users.westnet.gr/~cgian/statement.htm (accessed June 2005): "Statement From Political Prisoners In Turkey." The statement reads, in part, "To Our Peoples: . . . Remzi Basalak: He was arrested by Adana police on October 23, 1992. He exercised his right to silence. He was shown to the press as alive and handcuffed but he was murdered during torture. His tongue was cut off."

55. Charles W. Chesnutt, "The Dumb Witness," in *The Conjurer Woman and Other Conjure Tales,* ed. Richard Brodhead (Durham, N.C.: Duke University Press, 1993). The protagonist, Malcolm, seems to want to cut out the tongue of his slave Viney: "I will put it out of your power to dip your tongue in where you are not concerned" (p. 160). Only at the end of the tale do we learn that he has not cut out Viney's tongue. "The Dumb Witness" was written in the 1890s and unpublished in Chesnutt's lifetime.

56. Among these deposed rulers were Martina (641 C.E.) and Justinian II (695 C.E.). See Edward Gibbon, *The History of the Decline and Fall of the Roman Empire,* 6 vols. (1776–1788), ch. 48. See also the comments on Shakespeare's *Henry V* in Marc Shell, *Language Wars* (forthcoming).

57. The ventriloquist-dummy relationship is clearly relevant to such plays as *Titus Andronicus.* Marcus, for example, would be the ventriloquist to Lavinia the dummy ("Shall I speak for thee? shall I say 'tis so? / O, that I knew thy heart"; 2.4); and Lucius seeks such a ventriloquist ("O, say thou for her, who hath done this deed?"; 3.1). Worse than Philomel, Lavinia has also lost her hands ("Fair Philomel, why she but lost her tongue"; 2.4).

58. With the letter informing Charlemagne that he had been unanimously elected pope, Leo sent him the keys of the confession of Saint Peter, and the standard of the city. He did this to

show that he regarde
Holy See. In return,
congratulation and a g
had captured from the
(among other assets) enabl
churches and charitable ins
relatives of Pope Adrian I fo
hold his sacred office. On A
making his way toward the Fla
sion of the Greater Litanies, he w
men. He was thrown to the grou
root out his tongue and tear out hi
for a time bleeding in the street, he
the monastery of Saint Erasmus on th
seemed a miraculous manner, he recove
and tongue. Escaping from the monaster
Charlemagne, accompanied by many R
Day in the year 800, Pope Leo III crowne
king of the Franks, as emperor. Charlemagne
from the ruler at Byzantium, but the Byzanti
principle of imperial unity and regarded Charl
truder. See *Catholic Encyclopedia* (1907–1912), vo

59. On one trick for making people believe in
ration miracles, see B. Premanand, "The Miracle o
Tongue and Restoring It," *Gesellschaft zur Wissensch*
tersuchung von Parawissenschaften e.V. (Rossdorf, Germa
12, 1989).

60. See Luther Robinson, *We Made Peace with Polio*
ville, Tenn.: Broadman, 1960).

61. See Anonymous, "A Stuttering Philosopher (Sculpt
Chicago Historical Society, 20, nos. 1–2 (1934–1935): 45.

62. Edgar Bergen, "Meet Charlie McCarthy!" in *True Com*
14 (July 1942): 3–6. The Charlie McCarthy routine was firs
heard on the radio (*The Rudy Vallee Program,* December 17,
1936). Thereafter, Edgar Bergen and Charlie McCarthy had a

ally difficult, I exaggerate it and get everyone on the set to laugh with me. A stutter can really be quite charming. We are human and not perfect." Peter Bonerz (Jerry the dentist on *The Bob Newhart Show* and director of *Friends, Murphy Brown,* and *Home Improvement*), in an interview reported in Polly Drew, "A Stutter Needn't Stop You," *Milwaukee Journal Sentinel* (July 27, 1997). Also at www.jsonline.com/news/sunday/lifestyle/0727polly .stm (accessed June 2005).

68. Willis' character, a Manhattan psychotherapist, calls a teenager a "nut case" for using violence when someone makes fun of the teen's stuttering. On Palin, see Michael Palin, Foreword, in Lena Rustin, Frances Cook, Willie Botterill, Cherry Hughes, and Elaine Kelman, *Stammering: A Practical Guide for Teachers and Other Professionals* (London: David Fulton, 2001).

69. John Updike, "Getting the Words Out," in Updike, *Self-Consciousness: Memoirs* (New York: Knopf, 1989), p. 87.

70. "Psellism," in *Household Words,* 348 (November 22, 1856): 464–469; quoted from *Household Words: A Weekly Journal Conducted by Charles Dickens,* 14, nos. 330–353 and the number-and-a-half for Christmas, July 19, 1856, to December 27, 1856 (London: Office 16, Wellington Street North, 1856).

71. Groucho Marx, "Why Harpo Doesn't Talk." Robert Marx is quoted from an interview in Louvish, *Monkey Business,* p. 75. Two of Gummo's poems were published in *Variety* (December 1915 and April 1916). The manuscript of Gummo's *Adam's Apple* (1919) is in the Library of Congress, Washington, D.C. "Breath-holding, whisper-, and voice-making instrument": John Rupert Firth, *The Tongues of Men* (London: Watts, 1937), p. 40. "From a superstitious notion": John Craig, *A New Universal Etymological, Technological, and Pronouncing Dictionary of the English Language* (London: Henry George Collins, 1849). "Mutism": Thomas Clifford Allbutt, ed., *A System of Medicine* (New York: Macmillan, 1899), 7:418, on "the leading peculiarities of hysterical mutism." On the term *elective,* see D. J. Salfield, "Observations of Elective Mutism in Children," *Journal of Mental Science,* 96

(1950): 1024. "Silent Panic" (1960) was an episode of *The June Alyson Show,* written by Arthur Drake; see Louvish, *Monkey Business,* p. 385.

72. J. Kalinowski, A. Stuart, S. Sark, and J. Armson, "Stuttering Amelioration at Various Auditory Feedback Delays and Speech Rates," *European Journal of Disorders of Communication,* 31 (1996): 259–269.

73. I noted also that Porky hardly ever wears pants—except when he comes out of the shower, in such films as *Porky's Bear Facts* (1941). I wondered whether Porky's corkscrew tail might recall the corkscrew penises of real pigs. Andrew Ferguson Fraser, *Reproductive Behavior in Ungulates* (London: Academic Press, 1968), discusses the "spiral glans penis" of the pig.

74. In *Hamateur Night,* the fox recites Hamlet's famous soliloquy "To be or not to be." As early as 1933, the RKO Film Company was releasing its "Aesop's Fables" series of talking-animal cartoons, which included titles like *Fresh Ham.*

7. Last Stop

1. Thomas Carlyle, *Sartor Resartus: The Life and Opinions of Herr Teufelsdröckh* (London, 1831), II.ix: "In what words . . . [can we] speak even afar-off of the unspeakable?"

2. Both Old and New Testament traditions outlaw the uttering of certain words. Saint Paul writes, "He . . . heard unspeakable words, which it is not lawful for a man to utter" (2 Corinthians 12:4, translation of 1611).

3. Sometimes the forbidden term becomes confused with the supposedly profane thing or person to which it refers; thus, Carlyle refers to the "unspeakable Turk" and Crosland to the "unspeakable Scot." See Thomas Carlyle, *Westminster Review* (July 6, 1831): "How they sailed . . . into Paynim land; fought with that unspeakable Turk, King Machabol"; and T. W. H. Crosland (Thomas William Hodgson), *That Unspeakable Scot* (London: G. Richards, 1902).

long career on TV, running almost continuously, with various sponsors and on different networks, from 1937 to 1956. On the visits to Rancho los Amigos, see Virginia Lee Counterman Acosta, *Polio Tragedy of 1941* (n.p., 1999), p. 19.

63. Edgar Allan Poe, "The Premature Burial" (1844), in *The Works of the Late Edgar Allan Poe,* ed. N. P. Willis, J. R. Lowell, and R. W. Griswold (New York: Redfield, 1850), 1:325–338.

64. Jane Boyle Needham, *Looking Up,* as told to Rosemary Taylor (New York: Putnam, 1959), p. 54.

65. Gummo eventually dropped out of the act with the other Marx brothers, Groucho, Harpo, Chico, and Zeppo. He appeared with his uncle Heine Schoenberg (Harry Shean) in a ventriloquism act. One version of the story goes as follows: Gummo would sit on his uncle's knee while wearing a papier-mâché head and answering his uncle's jokes. "His uncle would stuff both of Gummo's legs into one leg of the dummy's pants. He would then stab the other one with a long hat-pin." Gummo (Milton) Marx also says that he and his uncle Harry Shean "concocted an act which consisted of a ventriloquist's dummy, in which I was inside. The head was over my head and I operated the mechanical part as well as speaking. Uncle Harry just stood there." Quoted from an interview in Richard Anobile, with Groucho Marx, *The Marx Brothers' Scrapbook* (New York: Darien House, 1973); and Simon Louvish, *Monkey Business: The Lives and Legends of the Marx Brothers* (London: Faber and Faber, 1999), p. 45. See also Groucho Marx, "Why Harpo Doesn't Talk," *Los Angeles Times* (December 12, 1948).

66. J. G. Hamann to Immanuel Kant, Late December 1759, in Kant, *The Cambridge Edition of the Works of Immanuel Kant,* trans. and ed. Arnulf Zweig (Cambridge: Cambridge University Press, 1999), p. 62: "I don't like wine for its own sake but because it loosens my tongue enough to tell you the truth as I sit drunkenly on my donkey." See also ibid., p. 65.

67. "I'm fifty-eight years old, and if I stutter while giving Candice Bergen a direction, who cares? If [the stuttering] is re-

show that he regarded the Frankish king as the protector of the Holy See. In return, he received from Charlemagne letters of congratulation and a great part of the treasure which the king had captured from the Avars. The acquisition of this wealth (among other assets) enabled Leo to be a great benefactor to the churches and charitable institutions of Rome. A number of the relatives of Pope Adrian I formed a plot to render Leo unfit to hold his sacred office. On April 25, 799, when the pope was making his way toward the Flaminian Gate during the procession of the Greater Litanies, he was attacked by a body of armed men. He was thrown to the ground, and an effort was made to root out his tongue and tear out his eyes. After he had been left for a time bleeding in the street, he was hurried off by night to the monastery of Saint Erasmus on the Coelian. There, in what seemed a miraculous manner, he recovered the full use of his eyes and tongue. Escaping from the monastery, he sought refuge with Charlemagne, accompanied by many Romans. On Christmas Day in the year 800, Pope Leo III crowned Charles the Great, king of the Franks, as emperor. Charlemagne sought recognition from the ruler at Byzantium, but the Byzantines adhered to the principle of imperial unity and regarded Charlemagne as an intruder. See *Catholic Encyclopedia* (1907–1912), vol. 9, "Leo III."

59. On one trick for making people believe in tongue-restoration miracles, see B. Premanand, "The Miracle of Cutting the Tongue and Restoring It," *Gesellschaft zur Wissenschaftlichen Untersuchung von Parawissenschaften* e.V. (Rossdorf, Germany, March 12, 1989).

60. See Luther Robinson, *We Made Peace with Polio* (Nashville, Tenn.: Broadman, 1960).

61. See Anonymous, "A Stuttering Philosopher (Sculpture)," *Chicago Historical Society,* 20, nos. 1–2 (1934–1935): 45.

62. Edgar Bergen, "Meet Charlie McCarthy!" in *True Comics,* 14 (July 1942): 3–6. The Charlie McCarthy routine was first heard on the radio (*The Rudy Vallee Program,* December 17, 1936). Thereafter, Edgar Bergen and Charlie McCarthy had a

Laokoön Revisited," in idem, *The Play and Place of Criticism* (Baltimore, Md.: Johns Hopkins University Press, 1967). This essay is incorporated in Krieger, *Ekphrasis: The Illusion of the Natural Sign* (Baltimore, Md.: Johns Hopkins University Press, 1992).

54. See http://users.westnet.gr/~cgian/statement.htm (accessed June 2005): "Statement From Political Prisoners In Turkey." The statement reads, in part, "To Our Peoples: . . . Remzi Basalak: He was arrested by Adana police on October 23, 1992. He exercised his right to silence. He was shown to the press as alive and handcuffed but he was murdered during torture. His tongue was cut off."

55. Charles W. Chesnutt, "The Dumb Witness," in *The Conjurer Woman and Other Conjure Tales,* ed. Richard Brodhead (Durham, N.C.: Duke University Press, 1993). The protagonist, Malcolm, seems to want to cut out the tongue of his slave Viney: "I will put it out of your power to dip your tongue in where you are not concerned" (p. 160). Only at the end of the tale do we learn that he has not cut out Viney's tongue. "The Dumb Witness" was written in the 1890s and unpublished in Chesnutt's lifetime.

56. Among these deposed rulers were Martina (641 C.E.) and Justinian II (695 C.E.). See Edward Gibbon, *The History of the Decline and Fall of the Roman Empire,* 6 vols. (1776–1788), ch. 48. See also the comments on Shakespeare's *Henry V* in Marc Shell, *Language Wars* (forthcoming).

57. The ventriloquist-dummy relationship is clearly relevant to such plays as *Titus Andronicus.* Marcus, for example, would be the ventriloquist to Lavinia the dummy ("Shall I speak for thee? shall I say 'tis so? / O, that I knew thy heart"; 2.4); and Lucius seeks such a ventriloquist ("O, say thou for her, who hath done this deed?"; 3.1). Worse than Philomel, Lavinia has also lost her hands ("Fair Philomel, why she but lost her tongue"; 2.4).

58. With the letter informing Charlemagne that he had been unanimously elected pope, Leo sent him the keys of the confession of Saint Peter, and the standard of the city. He did this to

"What Shall We Do about Claudius?" Derek Jacobi, who played Claudius in the TV series, also played the stuttering codebreaker Allan Turing in the stageplay *Breaking the Code* (1986; film version, 1996). Alan Turing was the British mathematician who broke the Enigma Code during World War II.

49. In the seventh and sixth centuries B.C.E, the Etruscans controlled the major part of the Italian peninsula, living in walled city-states set on hilltops. Their art shows influences of earlier Italic cultures, the eastern Mediterranean, and Greece, but their style is unique.

50. That is how Immanuel Kant puts a similar matter in "What Is Enlightenment?" in Kant, *On History,* ed. Lewis White Beck, trans. Lewis White Beck, Robert E. Anchor, and Emil L. Fackenheim (Indianapolis: Bobbs-Merrill, 1963), p. 8.

51. Concerning Claudius' Shavian-like alphabet reforms, Suetonius ("Claudius," 41.3) references their appearance and indicates their adoption, though the precise nature of the biographer's distinctions remains somewhat elusive. Claudius, he says, "invented three new letters, and added them to the alphabet, maintaining that they were greatly needed; he published a book on their theory when he was still in private life, and when he became emperor had no difficulty in bringing about their general use. These characters may still be seen in numerous books, in the daily gazette, and in inscriptions on public buildings." *The Lives of the Twelve Caesars,* trans. J. C. Rolfe (London: Heinemann, 1914).

52. See W. J. T. Mitchell, "Ekphrasis and the Other," in Mitchell, *Picture Theory: Essays on Verbal and Visual Representation* (Chicago: University of Chicago Press, 1994).

53. As Mitchell points out, the tongue was not the only organ that the mutes in Turkish seraglios were missing. Gotthold Lessing's fear of literary emulation of the visual arts is not only fear of muteness or loss of eloquence, but also fear of castration, a threat which is re-echoed in the transformation from "superior being" to "doll," a mere feminine plaything. See Murray Krieger, "The Ekphrastic Principle and the Still Moment of Poetry; or,

ally difficult, I exaggerate it and get everyone on the set to laugh with me. A stutter can really be quite charming. We are human and not perfect." Peter Bonerz (Jerry the dentist on *The Bob Newhart Show* and director of *Friends, Murphy Brown,* and *Home Improvement*), in an interview reported in Polly Drew, "A Stutter Needn't Stop You," *Milwaukee Journal Sentinel* (July 27, 1997). Also at www.jsonline.com/news/sunday/lifestyle/0727polly .stm (accessed June 2005).

68. Willis' character, a Manhattan psychotherapist, calls a teenager a "nut case" for using violence when someone makes fun of the teen's stuttering. On Palin, see Michael Palin, Foreword, in Lena Rustin, Frances Cook, Willie Botterill, Cherry Hughes, and Elaine Kelman, *Stammering: A Practical Guide for Teachers and Other Professionals* (London: David Fulton, 2001).

69. John Updike, "Getting the Words Out," in Updike, *Self-Consciousness: Memoirs* (New York: Knopf, 1989), p. 87.

70. "Psellism," in *Household Words,* 348 (November 22, 1856): 464–469; quoted from *Household Words: A Weekly Journal Conducted by Charles Dickens,* 14, nos. 330–353 and the number-and-a-half for Christmas, July 19, 1856, to December 27, 1856 (London: Office 16, Wellington Street North, 1856).

71. Groucho Marx, "Why Harpo Doesn't Talk." Robert Marx is quoted from an interview in Louvish, *Monkey Business,* p. 75. Two of Gummo's poems were published in *Variety* (December 1915 and April 1916). The manuscript of Gummo's *Adam's Apple* (1919) is in the Library of Congress, Washington, D.C. "Breath-holding, whisper-, and voice-making instrument": John Rupert Firth, *The Tongues of Men* (London: Watts, 1937), p. 40. "From a superstitious notion": John Craig, *A New Universal Etymological, Technological, and Pronouncing Dictionary of the English Language* (London: Henry George Collins, 1849). "Mutism": Thomas Clifford Allbutt, ed., *A System of Medicine* (New York: Macmillan, 1899), 7:418, on "the leading peculiarities of hysterical mutism." On the term *elective,* see D. J. Salfield, "Observations of Elective Mutism in Children," *Journal of Mental Science,* 96

(1950): 1024. "Silent Panic" (1960) was an episode of *The June Alyson Show,* written by Arthur Drake; see Louvish, *Monkey Business,* p. 385.

72. J. Kalinowski, A. Stuart, S. Sark, and J. Armson, "Stuttering Amelioration at Various Auditory Feedback Delays and Speech Rates," *European Journal of Disorders of Communication,* 31 (1996): 259–269.

73. I noted also that Porky hardly ever wears pants—except when he comes out of the shower, in such films as *Porky's Bear Facts* (1941). I wondered whether Porky's corkscrew tail might recall the corkscrew penises of real pigs. Andrew Ferguson Fraser, *Reproductive Behavior in Ungulates* (London: Academic Press, 1968), discusses the "spiral glans penis" of the pig.

74. In *Hamateur Night,* the fox recites Hamlet's famous soliloquy "To be or not to be." As early as 1933, the RKO Film Company was releasing its "Aesop's Fables" series of talking-animal cartoons, which included titles like *Fresh Ham.*

7. Last Stop

1. Thomas Carlyle, *Sartor Resartus: The Life and Opinions of Herr Teufelsdröckh* (London, 1831), II.ix: "In what words . . . [can we] speak even afar-off of the unspeakable?"

2. Both Old and New Testament traditions outlaw the uttering of certain words. Saint Paul writes, "He . . . heard unspeakable words, which it is not lawful for a man to utter" (2 Corinthians 12:4, translation of 1611).

3. Sometimes the forbidden term becomes confused with the supposedly profane thing or person to which it refers; thus, Carlyle refers to the "unspeakable Turk" and Crosland to the "unspeakable Scot." See Thomas Carlyle, *Westminster Review* (July 6, 1831): "How they sailed . . . into Paynim land; fought with that unspeakable Turk, King Machabol"; and T. W. H. Crosland (Thomas William Hodgson), *That Unspeakable Scot* (London: G. Richards, 1902).

4. Charles Sidney Bluemel, *The Riddle of Stuttering* (Danville, Ill.: Interstate Publishing, 1957). John Gavin Andrews and Mary Harris, with Roger Garside and David Kay, *The Syndrome of Stuttering* (London: Spastics Society Medical Education and Information Unit, in association with Heinemann Medical Books, 1964).

5. Jason Gay, "Sweet Relief," on Gay, *The Singer and the Song,* CD (Eagle Lake, Minn.: Now and Then Records, 1997). Reprinted by permission. Complete lyrics at www.jasongay.com.

6. "Elles se montrent surtout chez les adultes, et particulièrement chez ceux qui prennent au tragique leur bégayement, soit parce qu'il est un obstacle à l'exercice de leur profession ou de leurs relations sociales, soit que, par une tendance naturelle de l'esprit, ils soient portés à s'exagérer leurs maux. . . . Le phobique verbal a peur de certaines lettres qui le plus souvent sont des consonnes, . . . et une fois qu'il est persuadé que telle lettre est difficile, il éprouve une véritable angoisse chaque fois que cette lettre apparaît au cours de ses conversations." Arthur Chervin, *Des Phobies verbales* (Paris: Société d'Editions Scientifiques, 1895), pp. 2–3, quoted in René Bernard, *Le Bègue sur la scène française* (Paris: Droz, 1945; facsimile rpt. Geneva: Slatkine, 1977), p. 30.

7. Robert A. Aronowitz, *Making Sense of Illness: Science, Society, and Disease* (Cambridge: Cambridge University Press, 1998).

8. David B. Rosenfield, private communication, January 2004. See also Rosenfield, "Stuttering," in S. C. Schachter and O. Devinsky, eds., *Behavioral Neurology and the Legacy of Norman Geschwind* (Philadelphia: Lippincott-Raven, 1997), pp. 101–111.

9. "La manière de penser du bègue par rapport à son langage (et en général, ajouterons nous, de ceux qui sont affectés de défauts de prononciation) se différencie remarquablement de celle d'un homme sain. Alors que celui-ci ne s'intéresse aucunement à son parler, . . . le bègue accorde au sien une attention extraordinaire et morbide. Il se prépare d'avance à toute conversation, il redoute la prononciation de certains mots. Il se sent obsédé, jusque dans son rêve, par ces mots, par ces lettres." S.

Loew, *Nouvelles Voies pour la guérison du bégayement et de la crainte de parler* (Tel Aviv: Editions de La Méthode Dr. Loew, 1936), p. 15, cited in René Bernard, *Le Bègue sur la scène française* (Paris: Droz, 1945), p. 30.

10. Jean Métellus, *La Parole prisonnière* (Paris: Gallimard, 1986), pp. 156–157.

11. Abraham Herbert Kanter and Abe Samuel Kohn, *—And the Stutterer Talked* (Boston: Bruce Humphries, 1938). Ernest Tompkins, "Stammering and Its Extirpation," pamphlet (Los Angeles, 1916), reprinted from *The Pedagogical Seminary,* 23 (June 1916): 153–174.

12. Kanter and Kohn, *—And the Stutterer Talked,* pp. 72–73.

13. Tam Hoskyns, *The Talking Cure* (London: Hamish Hamilton, 1997).

14. See Oliver Bloodstein, "The Psychoanalysis of Stuttering," in Jon Eisenson, ed., *Stuttering: a Symposium,* introd. Wendell Johnson (New York: Harper, 1958).

15. P. G. Wodehouse, "The Truth about George," in idem, *Meet Mr. Mulliner* (London: Herbert Jenkins, 1930), pp. 11–14. The story was adapted for TV in 1975, appearing on the BBC's *Wodehouse Playhouse* (produced by David Askey), with Wodehouse himself doing the introduction, John Alderton as George Mulliner, and Pauline Collins as Susan Blake.

16. The stutterer's inability to take the talking cure was likewise the gist (in a more serious vein) of Rudolf Denhardt's pre-Freudian work, *Das Stottern: Eine Psychose* [Stuttering: A Psychosis] (Leipzig: E. Keil's Nachfolger, 1890).

17. See the research done by Drs. A. R. Braun, C. L. Ludlow, and S. Stager at the National Institutes of Health (Bethesda, Md.) and the research by Dr. Gerald Maguire at the University of California, Irvine. Delayed auditory feedback is referred to as DAF or DA. One manual for teachers describes the technique: "Introduce the concept that some children stutter. . . . Sometimes these children go to special teachers called Speech Pathologists. . . . The teacher should have one group of students use a special ma-

chine called a Delayed Auditory Feedback Device, or a DAF. When the children talk into the DAF machine, a little time will pass before they actually hear themselves in the headphones. A knob on the DAF machine will allow you to set the appropriate amount of time from when you talk to when you hear yourself in the headset." Lesson 29: "Voice, Hearing, and Stuttering," Grades 3–4 (Utah State University, Junior Engineering, 1997). See http://juniorengineering.usu.edu/lessons/voice/voice.php (accessed January 2005). See also www.ecu.edu/csd/Stutt.html, where Dr. Joe Kalinowski and his colleagues at East Carolina University report on a similar technique which they call Altered Auditory Feedback (AAF). J. Kalinowski, T. Saltuklaroglu, V. Guntupalli, and A. Stuart, "Gestural Recovery and the Role of Forward and Reversed Syllabic Repetitions as Stuttering Inhibitors in Adults," *Neuroscience Letters,* 363 (2004): 144–149.

18. See www.rickywburk.org/speech/therapy.htm (accessed January 2005).

19. Kanter and Kohn, —*And the Stutterer Talked,* p. 79.

20. The Five Scamps, "Stuttering Blues," recorded for OKeh Records, 1951; collected on *The OKeh Rhythm and Blues Story, 1949–1957,* 3-CD set (Epic/OKeh/Legacy, 1993).

21. David F. Newton, quoted in Benjamin Nathaniel Bogue, *Stammering: Its Cause and Cure* (Indianapolis: B. N. Bogue, 1920), p. 151.

22. For an early statistical claim, see ibid., esp. ch. 7. The theorist Charles Van Riper, a stutterer, has written about his own suicide attempts as well as those of other stutterers.

23. "Bad character": Stereotypes include the widely accepted impression that stutterers are nervous, shy, quiet, self-conscious, withdrawn, tense, anxious, fearful, reticent, and guarded. See M. L. Hurst and E. B. Cooper, "Employer Attitudes toward Stuttering," *Journal of Fluency Disorders,* 8 (1983): 1–12; P. A. White and S. R. C. Collins, "Stereotype by Inference: A Possible Explanation for the 'Stutterer' Stereotype," *Journal of Speech and Hearing Research,* 27 (1984): 567–570; C. L. Woods and D. E.

Williams, "Speech Clinicians' Conception of Boys and Men Who Stutter," *Journal of Speech and Hearing Disorders,* 36 (1971): 225–234; and C. L. Woods and D. E. Williams, "Traits Attributed to Stuttering and Normally Fluent Males," *Journal of Speech and Hearing Research,* 19 (1976): 267–278.

"Low intelligence": see LaVange Hunt Richardson, *The Personality of Stutterers* (Evanston, Ill.: American Psychological Association, 1944).

24. Kanter and Kohn, *—And the Stutterer Talked,* p. 130.

25. On the experience of isolation: "Many children who stutter refuse to accept that there are other people like them; and even older stutterers, Mrs. [Lee] Caggiano points out, often lack the necessary language for connection, conditioned (as they are) to believing that 'stuttering must be so horrible we can't talk about it, since we talk about everything but this.'" David L. Ulin, "Finding the Words: How Some Stutterers Are Talking Their Way Out of Isolation," *Chicago Tribune* (September 24, 2000).

In "Wenn die Grazie misslingt: Zur psychosozialen Situation stotternder Menschen" [When Grace Fails: On the Psychosocial Situation of the Stutterer] (Regensburg, Germany, 1993), Jürgen Benecken discusses how people generally belittle and deny "the severity of social stigmatization" and "the life-threatening isolation" that stutterers often experience.

26. Oliver Sacks, *Seeing Voices: A Journey into the World of the Deaf* (Berkeley: University of California Press, 1989). Carol Padden, *Deaf in America: Voices from a Culture* (Cambridge, Mass.: Harvard University Press, 1990).

27. On talkies, see Nicholas Mirzoeff, *Silent Poetry: Deafness, Sign, and Visual Culture in Modern France* (Princeton, N.J.: Princeton University Press, 1995). On education: Donald F. Moores, *Educating the Deaf,* 4th ed. (Boston: Houghton Mifflin, 1995). On family structure: Lou Ann Walker, *Loss for Words: The Story of Deafness in a Family* (New York: HarperCollins, 1987).

28. Edward Wheeler Scripture, *Stuttering, Lisping, and Correction of the Speech of the Deaf,* 2nd rev. ed. (New York: Macmillan,

1923). This work set an early standard, from the viewpoint of cure.

29. Benjamin Constant, *Mémoires sur les Cent-Jours, en forme de lettres* (Paris: Béchet, 1820–1822), vol. 1. A sample anecdote: "Several foreigners were assembled in [Prince] Eugène [de Beauharnais]'s apartment [in Paris in 1799], the rôles were distributed and learned in advance, and the two victims designated. When they were all seated at table, Dugazon, pretending to be a stutterer, addressed some remark to Thiémet [a famous ventriloquist of the period], who, having a similar rôle, replied by stuttering also. Then each of the two pretended to believe that the other was mocking him, and there ensued a quarrel of stutterers; the angrier they grew, the harder they found it to express themselves. Thiémet, who besides playing the stutterer had also assumed the character of a deaf man, turned to his neighbor, his ear-trumpet at his ear, and asked: 'Wh-wh-what i-i-is he s-s-saying?' 'Nothing,' responded the officious neighbor, who wanted to prevent a quarrel and take his stutterer's side. 'Y-y-yes, he i-i-s m-m-mock-mock-ing me.' Then the quarrel grew more lively; they were about to come to blows, and each of the two stutterers had seized a carafe to throw at his antagonist's head, when a generous splashing from the water contained in the carafes made their officious neighbors comprehend the danger of attempts at conciliation. The two stutterers, however, continued shouting like deaf men until the last drop of water was spilled; and I remember that Eugène, who was the author of this plot, was in fits of laughter the whole time it lasted. People dried themselves, and everyone was presently composed, glass in hand. Eugène, whenever he got up a joke of this kind, never failed to relate it to his mother, and sometimes even to his stepfather. They were greatly amused by it, Joséphine [Mme. Bonaparte] especially." (Trans. Casiana Ionita.)

30. George Adams Fisher, "The Biter Bit: A Tale of Two Stutterers," *The Boy's Own Paper,* 34, no. 12 (December 23, 1911).

31. Wodehouse, "The Truth about George," pp. 16–17.

32. Malezieu's play is included in *Les Divertissements de Seaux* (Trévoux, 1762), vol. 1, p. 234. All are mentioned in Bernard, *Le Bègue sur la scène française.*

33. On caesura in song: Andrew Kirkman and Dennis Slavin, eds., *Binchois Studies* (New York: Oxford University Press, 2000); John Andrew Bailey and Beth Anne Lee–De Amici, "Bridging the Medial Caesura: The Wraparound Rondeau," in Andrew Kirkman and Dennis Slavin, eds., *Binchois Studies* (Oxford: Oxford University Press, 2000). On modern music: Bruce Cole, *Caesura,* score for a sextet (London: Boosey and Hawkes, 1976). On jazz and dance: Chan Parker, *Ma vie en mi bemol* (Columbia: University of South Carolina Press, 1998), esp. the section called "Caesura." On religion: Philippe Lacoue-Labarthe, "The Caesura of Religion," in David J. Levin, ed., *Opera through Other Eyes* (Stanford, Calif.: Stanford University Press, 1993); and Philippe Lacoue-Labarthe, "The Caesura of the Speculative," in Lacoue-Labarthe, *Typography: Mimesis, Philosophy, Politics,* introd. Jacques Derrida, ed. Christopher Fynsk (Cambridge, Mass.: Harvard University Press, 1989). On caesura in versification: Gotthard Stephan, *Die Ausdruckskraft der Caesura Media im iambischen Trimeter der attischen Tragödie* (Königstein: Hain, 1981); Hans Reger, *Die epische Caseura in der Chaucerschule* (Bayreuth: Ellwanger, 1910).

34. These terms are synonymous with *gobbling*—an echoic word that indicates the sound of the turkey. *OED,* s.v. "turkey."

35. Philip Larkin, "Next, Please," from *The Less Deceived* (Hessle, East Yorkshire: Marvell, 1955), reprinted in Larkin, *Collected Poems,* ed. Anthony Thwaite (London: Marvell, 1988). See Tim Trengove-Jones, "Larkin's Stammer," *Essays in Criticism,* 40 (1990): 322–338.

Index